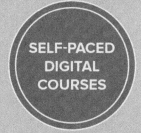
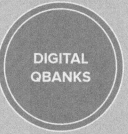
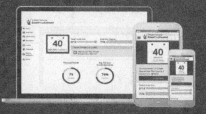

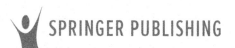

MEDICAL-SURGICAL NURSING CERTIFICATION EXPRESS REVIEW

MEDICAL-SURGICAL NURSING CERTIFICATION EXPRESS REVIEW

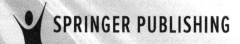
SPRINGER PUBLISHING

Springer Publishing Company, LLC
11 West 42nd Street, New York, NY 10036
www.springerpub.com

Acquisitions *Editor*: Elizabeth Nieginski
Compositor: diacriTech

ISBN: 978-0-8261-5951-9
ebook ISBN: 978-0-8261-5952-6
DOI: 10.1891/9780826159526

Printed by BnT

The author and the publisher of this Work have made every effort to use sources believed to be reliable to provide information that is accurate and compatible with the standards generally accepted at the time of publication. The author and publisher shall not be liable for any special, consequential, or exemplary damages resulting, in whole or in part, from the readers' use of, or reliance on, the information contained in this book. The publisher has no responsibility for the persistence or accuracy of URLs for external or third-party Internet websites referred to in this publication and does not guarantee that any content on such websites is, or will remain, accurate or appropriate.

CMSRN® is a registered service mark of the Medical-Surgical Nursing Certification Board (MSNCB). MSNCB does not sponsor or endorse this resource, nor does it have a proprietary relationship with Springer Publishing.

MEDSURG-BC™ is a registered service mark of the American Nurses Credentialing Center (ANCC). ANCC does not sponsor or endorse this resource, nor does it have a proprietary relationship with Springer Publishing.

Library of Congress Control Number: 2022941709

Contact sales@springerpub.com to receive discount rates on bulk purchases.

Publisher's Note: **New and used products purchased from third-party sellers are not guaranteed for quality, authenticity, or access to any included digital components.**

Printed in the United States of America.

CONTENTS

PREFACE

If you have purchased this *Express Review*, you are likely well into your exam prep journey to certification. This book was designed to be a high-speed review—a last-minute gut check before your exam day. We created this review, which is a quick summary of the key topics you'll encounter on the exam, to supplement your certification preparation studies. We encourage you to use it in conjunction with other study aids to ensure you are as prepared as possible for the exam.

This book follows the most recent exam content outlines from the Certified Medical-Surgical Registered Nurse (CMSRN®) Certification Examination and the Medical-Surgical Nursing Board Certification Examination blueprints and uses a succinct, bulleted format to highlight what you need to know. The aim of this book is to help you solidify your retention of information in the month or so leading up to your exam. It is written by certified medical-surgical nurses who are familiar with the exam and the content you need to know. Special features appear throughout the book to call out important information, including:

- **Complications:** Problems that can arise with certain disease states or procedures
- **Nursing Pearls:** Additional patient care insights and strategies for knowledge retention
- **Alerts:** Need-to-know details on how to handle emergency situations or when to transfer care
- **Pop Quizzes:** Critical-thinking questions to test your ability to synthesize what you've learned (answers in Chapter 16)
- **List of Abbreviations:** A useful appendix to help guide you through the alphabet soup of clinical terms

We know life is busy. Being able to prepare for your exam efficiently and effectively is paramount, which is why we created this *Express Review*. You have come to the right place as you continue on your path of professional growth and development. The stakes are high, and we want to help you succeed. Best of luck to you on your certification journey. You've got this!

PASS GUARANTEE

If you use this resource to prepare for your exam and you do not pass, you may return it for a refund of your full purchase price. To receive a refund, you must return your product along with a copy of your original receipt and exam score report. Product must be returned and received within 180 days of the original purchase date. Excludes tax, shipping, and handling. One offer per person and address. Refunds will be issued within 8 weeks from acceptance and approval. This offer is valid for U.S. residents only. Void where prohibited. To begin the process, please contact customer service at CS@springerpub.com.

GENERAL EXAMINATION INFORMATION

OVERVIEW

This chapter reviews examination information for certification as a medical-surgical nurse through MSNCB and ANCC. Each credential is valid for 5 years. Although the exams differ in application requirements and format, they are similar in content (Table 1.1).

Table 1.1 Comparison of MSNCB and ANCC	CMSRN	RN-BC
Credential	CMSRN	RN-BC
Certifying body	MSNBC	ANCC
Cost	$375	$395
Member cost	$255 for AMSN member	$295 for ANA member
Recognized for Magnet status?	Yes	Yes
Number of questions	150 (125 scored)	150 (125 scored)
Computer-based exam?	Yes	Yes
Work experience requirement	2 years	2 years
Need active RN license?	Yes	Yes
Minimum time worked as RN	2,000 hours in last 3 years	2,000 hours in last 3 years
Continuing education required	None	30 hours in the last 3 years
Type of practice	Clinical, management, or educational	Clinical
Certification duration	5 years	5 years

BENEFITS OF CERTIFICATION

- Indicates expert knowledge in area of practice
- Helps to ensure quality patient care
- Builds trust on the part of the patient and facility
- Establishes a high level of standards within healthcare
- Strengthens the nurse's resume and job qualifications
- Increases potential for earning power

MEDICAL-SURGICAL NURSING CERTIFICATION BOARD

Exam Format

- The exam is a CBT.
- The exam consists of 150 questions; 125 are scored, and 25 are experimental.
- The time to complete the exam is 3 hours.
- A passing score is 95 out of 125 questions correct, or 71%.
- A successful candidate will earn a CMSRN certification.
- Accommodations can be made for candidates with disabilities. Contact MSNCB at certification @msncb.org to request assistance.

Exam Content

Seven domains of medical-surgical nursing practice are covered on the exam:
- Diagnostic/patient monitoring
- Teaching/coaching
- Helping role
- Administering nursing intervention
- Managing emergency
- Ensuring quality
- Organization/work role competency

Six areas of patient problems are covered on the exam:
- Gastrointestinal: 24 to 27 questions (16%–18%)
- Pulmonary: 22 to 26 questions (15%–17%)
- Cardiovascular/hematological: 24 to 27 questions (16%–18%)
- Diabetes (type 1 and 2)/other endocrine/immunological: 27 to 30 questions (18%–20%)
- Urological/renal: 21 to 24 questions (14%–16%)
- Musculoskeletal/neurological/integumentary: 22 to 26 questions (15%–17%)

Eligibility

To apply for the MSNCB exam, a candidate must meet the following qualifications:
- Hold an active, unencumbered RN license in the United States, U.S. territories, or Canada
- Have 2 years of practice in a medical-surgical setting
- Have a minimum of 2,000 hours of practice, including clinical, management, or education in a medical-surgical setting in the last 3 years

How to Apply

- Meet all of the eligibility criteria.
- Visit msncb.org.
- Pay fee for exam: $375, or $255 for current AMSN members.
- Receive an authorization to test.
- Schedule exam within 90 days.

MSNCB Contact Information

Details of the exam are subject to change. For the most up-to-date information, please contact MSNCB:
PO Box 56
Pitman, NJ 08071
Toll-free phone number: 866-877-2676
Fax: 856-589-7463
Email: certification@msncb.org
Website: www.msncb.org

AMERICAN NURSES CREDENTIALING CENTER

Exam Format

- The exam is a CBT.
- The exam consists of 150 questions; 125 are scored, and 25 are experimental.
- Candidates are given 3 hours to complete the exam.
- A passing score is 350 out of 500 points (70%).
- A successful candidate will earn a certification of RN-BC.
- Accommodations can be made for candidates with disabilities. Contact ANCC before scheduling the exam at certification@ana.org if assistance is required.

Exam Content

Three domains of medical-surgical nursing practice are covered on the exam:
- Assessment and diagnosis: 52 questions (42%)
  - Health history collection
  - Physical assessment
  - Psychosocial assessment
  - Cognitive assessment
  - Diagnostic and laboratory testing
  - Nursing diagnosis identification and prioritization
  - Fluids and electrolytes
- Planning, implementation, and evaluation: 58 questions (46%)
  - Nursing care planning
  - Postoperative complication prevention and management
  - Patient teaching
  - Education topics
  - Patient safety measures
  - Nonpharmacologic treatments
  - Medication interactions and adverse effects
  - Health and wellness promotion
- Professional role: 15 questions (12%)
  - Therapeutic communication
  - Nursing ethics

Eligibility

To apply for the ANCC exam, a candidate must meet the following qualifications:
- Hold an active, unencumbered RN license in a U.S. state or territory or the equivalent legally recognized certification in another country
- Have 2 years of practice in a medical-surgical setting
- Have a minimum of 2,000 hours of practice in a medical-surgical setting in the last 3 years
- Have a minimum of 30 hours of continuing education credits in medical-surgical nursing within the last 3 years

How to Apply

- Meet all of the eligibility criteria.
- Visit www.nursingworld.org/our-certifications/medical-surgical-nurse/.
- Pay fee for exam: $395, or $295 for current ANA members.
- Receive an authorization to test.
- Schedule exam within 90 days.

Contact Information for ANCC

Details of the exam are subject to change. For the most up-to-date information, please contact ANCC:

    8515 Georgia Avenue, Suite 400
    Silver Spring, MD 20910-4392
    Toll-free phone number: 800-284-2378
    Email: certification@ana.org
    Website: www.nursingworld.org

RESOURCES

American Nurses Association. (n.d.). *Medical-Surgical Nursing Certification (MEDSURG-BC™)*. https://www.nursingworld.org/our-certifications/medical-surgical-nurse/

Medical-Surgical Nursing Certification Board. (n.d.). *Why become a certified medical-surgical registered nurse (CMSRN)?* https://www.msncb.org/medical-surgical/get-certified

2

CARDIOVASCULAR SYSTEM

ACUTE CORONARY SYNDROME

Overview

- *Acute coronary syndrome* is the result of a blockage in one of the coronary arteries.
- Acute coronary syndrome includes:
  - Unstable angina
  - NSTEMI
  - STEMI

ANGINA

Overview

- *Angina* is pain or pressure in the chest that is caused by an insufficient supply of blood to the myocardium. There is no elevation in cardiac enzymes with angina.
- Angina can be stable or unstable.
  - Stable angina is a result of atherosclerosis and is often caused by physical exertion when the narrowed coronary arteries cannot provide enough oxygenated blood to the myocardium. Pain lasts less than 15 minutes and is primarily relieved by nitroglycerin and rest.
  - Unstable angina occurs without any precipitating factors, and pain lasts more than 15 minutes. It is poorly controlled, or sometimes not controlled at all, with nitroglycerin and rest.

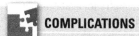 **COMPLICATIONS**

Inadequately treated unstable angina is more likely to lead to adverse cardiac events such as MI.

Signs and Symptoms

- Chest pressure or pain
- Diaphoresis
- Dizziness
- Nausea
- Palpitations
- Shortness of breath

Diagnosis

Labs

- BNP: abnormal if greater than 100 pg/mL
- CBC
- CK-MB: cardiac enzymes elevated in MI
- CMP: may reflect electrolyte abnormalities
- CRP: marker of inflammation in the heart; would be elevated
- Lipids
- Magnesium: low levels may cause arrythmias
- Troponin: if elevated, indicates heart muscle damage

Diagnostic Testing
- 12-lead EKG
- Chest x-ray
- Echocardiogram

Treatment

- Aspirin: chewable or non–enteric coated
- Nitroglycerin (Appendix 2.1 at the end of this chapter)
  - First-line treatment for stable angina
    - Short-acting sublingual nitroglycerin
    - Long-acting nitrates: oral isosorbide
  - Topical or transdermal nitrates: poor treatment for unstable angina
- Oxygen
- Pain medication

 ALERT!

Nitroglycerin is contraindicated for patients who have taken a phosphodiesterase inhibitor in the previous 24 to 48 hours. It is imperative to ask the patient if they have taken this medication in the last 24 to 48 hours.

Nursing Interventions

- Administer medications as ordered.
- Assess ABCs.
- Assess oxygenation level.
- Assess pain level.
- Ensure bed rest as ordered.
- Monitor telemetry for acute changes.
- Monitor vital signs.
- Obtain IV access.
- Provide emotional support.

 POP QUIZ 2.1

An older adult patient is admitted with a substernal chest pain rating of 9/10. Admission vitals are HR 89, BP 104/56, RR 19, and pulse oximetry 89%. What interventions should the nurse initiate, and what orders should the nurse anticipate from the provider?

Patient Education

- Begin a smoking cessation plan, as needed.
- Exercise as tolerated.
- Follow a heart-healthy diet.
- Maintain a healthy weight.
- Manage stress.
- Take medications as prescribed.

MYOCARDIAL INFARCTION

Overview

- An *MI* is the result of one or more of the coronary arteries that supply blood to the heart becoming completely blocked, cutting off the blood supply to the myocardium.
- There are two types of MI: STEMI and NSTEMI.
  - *STEMI*: complete occlusion of one or more of the coronary arteries; ST segment of patient's 12-lead EKG appears elevated.
  - *NSTEMI*: partial occlusion of one or more of the coronary arteries; ST segment of patient's 12-lead EKG does not appear elevated.

Signs and Symptoms

- Anxiety
- Diaphoresis
- Dizziness
- Nausea

NURSING PEARL

All chest pain should be assumed to be cardiac in nature until proven otherwise. Atypical chest pain can include epigastric pain, including indigestion.

(continued)

Signs and Symptoms *(continued)*

- Pain that spreads to the shoulders, neck, left arm, or jaw (unrelieved by nitroglycerin)
- Pallor
- Palpitations

Diagnosis

Labs

- BNP
- CBC
- CK-MB: elevated in MI
- CMP: may reflect electrolyte abnormalities
- CRP: c-reactive protein is elevated; the higher the level, the greater the severity of disease
- Lipids
- Myoglobin: if elevated, indicates heart muscle damage
- Troponin: if elevated, indicates heart muscle damage

Diagnostic Testing

- 12-lead EKG
- Cardiac catheterization
- Chest x-ray
- Dobutamine stress test
- Echocardiogram
- MUGA scan

Treatment

- ACE inhibitors
- Analgesics (including morphine)
- Anticoagulants
- Aspirin
- Beta-blockers
- Nitroglycerin
- Oxygen
- Statin drugs
- Thrombolytics
- Vasodilators

Nursing Interventions

- Assess ABC.
- Assess the need for oxygen.
- Assess vital signs.
- Administer medications as ordered.
- Monitor telemetry for acute changes.
- Obtain IV access.

Patient Education

- Begin a smoking cessation plan, if needed.
- Follow a heart-healthy diet.
- Exercise as tolerated.
- Manage stress.
- Take medications as prescribed.

ANEURYSM

Overview

- *Aortic aneurysm* occurs when the vessel wall becomes weakened, causing it to become distended or enlarged.
- Aortic aneurysm can occur in the thoracic cavity or in the abdominal cavity.

Signs and Symptoms

- Abdominal
  - Abdominal pain
  - Back pain
  - Can be asymptomatic
  - Feeling of pulsation in the abdomen
- Thoracic
  - Dry cough
  - Dysphagia
  - Severe chest pain

Diagnosis

Labs

- CBC: hemoglobin may be low, indicating internal bleeding

Diagnostic Testing

- Abdominal and chest x-ray
- Abdominal ultrasound
- CT with contrast
- Echocardiogram
- MRI

Treatment

- Medications including antihypertensives (see Appendix 2.1)
- Surgical intervention

Nursing Interventions

- Assess ABC.
- Assess for worsening symptoms.
- Administer medications as ordered by the provider.
- Monitor vital signs.
- Obtain IV access.

Patient Education

- Adhere to surveillance schedule to monitor aneurysm.
- Begin a smoking cessation plan, as needed.
- Monitor blood pressure closely to maintain prescribed range.
- Take medications as prescribed.

 POP QUIZ 2.2

An adult patient is admitted with abdominal pain that radiates to the back. The patient states that they have a previous diagnosis of abdominal aortic aneurysm. The patient has forgotten to take their antihypertensive medications for the last week. Admission vitals are HR 100, BP 189/99, RR 22, and pulse oximetry 95%. What should the nurse anticipate, and what interventions should the nurse begin?

ARRHYTHMIAS

Overview

- An *arrhythmia* is an abnormality in the heart's rhythm or heartbeat pattern.
- Arrhythmias occur when the heartbeat starts in an irregular part of the heart, an abnormal rate or rhythm develops, or the electrical signal is blocked from traveling down the normal pathway.

Signs and Symptoms

- Altered mental status
- Can be asymptomatic
- Chest pain
- Diaphoresis
- Increasing oxygen requirements
- Palpitations
- Shortness of breath

Diagnosis

Labs

- BMP: many reflect electrolyte abnormalities
- Cardiac enzymes: levels include CK, CK-MB, troponin, and myoglobin, elevated with cardiac damage

Diagnostic Testing

- 12-lead EKG
- Echocardiogram
- Electrophysiology studies
- Stress testing

Treatment

- Ablation
- Cardioversion
- Defibrillation
- Medications (see Appendix 2.1)
  - Antiarrhythmic agents
  - Beta-blockers
  - Calcium channel blockers
- Pacemaker placement

Nursing Interventions

- Assess ABC.
- Assess vital signs.
- Administer medications as ordered.
- Monitor telemetry for acute changes.

Patient Education

- Follow up as indicated by the provider.
- Learn about pacemaker regimen if one is present.
- Take medications as prescribed.

POP QUIZ 2.3

The nurse notices that a patient is experiencing sinus bradycardia on the telemetry monitor overnight. What assessments should the nurse initiate?

CARDIOMYOPATHY

Overview

- *Cardiomyopathy* is a chronic disease of the myocardium, in which the muscle is thickened, enlarged, or stiffened. The weakened heart muscle loses the ability to pump blood effectively, which can result in HF and arrhythmias.
- Cardiomyopathies occur in three major categories:
  - Dilated cardiomyopathy is the most common type. The heart cavity is dilated, which results in weak and slow pumping of the blood. Many patients with dilated cardiomyopathy develop HF.

(continued)

Overview (continued)

- Hypertrophic cardiomyopathy occurs when the muscle mass of the left ventricle enlarges, or hypertrophies. This type of cardiomyopathy is often genetic.
- Restrictive cardiomyopathy is the least common type. In this type, the heart muscle of the ventricles becomes rigid. Restrictive cardiomyopathy affects the diastolic function of the heart, resulting in less filling time between beats.

Signs and Symptoms

- Atrial fibrillation
- Cardiomegaly
- Chest pain
- Cough
- Dyspnea
- Fatigue
- Peripheral edema

Diagnosis

Labs

- ABG: may show hypoxemia
- BUN and creatinine: may be elevated due to reductions in renal flow from reduced cardiac output
- BMP: may reflect electrolyte imbalances
- Cardiac enzymes: levels include CK, CK-MB, troponin, and myoglobin, elevated with cardiac damage

Diagnostic Testing

- 12-lead EKG
- Cardiac catheterization
- Chest x-ray
- Echocardiogram

Treatment

- Fluid restrictions
- Medications (see Appendix 2.1)
  - ACE inhibitors
  - Antiarrhythmics
  - Beta-blockers
- Sodium restriction
- May progress to needing pacing or transplant

Nursing Interventions

- Assess ABC.
- Administer medications as ordered.
- Monitor vital signs.
- Monitor for acute changes in telemetry.
- Obtain IV access.

Patient Education

- Adhere to sodium- and fluid-restricted diet.
- Begin a smoking cessation plan, as needed.
- Begin alcohol and substance use cessation, as needed.
- Exercise as tolerated.
- Take medications as prescribed.
- Learn pacemaker regimen if one is present.

DEEP VEIN THROMBOSIS

Overview

A *DVT* is a blood clot in a major vein, most often in the lower extremities.

Signs and Symptoms

- Tenderness or pain in the calf or thigh
- Unilateral lower extremity edema
- Warmth in the calf or thigh

Diagnosis

Labs
D-dimer: screening test for possible presence of clot; less than 250 ng/mL indicates low DVT risk

Diagnostic Testing
- Ultrasound
- Venography
- Venous duplex scan

Treatment

- Compression garments
- IVC filter
- Medications (see Appendix 2.1)
  - Anticoagulants
  - Thrombolytics

Nursing Interventions

- Assess ABC.
- Monitor affected extremity, especially pulses.
- Monitor vital signs.
- Monitor for signs and symptoms of CVA or PE.
- Obtain IV access.

Patient Education

- Follow up as indicated by the provider.
- Monitor for signs and symptoms of bleeding if on anticoagulants.
- Reduce long periods of sitting or inactivity.
- Take medications as prescribed.

 POP QUIZ 2.4

A patient presents to the ED with left leg pain. The left leg is swollen, red, and painful. The patient reports massaging the left leg for pain relief. Which action should the nurse take?

ENDOCARDITIS

Overview

Endocarditis is an infection of the endocardium, or the inner layer of the heart muscle. It can also include infection of the heart's four valves.

Signs and Symptoms

- Arthralgias
- Chills
- Cough
- Dyspnea

(continued)

Signs and Symptoms *(continued)*

- Heart murmur
- Low-grade fever
- Weakness

Diagnosis

Labs
- CBC with differential: reduced RBCs and leukocytosis if endocarditis present
- Blood cultures

Diagnostic Testing
Echocardiogram

Treatment

- IV antibiotics
  - Lengthy course
  - Possible continuation at home if stable; dependent on overall health
- Surgical replacement of infected valves

Nursing Interventions

- Assess ABC.
- Administer medications as ordered.
- Monitor vital signs.
- Monitor for signs and symptoms of CVA or PE.
- Obtain IV access.

Patient Education

- Learn about the central line and its care, if discharged with IV antibiotics.
- Seek treatment or counseling for IV drug use as applicable.

HEART FAILURE

Overview

- *HF* is characterized by the ventricles of the heart not filling adequately or inefficiently ejecting blood, resulting in reduced circulation of oxygenated blood.
- Right-sided HF is characterized by difficulty with ventricles filling, while left-sided HF is characterized by difficulty with ventricles emptying.

Signs and Symptoms

- Cough
- Difficulty sleeping
- Dyspnea
- Crackles in auscultated lungs
- Edema
- Fatigue
- JVD
- Orthopnea
- Pulmonary edema
- S3 and S4 heart tones

Diagnosis

Labs

- BMP: may reflect electrolyte abnormalities or evidence of AKI
- BNP: elevated >100 mL in HF; the higher the result, the more severe the HF
- CBC with differential anemia is common in HF
- CRP: can be elevated in patients with comorbidities (e.g., COPD)
- Troponin

Diagnostic Testing

- 12-lead EKG
- Cardiac catheterization
- Chest x-ray
- Echocardiogram

Treatment

- Fluid restriction
- Medications (see Appendix 2.1)
  - ACE inhibitors
  - Aldosterone antagonists
  - ARBs
  - Beta-blockers
  - Digoxin
  - Diuretics
  - Vasodilators
- Oxygen
- Sodium restriction

Nursing Interventions

- Assess ABC.
- Assess fluid and electrolyte imbalances; peripheral or pulmonary edema is a sign of fluid overload.
- Assess vital signs.
- Administer medications as ordered.
- Elevate the head of the bed if the patient has orthopnea.
- Elevate lower extremities if the patient is experiencing peripheral edema.
- Monitor weight daily. Report weight gain greater than 2 lb in 24 hours or 5 lb in 1 week to the provider, as this may indicate fluid overload.
- Obtain IV access.

Patient Education

- Adhere to fluid restrictions as ordered by the provider.
- Adhere to sodium restrictions as ordered by the provider.
- Exercise as tolerated.
- Take medications as prescribed.

POP QUIZ 2.5

An older adult patient presents with a history of HF. The patient states that they have not taken their cardiac medications. The patient's vital signs are BP 165/70, HR 89, RR 22, and pulse oximetry 92% on room air. BNP is >200 pg/mL. What other signs of HF would the nurse expect, and what would be the first medication the nurse would administer with the provider orders?

HYPERLIPIDEMIA

Overview

Hyperlipidemia is characterized by high levels of lipids in the blood.

Signs and Symptoms

There are often no signs of hyperlipidemia, and it is usually diagnosed through routine blood testing.

Diagnosis

Labs

Fasting lipid panel (normal values):
- Total cholesterol less than 200 mg/dL
- LDL cholesterol less than 100 mg/dL
- HDL cholesterol greater than 40 mg/dL
- Triglycerides less than 150 mg/dL

Diagnostic Testing

There are no diagnostic tests specific to diagnosing hyperlipemia.

Treatment

Medications: statins (see Appendix 2.1)

Nursing Interventions

- Administer medications as ordered.
- Assess vital signs.
- Encourage compliance with a low-fat diet.

Patient Education

- Adhere to a low-fat, heart-healthy diet.
- Exercise as tolerated.
- Take medications as prescribed.

HYPERTENSION

Overview

- *Hypertension* is a condition in which a person's blood pressure is elevated.
- Blood pressure categories:
  - Normal: less than 120 systolic and less than 80 diastolic
  - Elevated: 120 to 129 systolic and less than 80 diastolic
  - Hypertension stage 1: 120 to 129 systolic and 80 to 89 diastolic
  - Hypertension stage 2: 140 or higher systolic and 90 or higher diastolic
  - Hypertensive crisis: higher than 180 systolic and higher than 120 diastolic

Signs and Symptoms

- Blurred vision
- Dizziness
- Dyspnea
- Severe headaches
- Tinnitus

Diagnosis

Labs

- BMP: may reflect electrolyte abnormalities; evidence of kidney injury if elevated
- CBC: may detect anemia
- Fasting lipid profile
- TSH
- UA: may contain proteinuria (indicating kidney disease)

Diagnostic Testing
- 12-lead EKG
- Ophthalmic appointment to determine if hypertension has affected the eye
- Serial blood pressure readings

Treatment
- Medications: antihypertensives (see Appendix 2.1)

Nursing Interventions
- Administer medications as ordered.
- Assess ABC.
- Monitor vital signs.

Patient Education
- Adhere to fluid and sodium restrictions, if recommended by the provider.
- Avoid caffeine.
- Begin a smoking cessation plan, as needed.
- Exercise as tolerated.
- Reduce stress.
- Take medications as prescribed.

PERIPHERAL VASCULAR DISEASE

Overview
- PVD occurs when blood vessels become restricted or blocked.
- The most common cause of PVD is atherosclerosis.

Signs and Symptoms
- Coolness of extremities
- Decreased or absent pedal pulses
- Intermittent claudication
- Nonhealing wounds
- Skin changes, including hair loss to extremities and pale skin

Diagnosis
Labs
- Lipid panel

Diagnostic Testing
- Ankle-brachial index
- CT angiography
- Doppler duplex ultrasound
- MRA

Treatment
- Arterial stenting
- Bypass grafting
- Medications (see Appendix 2.1)
  - Anticoagulants
  - Antiplatelets
  - Thrombolytics
  - Vasodilators
- Thrombectomy

Nursing Interventions

- Assess ABC.
- Assess vital signs.
- Assess affected extremities for decreased perfusion.
- Assess skin for nonhealing wounds.
- Assess and treat pain.
- Administer medications as ordered.
- Perform postoperative graft management.

Patient Education

- Exercise as tolerated.
- Maintain a low-fat, heart-healthy diet.
- Monitor extremities for wounds.
- Begin a smoking cessation plan, as needed.
- Take medications as prescribed.

SHOCK

Overview

- *Shock* is the result of the body's organs and tissues not receiving an adequate flow of blood.
- *Cardiogenic shock* is a condition in which inadequate organ perfusion is primarily a result of cardiac dysfunction.
- *Hypovolemic shock* occurs as a result of large losses of blood or body fluids.

Signs and Symptoms

- Altered mental status
- Cool, mottled extremities
- Hypotension
- Oliguria
- Tachycardia
- Thready, rapid, or absent peripheral pulses

Diagnosis

Labs

- ABG: will show metabolic acidosis
- BMP: may reflect electrolyte abnormalities; evidence of kidney injury if elevated
- BNP: elevated
- CBC: may show elevated WBC counts, indicating possible infection
- CK-MB: increased to indicate cardiac muscle damage
- Lactate: will be elevated
- Troponin: may be elevated

Diagnostic Testing

- 12-lead EKG
- Cardiac catheterization
- Chest x-ray
- CT scan
- Echocardiogram

Treatment

- Medications (see Appendix 2.1)
  - Anticoagulants
  - Antiplatelet drugs
  - Inotropic agents
  - Vasopressors
  - Vasodilators
- Volume resuscitation with blood or fluids

Nursing Interventions

- Assess ABC.
- Assess for acute changes in telemetry.
- Assess for changes in mental status.
- Assess vital signs.
- Administer medications as ordered.
- Monitor fluid status.
- Obtain IV access.

Patient Education

- Manage cardiac illness leading to shock.
- Maintain appropriate fluid balance.

Appendix 2.1 Cardiovascular Medications

Indications	Mechanism of Action	Contraindications, Precautions, and Adverse Effects
ACE inhibitors (captopril, enalapril, lisinopril)		
• Left-sided HF • First-line treatment for hypertension	• Inhibit the conversion of angiotensin I to angiotensin II • Reduce vascular resistance • Dilate veins	• Use with caution in patients with CKD or AKI. • Cough is the most common side effect. • Medication can cause hyperkalemia.
ARBs (losartan, valsartan)		
• Left-sided HF • Second line antihypertensive, used if patient cannot tolerate ACE inhibitors	• Block the binding of angiotensin I to angiotensin II receptors	• Use with caution in patients with CKD or AKI.
Aldosterone antagonists (spironolactone)		
• Left- or right-sided HF • Treatment of fluid overload	• Block aldosterone, which blocks sodium reabsorption and causes diuresis	• Monitor for hyperkalemia. • Monitor for hypermagnesemia.
Antiarrhythmics, class III (amiodarone)		
• Rate control for tachyarrhythmias	• Delayed repolarization and depression of node automaticity, leading to slowed heart rate	• Use caution in patients with underlying heart block or hepatic impairment.

(continued)

Appendix 2.1 Cardiovascular Medications *(continued)*

Indications	Mechanism of Action	Contraindications, Precautions, and Adverse Effects
Anticoagulants (heparin)		
• DVT treatment and prophylaxis • Valvular heart disease • PVD	• Inhibit thrombin	• Use with caution in patients at risk for bleeding.
Antiplatelet agents (aspirin, clopidogrel)		
• A-fib/A-flutter • CAD, PVD • Acute coronary syndrome	• Decrease platelet aggregation	• Use caution in patients at risk for bleeding.
Beta-blockers (atenolol, labetalol metoprolol)		
• Left or right-sided HF	• Block the effects of epinephrine and norepinephrine, decreasing heart rate and contractility • Cause vasodilation	• Medication can cause bronchospasm. • Medication is contraindicated in patients with bradycardia and sick sinus syndrome.
Calcium channel blockers (diltiazem)		
• Rate control • Antihypertensive	• Block calcium influx across myocardial and smooth muscle • Slow AV conduction	• Use caution in patients with HF.
Cardiac glycosides (digoxin)		
• Left-sided symptomatic HF	• Slow conduction through the AV node to improve contractility	• Monitor for digoxin toxicity symptoms. • Use caution in patients with CKD or AKI.
Loop diuretics (furosemide)		
• Left-sided HF with fluid overload	• Inhibit sodium and chloride reabsorption, causing excretion of electrolytes and water	• Monitor for dehydration. • Monitor for electrolyte imbalance.
Vasodilators (isosorbide, nitroglycerin)		
• Acute HF or angina	• Dilate veins to reduce systemic vascular resistance	• Headache is a common side effect. • Do not use in hypotensive patients. • Medication is contraindicated if patient has used phosphodiesterase inhibitors 24 hours previously.

Note: All agents are contraindicated in the presence of hypersensitivity to the medication or one of its components.

RESOURCES

American Heart Association. (2022). *Understanding blood pressure readings*. https://www.heart.org/en/health-topics/high-blood-pressure/understanding-blood-pressure-readings?gclid=CjwKCAiAgbiQBhAHEiwAuQ6Bk m81ukM0oiY_jdw8rlsmdJVl3X_9sxhZ4fr8G0q38lIsgN6R8LeuIxoCzRIQAvD_BwE

DuBrock, H. M., AbouEzzeddine, O. F., & Redfield, M. M. (2018). High-sensitivity C-reactive protein in heart failure with preserved ejection fraction. *PLoS One, 13*(8).

Harding, M., Roberts, D., Kwong, J., Hagler, D., & Reinisch, C. (2020). *Lewis's medical-surgical nursing* (11th ed.). Elsevier.

Longe, J. L. (Ed.). (2018). *The gale encyclopedia of nursing and allied health* (4th ed.). Gale. https://link.gale.com/apps/pub/07UZ/GVRL?u=kcls_main&sid=GVRL

Prescribers' Digital Reference. (n.d.[a]). *Amiodarone* [Drug information]. https://www.pdr.net/drug-summary/Amiodarone-Hydrochloride-Injection-amiodarone-hydrochloride-3234.8358

Prescribers' Digital Reference. (n.d.[b]). *Cozaar* [Drug information]. https://www.pdr.net/drug-summary/Cozaar-losartan-potassium-339.4526

Prescribers' Digital Reference. (n.d.[c]). *Digoxin* [Drug information]. https://www.pdr.net/drug-summary/Digoxin-digoxin-724

Prescribers' Digital Reference. (n.d.[d]). *Diltiazem* [Drug information]. https://www.pdr.net/drug-summary/Diltiazem-Hydrochloride-Injection-diltiazem-hydrochloride-725.1140#14

Prescribers' Digital Reference. (n.d.[e]). *Heparin* [Drug information]. https://www.pdr.net/drug-summary/Heparin-Sodium-Injection-heparin-sodium-1263

Prescribers' Digital Reference. (n.d.[f]). *Lasix* [Drug information]. https://www.pdr.net/drug-information/lasix?druglabelid=2594

Prescribers' Digital Reference. (n.d.[g]). *Lisinopril* [Drug information]. https://www.pdr.net/drug-summary/Zestril-lisinopril-2456.5955

Prescribers' Digital Reference. (n.d.[h]). Metoprolol [Drug information].https://www.pdr.net/drug-summary/Metoprolol-Tartrate-metoprolol-tartrate-3114.5976

Prescribers' Digital Reference. (n.d.[i]). *Nitroglycerin* [Drug information]. https://www.pdr.net/drug-summary/Nitroglycerin-in-5--Dextrose-nitroglycerin-1148

Prescribers' Digital Reference. (n.d.[j]). *Plavix* [Drug information]https://www.pdr.net/drug-summary/Plavix-clopidogrel-bisulfate-525.3952#11

Prescribers' Digital Reference. (n.d.[k]). *Spironolactone* [Drug informationhttps://www.pdr.net/drug-summary/Aldactone-spironolactone-978.2934

3

ENDOCRINE SYSTEM

ADRENAL INSUFFICIENCY (ADDISON'S DISEASE)

Overview

Adrenal insufficiency results from a hypoactive adrenal cortex, leading to limited production of cortisol and aldosterone. A lack of aldosterone causes the kidneys to excrete excess sodium and water while retaining potassium.

Signs and Symptoms

- Dehydration
- Dizziness
- Fatigue
- Nausea
- Polyuria
- Weakness

Diagnosis

Labs

- ACTH stimulation test
- BMP
- Cortisol level

Diagnostic Testing

- CT scan

Treatment

- Corticosteroids on a schedule to mimic the body's natural secretion of corticosteroids
- High-sodium diet

Nursing Interventions

- Monitor electrolytes.
- Monitor fluid balance.
- Monitor telemetry for acute changes.

Patient Education

- Increase sodium intake as instructed by provider.
- Take medications as prescribed.

DIABETES INSIPIDUS

Overview

- *DI* is a condition in which the pituitary gland fails to make sufficient quantities of ADH, or the kidneys fail to respond appropriately to the ADH that is produced. As a result, the body creates large amounts of dilute urine.
- In *central DI*, the pituitary gland fails to produce enough ADH. Central DI is caused by damage to the pituitary gland by trauma or disease. Other causes of central DI are excessive alcohol use and medications that reduce ADH production, such as the antiepileptic medication phenytoin.
- In *nephrogenic DI*, the kidneys fail to respond to ADH. Nephrogenic DI can be caused by hypercalcemia, pregnancy, or lithium use.

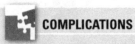

COMPLICATIONS

The most common complication of DI is dehydration resulting from large-volume urine output.

Signs and Symptoms

- Electrolyte derangement
- Extreme thirst
- Large-volume urine output

Diagnosis

Labs

- ADH
  - Possible low level in central DI or normal level in nephrogenic DI
  - Random plasma sample greater than 287 mOsm/kg indicative of DI
- BMP: possible high sodium due to large-volume dilute urine output
- CBC: often elevated due to concentration of plasma
- Serum osmolality
- UA: two diagnostic criteria:
  - Urine specific gravity less than 1.005
  - Urine osmolality less than 200 mOsm/kg

Diagnostic Testing

- Brain MRI to assess for trauma and check for tumors
- Water deprivation test

Treatment

- Medical-surgical goal: Maintain adequate hydration and electrolyte balance.
- Limit sodium intake.
- Administer medications (Appendix 3.1 at the end of this chapter):
  - First-line treatment: desmopressin
  - Antidiuretics
  - Thiazide diuretics

Nursing Interventions

- Administer medications as ordered.
- Monitor fluid input and output.
- Monitor labs for electrolyte derangement.
- Monitor urine for specific gravity and osmolality to assess for dehydration.
- Notify provider if urine output is increasing to greater than 50 mL/kg/24 hr.

Patient Education

- Increase fluid intake.
- Take medications as prescribed.

POP QUIZ 3.1

A patient who weighs 90 kg is admitted to the medical-surgical unit with a new diagnosis of DI. In 24 hours, the patient has urine output of 8.5 L. What is the appropriate next step for the nurse?

DIABETES MELLITUS

Overview

- *Diabetes mellitus* is a condition in which the pancreas does not produce enough insulin or the body's cells stop responding to the insulin that is produced.
- In type 1 diabetes, the pancreas produces little to no insulin. Type 1 diabetes is sometimes referred to as insulin-dependent diabetes because all patients require supplementary insulin for the rest of their lives.
- Providers may order an antibody test or c-peptide test to differentiate between type 1 and type 2 diabetes.

COMPLICATIONS

Uncontrolled diabetes can lead to a host of complications including blindness, diabetic nephropathy, peripheral vascular insufficiency, poor wound healing, and diabetic neuropathy. It also increases the risk of infections, heart disease, and stroke.

- In type 2 diabetes, the pancreas may not produce enough insulin, and insulin sensitivity in cells is reduced. Other causes of type 2 diabetes include inappropriate hepatic glucose production or altered production of hormones and cytokines by adipose tissue. All oral medications for diabetes are for type 2 diabetes. However, patients with type 2 diabetes may also require insulin due to the progressive nature of the disease.
- Patients with type 1 diabetes make up about 5% of diabetes cases in the United States.
- Patients with type 2 diabetes make up about 91% of diabetes cases in the United States.

Signs and Symptoms

- 3 Ps:
  - Polydipsia: excessive thirst
  - Polyphagia: excessive hunger
  - Polyuria: frequent urination
- Blurred vision
- Fatigue
- Unexplained weight loss
- Weakness

Diagnosis

Labs

- C-peptide: to differentiate type 1 diagnosis from type 2 diagnosis
- Fasting blood glucose:
  - 100 to 125 mg/dL considered prediabetes
  - Greater than 125 mg/dL indicative of diabetes
  - Often performed 2 days in a row for definitive diagnosis
- HbA1C
  - Prediabetes: 5.7% to 6.5%
  - Diagnostic for diabetes: greater than 6.5%
- UA
  - To check for glucose in the urine
  - Any glucose: abnormal and indicative of diabetes
- Oral glucose tolerance test
  - Blood glucose greater than 200 mg/dL diagnostic for diabetes

ALERT!

Hypoglycemia is a life-threatening emergency. Common symptoms include:

- Confusion
- Diaphoresis
- Dizziness
- Hunger
- Irritability
- Lightheadedness
- Tachycardia

Hypoglycemia should be treated immediately by providing the patient a source of oral glucose, such as juice, if they are awake and alert. If the patient cannot safely swallow, give glucose via other means as directed by the provider.

Diagnostic Testing

There are no diagnostic tests specific to diagnosing type 1 or 2 diabetes.

Treatment

- Consistent carbohydrate diet for all patients with diabetes
- Maintenance of euglycemia
- Medications (see Appendix 3.1)
  - Insulin
    - Type 1 diabetes: only treatment
    - Type 2 diabetes: supplementary if uncontrolled with oral medications or if HbA1C greater than 9% at diagnosis
  - Noninsulin injectables: stimulate incretin hormone that is low in type 2 diabetes
  - Oral medications: first-line treatment for type 2 diabetes

Nursing Interventions

- Assess for wounds, paying careful attention to the feet to check for open or nonhealing wounds that the patient may have overlooked.
- Check blood glucose level as ordered by the provider.
- Monitor carbohydrate intake by counting grams of carbohydrates ingested.
- Monitor for signs and symptoms of hypoglycemia and hyperglycemia.

Patient Education

- Check blood glucose at least daily or more often if ordered by provider.
- Check feet for wounds daily.
- Count grams of carbohydrate intake.
- Eat regularly scheduled meals.
- Rotate site of insulin injections as applicable.
- Take medication as prescribed.
- Test blood sugar before and after exercise.
- Use caution if consuming alcohol.

DIABETIC KETOACIDOSIS

Overview

- When the body's cells are unable to access blood glucose when insulin levels are low, the body responds by converting fat and protein into glucose and releases acidic ketones into the bloodstream.
- The buildup of ketones can lead to DKA.
- DKA is most common with type 1 diabetes. DKA is rarely seen in type 2 diabetes because most patients with type 2 diabetes produce some insulin.

 NURSING PEARL

Alcohol must be used with caution by patients with diabetes, as it can cause both hypoglycemia and hyperglycemia. Signs of intoxication can be confused with, or mask, signs of hypoglycemia. Additionally, alcohol impairs the liver in regulating blood sugar, which can lead to hypoglycemia.

 NURSING PEARL

Teaching patients with diabetes thorough foot care is an important part of diabetes management. Diabetic peripheral neuropathy can lead to decreased sensation in the feet. Patients must inspect their feet daily to assess for any wounds. Nonhealing wounds can ultimately lead to amputation.

 POP QUIZ 3.2

The patient has an order for 10 units of insulin glargine to be given subcutaneously every night. When the nurse comes to administer the medication, the patient reports feeling lightheaded and sweaty. What should the nurse's next action be?

 COMPLICATIONS

The complications of DKA include low potassium, cardiac arrhythmias, cerebral edema, pulmonary edema, and AKI. Untreated DKA can be fatal.

Signs and Symptoms

- Abdominal pain
- Fatigue
- Fruity breath
- Hyperglycemia
- Muscle stiffness
- Nausea
- Polyuria
- Tachypnea
- Thirst
- Vomiting

NURSING PEARL

All patients with type 1 diabetes should have ketone testing strips at home. They should test their urine if they have signs or symptoms of DKA.

Diagnosis

Labs

- BMP to monitor electrolytes, anion gap, and renal function: chloride greater than 8 mEq diagnostic criterion for DKA
- Serum glucose: blood glucose greater than 250 mg/dL diagnostic criterion for DKA
- UA to assess for ketones
- Venous or ABG to monitor blood pH: pH less than 7.3 diagnostic criterion for DKA

Diagnostic Testing

- EKG or continuous telemetry monitoring may be necessary to monitor the potential for cardiac arrhythmias due to hypokalemia complications.

Treatment

- Electrolyte replacement when applicable
- Institutional policy for when to reintroduce subcutaneous insulin
- Intravenous insulin (see Appendix 3.1)
- Intravenous hydration (see Appendix 3.1)
- Oral or intravenous bicarbonate

Nursing Interventions

- Administer insulin as ordered to maintain euglycemia.
- Monitor blood glucose level according to institution policy.
- Monitor oral carbohydrate intake by counting grams of carbohydrates ingested.
- Monitor potassium levels, as IV insulin can decrease potassium. Consider treating hypokalemia first, before hyperglycemic issue.
- Patients receiving IV insulin may be kept NPO for strict glucose control.

Patient Education

- Check blood glucose at least daily, or more often as instructed by provider.
- Count grams of carbohydrate intake daily.
- If DKA is suspected, check urine for ketones using urine dipstick.
- Monitor for signs and symptoms of hypoglycemia, including shakiness, dizziness, hunger, tachycardia, diaphoresis, confusion, and irritability.
- Monitor for signs and symptoms of hyperglycemia, including nausea, weakness, dry mouth, frequent urination, excessive thirst, excessive hunger, headache, and shortness of breath.
- Rotate sites of insulin injection. Repeated injections in the same area can lead to lipohypertrophy.
- Take medication as prescribed.

NURSING PEARL

All patients with type 1 diabetes should know signs and symptoms of DKA and that DKA is a life-threatening emergency.

POP QUIZ 3.3

A patient receives intravenous insulin overnight. Which electrolyte should the nurse expect to be low on the patient's morning labs?

HYPOGLYCEMIA

Overview

Hypoglycemia occurs when blood glucose falls below the level necessary to properly support the body's need for energy and stability throughout its cells.

Signs and Symptoms

- Confusion
- Dizziness
- Drowsiness
- Fatigue
- Hunger
- Irritability

Diagnosis

Labs
- Blood glucose

Diagnostic Testing
There are no diagnostic tests specific to diagnosing hypoglycemia.

Treatment

- If awake and alert, the patient should consume a source of oral glucose, such as juice.
- If unable to safely swallow, the patient should be given IV dextrose as ordered by the provider.

Nursing Interventions

- Monitor for signs and symptoms of hypoglycemia.

Patient Education

- Check blood glucose as ordered by the provider, at least daily.
- Have sources of oral glucose readily available.
- Monitor for symptoms of hypoglycemia.

> **POP QUIZ 3.4**
>
> The nurse is preparing a patient with insulin-dependent diabetes for surgery the following morning, including keeping the patient NPO per order. The patient states that they self-administered their scheduled long-acting insulin before coming to the hospital. What are the appropriate nursing actions to prevent hypoglycemia?

HYPERTHYROIDISM

Overview

- Hyperthyroidism results from an excess of the hormones T3 and T4 being released into the bloodstream.
- The most common cause of hyperthyroidism is Graves' disease, an autoimmune condition that causes excessive thyroid hormone to be released.

Signs and Symptoms

- Bulging eyes (Graves' ophthalmopathy)
- Enlarged thyroid gland (goiter)
- Heat intolerance
- Nervousness
- Tachycardia
- Tremors
- Weight loss

Diagnosis

Labs
- T3
- T4
- TSH

Diagnostic Testing
- Thyroid ultrasound

Treatment

- Medications to block hormone synthesis (Appendix 3.2 at the end of this chapter):
  - First-line treatment: thioamides
  - Beta-blockers
- Surgical resection of all or part of the thyroid gland

Nursing Interventions

- Monitor for tachycardia.
- Monitor for increased blood pressure.

Patient Education

- Take medications as prescribed.

POP QUIZ 3.5

A patient presents to the medical-surgical floor with bulging eyes and enlarged thyroid. The patient experiences new-onset weakness and seizure. What should the nurse immediately do for this complication?

HYPOTHYROIDISM

Overview

Hypothyroidism results from insufficient or inadequate production of the hormones T3 and T4.

Signs and Symptoms

- Bradycardia
- Cold intolerance
- Constipation
- Difficulty concentrating
- Fatigue
- Weight gain

Diagnosis

Labs
- TSH
- T4
- T3

Diagnostic Testing
- Thyroid ultrasound

Treatment

- Thyroid hormone replacement with medication

Nursing Interventions

- Monitor for signs and symptoms of hyperthyroidism resulting from overmedication.

Patient Education

- Take medications as prescribed.

HYPERFUNCTION OF THE ADRENALS (CUSHING'S DISEASE)

Overview

Cushing's disease results from overproduction of cortisol by the adrenal cortex.

Signs and Symptoms

- Fatigue
- Hirsutism in female patients
- Hyperglycemia
- Infertility in male patients
- Irritability
- Muscle wasting

Diagnosis

Labs

- Blood glucose
- Cortisol level

Diagnostic Testing

- CT scan to assess adrenal glands

Treatment

- Medications to block or decrease cortisol levels

Nursing Interventions

- Give medications as ordered.
- Monitor blood glucose.

Patient Education

- Take medications as ordered.

POLYCYSTIC OVARIAN SYNDROME

Overview

- *PCOS* is a condition in which the ovaries produce abnormal amounts of androgens.
- The ovaries develop multiple small, fluid-filled cysts.

Signs and Symptoms

- Acne
- Higher body mass index
- Hirsutism
- Menstrual irregularity

Diagnosis

Labs

- Androgen testing

Diagnostic Testing

- Pelvic or vaginal ultrasound
- Vaginal exam

Treatment

- First-line treatment: birth control pills for patients who are not actively trying to get pregnant
- Hormones to regulate menstruation

Nursing Interventions

Assess patient for symptoms of related disorders:
- Diabetes
- Heart disease
- Inflammation
- Insulin resistance
- Mood disorder
- Obstructive sleep apnea

Patient Education

- Exercise regularly.
- Take medications as prescribed.

SYNDROME OF INAPPROPRIATE ANTIDIURETIC HORMONE

Overview

SIADH is a condition in which the body makes too much ADH, causing the body to retain too much water.

Signs and Symptoms

- Confusion
- Headache
- Nausea
- Vomiting
- Weakness

Diagnosis

Labs
- BMP to check sodium
- Urine osmolality

Diagnostic Testing
There are no diagnostic tests specific to diagnosing SIADH. However, imaging may be ordered to find causes, such as a tumor.

Treatment

- Fluid restriction
- Hypertonic saline
- Loop diuretics
- Treatment of underlying cause

Nursing Interventions

- Monitor fluid and electrolytes.

Patient Education

- Adhere to fluid restrictions and dietary restrictions as ordered by the provider.

Appendix 3.1 Diabetes Medications

Indications	Mechanism of Action	Contraindications, Precautions, and Adverse Effects
Alpha-glucosidase inhibitors (acarbose, miglitol)		
• Taken with meals to prevent hyperglycemia by slowing digestion	• Delay carbohydrate digestion and absorption	• Medication is contraindicated in patients with chronic intestinal disease. • Medication is contraindicated in patients with serum creatinine greater than 2 mg/dL.
Amylin mimetic (pramlintide acetate)		
• Hyperglycemia • May be administered in combination with insulin	• Improves glycemic control • Slows gastric emptying • Suppresses postprandial glucagon secretion	• Medication is contraindicated in patients with gastroparesis or renal failure.
Antidiuretics (carbamazepine, chlorpropamide, clofibrate)		
• Central DI • Antidiuretic agent often combined with hydrochlorothiazide	• Increase release of ADH	• Hypoglycemia is a common side effect. Serum glucose must be closely monitored.
Biguanide (metformin)		
• Antihyperglycemic agent • First-line treatment for type 2 diabetes	• Improves glucose tolerance • Decreases hepatic gluconeogenesis production • Decreases intestinal absorption of glucose • Improves insulin sensitivity by increasing glucose uptake	• The medication is contraindicated in patients with renal or liver failure, unstable HF, acidosis, or severe alcohol misuse. • It decreases B12 levels. • Hold medications 48 hours before and after CT scan with IV contrast. • Metformin is not a cause of hypoglycemia.
Bile acid sequestrant (colesevelam)		
• Taken to prevent hyperglycemia	• Traditionally used to lower cholesterol but can also lower blood glucose; studies under way to understand the mechanism	• Medication is contraindicated in patients with history of bowel obstruction or motility disorders. • Use carefully in combination with medications that have a narrow therapeutic window, as absorption may be decreased.
Desmopressin (DDAVP)		
• Central DI • First-line treatment for DI • Synthetic analogue of ADH	• Increase water resorption in the central collecting duct of the kidneys	• Electrolyte excretion is not affected by this medication, so close monitoring of blood chemistries is required.

(continued)

Appendix 3.1 Diabetes Medications *(continued)*

Indications	Mechanism of Action	Contraindications, Precautions, and Adverse Effects
Dipeptidyl peptidase-IV inhibitors (alogliptin, sitagliptin)		
• Taken daily to prevent hyperglycemia by increasing insulin production	• Stimulate insulin secretion and suppress glucagon secretion • Inhibit gastric emptying	• Medication is contraindicated in patients with pancreatitis.
Dopamine agonist (bromocriptine)		
• Taken to prevent hyperglycemia	• Believed to decrease insulin resistance by inhibiting overactive sympathetic CNS, thereby reducing glucose production in the liver	• Medication is contraindicated in patients with severe psychotic disorders. • Do not use with strong CYP3A4 inhibitors (e.g., azole antimycotics, HIV PIs). • Medication is contraindicated in patients with cardiac disease. • Use with caution in patients with renal or hepatic impairment. • Do not use for pregnant patients.
GLP-1 receptor agonist (short and long acting) (dulaglutide, exenatide, lixisenatide, semaglutide)		
• Incretin mimetic • Hyperglycemia • Type 2 diabetes	• Potentiates glucose-dependent insulin secretion, increasing insulin levels • Delays gastric emptying	• Medication is contraindicated in patients with thyroid cancers. • Medication should not be used in patients with renal impairment.
Intermediate-acting insulin (neutral protamine hagedorn)		
• Hyperglycemia • Used in patients who are prone to hypoglycemia	• Binds to a glycoprotein receptor specific to insulin on the surface of target cells • Onset of 1–2 hours • Duration of 12 hours	• Hypoglycemia is the most common side effect. • Long-term use may cause lipohypertrophy.
Long-acting insulin (detemir, glargine)		
• Hyperglycemia • Once-daily dosing	• Binds to a glycoprotein receptor specific to insulin on the surface of target cells • Duration of 12–24 hours	• Hypoglycemia is the most common side effect. • Long-term use may cause lipohypertrophy.
Meglitinides (nateglinide, repaglinide)		
• Taken with meals to prevent hyperglycemia by stimulating the body to produce more insulin	• Stimulate insulin secretion by the pancreatic beta cells	• This medication class can cause hypoglycemia. • Use caution in patients with liver dysfunction.

(continued)

Appendix 3.1 Diabetes Medications *(continued)*

Indications	Mechanism of Action	Contraindications, Precautions, and Adverse Effects
Rapid-acting insulin (lispro, aspart)		
• Hyperglycemia • Correct high blood sugar before meals or preemptively before carbohydrate intake	• Binds to a glycoprotein receptor specific to insulin on the surface of target cells • Onset 5–15 minutes • Duration 4–6 hours	• Hypoglycemia is the most common side effect. • Long-term use may cause lipohypertrophy.
Short-acting insulin (regular)		
• Hyperglycemia • Given to correct high blood sugar before meals or preemptively before carbohydrate intake • In DKA, used as intravenous insulin infusion	• Binds to a glycoprotein receptor specific to insulin on the surface of target cells • Onset of 30–60 minutes • Duration of 6–8 hours	• Hypoglycemia is the most common side effect. • Long-term use may cause lipohypertrophy.
Sodium-glucose co-transporter-2 inhibitors (dapagliflozin, ertugliflozin)		
• Taken to prevent hyperglycemia by causing excess glucose to be excreted in urine	• Reabsorb the majority of the filtered glucose entering the kidneys • Cause excess glucose to be excreted in urine	• Dose adjustments are needed in patients with impaired renal function. • Medication does not cause hypoglycemia.
Sulfonylureas (glipizide, glyburide)		
• Hyperglycemia • Second-line treatment for type 2 diabetes	• Stimulate insulin secretion by the pancreatic beta cells	• This medication class can cause hypoglycemia. • Medication is contraindicated in patients with sulfa allergy. • Patients with renal failure may need lower dosage.
Thiazolidinediones (pioglitazone, rosiglitazone)		
• Hyperglycemia • Third-line treatment for type 2 diabetes	• Reduce insulin resistance and improve insulin sensitivity	• Medication is contraindicated in patients with NYHA Class III or IV HF. • Do not use in patients with active bladder cancer or a history of bladder cancer. • Medication does not cause hypoglycemia.
Thiazide diuretics (chlorothiazide, hydrochlorothiazide)		
• Nephrogenic DI • Create mild hypovolemia that increases sodium and water uptake in the proximal tubule	• Increase renal sodium excretion	• Use with caution in patients with impaired renal function.

Note: All medications are contraindicated in patients with sensitivity or allergy to the medication or its ingredients.

Appendix 3.2 Other Endocrine Medications

Indications	Mechanism of Action	Contraindications, Precautions, and Adverse Effects
Corticosteroids (cortisone)		
• Replacement of cortisol for patients with adrenal insufficiency	• Synthetic analog of cortisol	• Long-term steroid use can cause osteopenia. • Steroid use can cause hyperglycemia.
Loop diuretics (furosemide)		
• Used to decrease fluid volume in SIADH	• Inhibit sodium and chloride reabsorption, causing excretion of electrolytes and water	• Monitor for dehydration. • Monitor for electrolyte imbalance.
Thioamides (methimazole)		
• Treatment of hyperthyroidism	• Inhibit thyroid hormone production	• Medication is contraindicated in early pregnancy.
Thyroid hormones (levothyroxine)		
• Treatment of hypothyroidism	• Synthetic analog of T4	• Monitor TSH to ensure patient does not receive too much T4.

RESOURCES

Harding, M., Kwong, J., Robert, D., Hagler, D., & Reinisch, C. (2020). *Lewis's medical-surgical nursing* (11th ed.). Elsevier.

National Institutes of Health. (2017). *Polycystic ovary syndrome*. U.S. Department of Health and Human Services, National Institutes of Health. https://www.nichd.nih.gov/health/topics/pcos/more_information/FAQs/conditions-associated

Prescribers' Digital Reference. (n.d.[a]). *Avandia* [Drug information]. https://www.pdr.net/drug-summary/Avandia-rosiglitazone-maleate-175.404

Prescribers' Digital Reference. (n.d.[b]). *Carbamazepine* [Drug information]. https://www.pdr.net/drug-summary/Carbamazepine-carbamazepine-3186.4261

Prescribers' Digital Reference. (n.d.[c]). *Chlorothiazide* [Drug information]. https://www.pdr.net/drug-summary/Chlorothiazide-chlorothiazide-1960.1467

Prescribers' Digital Reference. (n.d.[d]). *Cortisone* [Drug information]. https://www.pdr.net/drug-summary/Cortisone-Acetate-cortisone-acetate-3309.2392

Prescribers' Digital Reference. (n.d.[e]). *Cycloset* [Drug information]. https://www.pdr.net/drug-summary/Cycloset-bromocriptine-mesylate-1309.4327

Prescribers' Digital Reference. (n.d.[f]). *DDAVP injection* [Drug information]. https://www.pdr.net/drug-summary/DDAVP-Injection-desmopressin-acetate-1901.319

Prescribers' Digital Reference. (n.d.[g]). *Farxiga* [Drug information]. https://www.pdr.net/drug-summary/Farxiga-dapagliflozin-3427.8279

Prescribers' Digital Reference. (n.d.[h]). *Glucophage* [Drug information]. https://www.pdr.net/drug-summary/Glucophage-Glucophage-XR-metformin-hydrochloride-892.4068

Prescribers' Digital Reference. (n.d.[i]). *Glucotrol* [Drug information]. https://www.pdr.net/drug-summary/Glucotrol-glipizide-1635.1620

Prescribers' Digital Reference. (n.d.[j]). *Humalog* [Drug information]. https://www.pdr.net/drug-summary/Humalog-insulin-lispro-291.3757

Prescribers' Digital Reference. (n.d.[k]). *Humalin R* [Drug information]. https://www.pdr.net/drug-summary/Humulin-R-regular--human-insulin--rDNA-origin--2912.3423

Prescribers' Digital Reference. (n.d.[l]). *Humalin N* [Drug information]. https://www.pdr.net/drug-summary/Humulin-N-NPH--human-insulin-isophane--rDNA-origin--2911.4411

Prescribers' Digital Reference. (n.d.[m]). *Januvia* [Drug information]. https://www.pdr.net/drug-summary/Januvia-sitagliptin-362.5870

Prescribers' Digital Reference. (n.d.[n]). *Lantus* [Drug information]. https://www.pdr.net/drug-summary/Lantus-insulin-glargine-520.3961

Prescribers' Digital Reference. (n.d.[o]). *Pramlintide acetate* [Drug information]. https://www.pdr.net/drug-summary/Symlin-pramlintide-acetate-62.3437

Prescribers' Digital Reference. (n.d.[p]). *Prandin* [Drug information]. https://www.pdr.net/drug-summary/Prandin-repaglinide-1005.736

Prescribers' Digital Reference. (n.d.[q]). *Precose* [Drug information]. https://www.pdr.net/drug-summary/Precose-acarbose-1315

Prescribers' Digital Reference. (n.d.[r]). *Synthroid* [Drug information]. https://www.pdr.net/drug-summary/Synthroid-levothyroxine-sodium-26.643

Prescribers' Digital Reference. (n.d.[s]). *Tapazole* [Drug information]. https://www.pdr.net/drug-summary/Tapazole-methimazole-1493

Prescribers' Digital Reference. (n.d.[u]). *Welchol* [Drug information]. https://www.pdr.net/drug-summary/Welchol-colesevelam-hydrochloride-2136

Swartout-Corbeil, D. M., & Oberleitner, M. G. (2018). Diabetes mellitus. In J. L. Longe (Ed.), *The Gale encyclopedia of nursing and allied health* (4th ed.). Gale.

EYES, EARS, NOSE, AND THROAT DISORDERS

CATARACTS

Overview

- Cataracts occur when the natural lens of the eye becomes opaque and interferes with the transmission of light to the retina.
- Proteins in the eye's lens disintegrate, and everything appears blurry, hazy, or less colorful.
- Cataracts are the most common cause of age-related vision loss in the world, affecting most older adults.

COMPLICATIONS

Complications of cataract surgery include bleeding, pain, risk of infection, and new or worsening vision problems, including double vision, dry eyes, and floaters.

Signs and Symptoms

- Blurred vision
- Double vision
- Opacity of the lens
- Seeing bright colors as faded or yellowed
- Sensitivity to light and glare
- Trouble seeing at night

Diagnosis

Labs
There are no labs specific to diagnosing cataracts.

Diagnostic Testing
Comprehensive eye exam, including:
- Pupil dilation
- Refraction and visual acuity test
- Retinal exam
- Slit-lamp exam

Treatment

- First-line treatment: prescription glasses to help improve vision
- Cataracts: removal only with surgery
  - Cloudy lens removed and replaced with artificial intraocular lens
  - Hazy vision: may return eventually; capsulotomy to restore clear vision

Nursing Interventions

- Assess the patient's vision (Figure 4.1).
- Encourage yearly ophthalmology visits.

(continued)

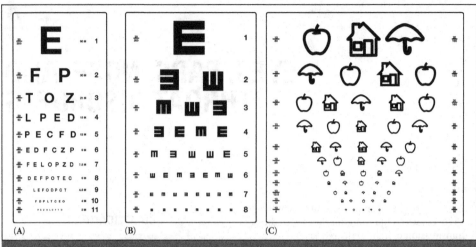

Figure 4.1 Charts for assessing visual acuity. (**A**) Snellen chart, used for patients ages 5 years and older. (**B**) Snellen "tumbling E" chart, used for patients ages 3 to 5 years and for those who cannot recognize the alphabet. (**C**) Allen cards, used for toddlers.

Source: Gawlik, K. S., Melnyk, B. M., and Teall, A. M. (2020). *Evidence-based physical examination best practices for health & well-being assessment.* Springer Publishing Company.

Nursing Interventions *(continued)*

- Encourage the patient to maintain a nutritious diet.
- Encourage the patient to wear prescription eyewear properly.
- If indicated, prepare the patient for surgery.

Patient Education

- Begin a smoking cessation program if needed.
- Eat a nutritious diet full of green, leafy vegetables; antioxidant-rich foods; and fruits. Nutritious diets may lessen the likelihood of developing age-related cataracts.
- Have a comprehensive eye exam at least every 2 years.
- Wear sunglasses and a hat with a brim to protect against sunlight.

 POP QUIZ 4.1

A patient arrives from the ED to the medical-surgical floor. The patient states that they have cataracts and need to make sure their eye drops are prescribed and given while they are hospitalized. What other nursing interventions are important for this patient?

DIABETIC RETINOPATHY

Overview

- *Diabetic retinopathy* is a complication of diabetes that results in vision loss.
- Diabetic retinopathy occurs when high blood sugar levels cause damage to the retina. This damage can occur when blood vessels:
  - Close and prevent passage of blood
  - Grow underneath the retina
  - Swell and leak

 COMPLICATIONS

Unmanaged hypertension and unmanaged hyperlipidemia increase the risk of diabetic retinopathy.

(continued)

Overview *(continued)*

- This condition can develop in people who have type 1 or type 2 diabetes if blood sugar is left uncontrolled.
- There are two types of diabetic retinopathy:
  - *Nonproliferative* is usually asymptomatic. It is the more common type, and most people with diabetes eventually get it.
  - *Proliferative* is the less common type, but it is more severe.

Signs and Symptoms

- Asymptomatic in early stage
- Blank or dark areas in visual field
- Blurry vision
- Colors appearing faded
- Floaters
- Trouble seeing at night
- Vision loss

Diagnosis

Labs
- Blood glucose monitoring

Diagnostic Testing
- Comprehensive dilated eye examination
- Fluorescein angiography, which shows if abnormal blood vessels are underneath the retina
- OCT, which is a detailed retinal scan

Treatment

- Blood glucose control
- Laser surgery
- Vitrectomy

Nursing Interventions

- Administer medications as prescribed.
- Assess visual acuity (see Figure 4.1).
- Educate patient on lifestyle, including tight glycemic control.
- Monitor blood glucose levels to maintain euglycemia.

Patient Education

- Control hypertension and hyperlipidemia, if present.
- Eat a nutritious diet.
- Get yearly dilated eye examinations.
- Maintain blood sugar levels within range.
- Take medications as prescribed.

 POP QUIZ 4.2

The patient presents with a blood pressure of 152/88, and the nurse observes a large bruise to the patient's right arm. When questioned about the bruise, the patient states that they have been bumping into things a lot. The patient has a history of diabetes. When the nurse asks about blood sugar readings, the patient says the readings have been normal. What should the nurse do next?

GLAUCOMA

Overview

- Glaucoma is characterized by damage to the optic nerve, usually by a high IOP.
- There are two types of glaucoma: open-angle glaucoma (chronic) and closed-angle glaucoma (acute).
- Damage caused by glaucoma cannot be reversed, so it is important to maintain regular ophthalmology visits.
- Glaucoma is one of the leading causes of blindness in people age 60 years and older.
- Often, glaucoma is not identified until advanced stages because it can be asymptomatic.

COMPLICATIONS

Complications of glaucoma include chronic corneal edema leading to loss of transparency, changes in visual acuity, and changes in central and peripheral vision. Damage caused by glaucoma cannot be reversed.

Signs and Symptoms

- Open-angle
  - Asymptomatic
  - Constriction of visual fields (patchy spots in central and peripheral fields)
  - Cupping of the disc
  - Elevated IOP
- Closed-angle
  - Blurred vision
  - Dilated or fixed pupils
  - Extreme pain
  - Halos around lights

Diagnosis

Labs
There are no labs specific to diagnosing glaucoma.

Diagnostic Testing
- Comprehensive dilated eye examination
- Tonometry
  - Measures IOP
  - Screening recommended by age 40 years

Treatment

Treatment aimed at reducing IOP and slowing vision loss:
- Prescription eye drops (Appendix 4.1 at the end of this chapter)
- Oral medications (see Appendix 4.1)
- Laser treatment
- Surgery

Nursing Interventions

- Assess visual acuity (see Figure 4.1).
- Administer medicated eye drops as ordered.
- Encourage yearly ophthalmology visits.
- Teach patients how to manage visual deficits, such as by using proper lighting, decluttering home, and turning head to view objects.
- If indicated, prepare patient for surgery.

Patient Education

- Avoid activities that increase IOP: bending at the waist, blowing nose, sexual intercourse, lifting objects heavier than 10 lb, keeping head in dependent position, and wearing tight shirts and collars.
- Get regular, comprehensive, dilated eye examinations.
- Limit caffeine.
- Use eye drops as prescribed.
- Wear eye protection when there is potential for eye injuries because injuries can cause glaucoma.

MACULAR DEGENERATION

Overview

- Macular degeneration occurs when the macula, the central portion of the retina, is damaged.
- It is typically called AMD because it is more likely to occur as a person ages. It is the leading cause of vision loss in adults older than 50 years.
- There are two types of AMD:
  - *Dry form* is more common. With dry form, the macula thins with age, and drusen (tiny clumps of protein) grow, causing central vision loss.
  - *Wet form* is rare but more serious. Abnormal blood vessels grow underneath the retina and cause scarring of the macula. Vision loss is more rapid with wet form.

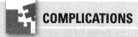 **COMPLICATIONS**

Macular degeneration leads to vision loss. This change in ability often leads to patients becoming depressed or anxious. Additionally, vision loss from macular degeneration can lead to hallucinations.

Signs and Symptoms

- Blurry vision
- Distorted vision
- Painless central vision loss

Diagnosis

Labs
There are no labs specific to diagnosing macular degeneration.

Diagnostic Testing
- Comprehensive dilated eye examination
- OCT
- Fluorescein angiography, which shows if abnormal blood vessels are underneath the retina
- Indocyanine green angiography, which looks at blood vessels in the choroid

Treatment

- Dry form
  - No treatment for dry form AMD
  - Possible slowing of vision loss with vitamins and supplement
- Wet form
  - Anti-VEGF drugs
  - Laser surgery

Nursing Interventions

- Assess visual acuity
- Administer medications as ordered.
- Encourage yearly ophthalmology visits.

(continued)

Nursing Interventions *(continued)*

- Encourage patients to maintain health with the daily recommended allowance of vitamin C, vitamin E, zinc, copper, and beta-carotene, or appropriate amounts of foods high in these nutrients.
- If indicated, prepare patient for surgery.

Patient Education

- Begin a smoking cessation program if needed.
- Get regular, comprehensive dilated eye examinations.
- Drive only during the day to avoid glare of headlights.

HEARING LOSS

Overview

- There are three types of hearing loss:
  - *Conductive hearing loss* is mechanical in nature and involves the outer or middle ear. It may be caused by an obstruction in the ear canal. It can be permanent but is most often temporary.
  - *Sensorineural hearing loss* occurs when the inner ear or auditory nerve is damaged. It is the most common form of hearing loss and is permanent.
  - *Mixed hearing loss* is a combination of both conductive and sensorineural hearing loss.

COMPLICATIONS

Hearing loss can have a significant effect on quality of life. Patients with hearing loss can feel depressed, anxious, or isolated.

Signs and Symptoms

- Asking others to repeat themselves
- Avoiding social gatherings that one previously enjoyed
- Difficulty communicating in noisy environments
- Difficulty understanding conversation
- Turning up television or music

Diagnosis

Labs
- Serum blood testing: only if needed to assess for underlying cause of hearing loss

Diagnostic Testing
- Audiometry
- CT scan, if cause is neurologic
- Otoscopic exam
- Neurologic exam
- Tuning fork tests: Rinne and Weber

Treatment

- Assistive listening devices: hearing aids, captioned phones, TV hearing devices
- Cochlear implants
- Removal of object that is affecting hearing conduction, such as cerumen
- Surgery

Nursing Interventions

- Administer medications as ordered.
- Use proper and effective communication:
  - Face the patient and ensure they can see your face when talking.

(continued)

Nursing Interventions *(continued)*

- Speak clearly.
- Do not shout.
- Use written communication if verbal communication is ineffective.
- Manage cerumen impaction.
- Give hearing device support, such as assisting patient with hearing aids or listening devices.

Patient Education

- Monitor medications for side effects of hearing loss.
- Notify others that hearing is impaired.
- Use ear protection when exposed to noisy environments.
- Use listening devices, such as hearing aids or headphones.

NURSING PEARL

Untreated hearing loss can lead to depression, anxiety, and social isolation.

POP QUIZ 4.3

A nurse is caring for a patient with bilateral ear hearing loss. The patient does not have hearing aids. What are some interventions the nurse can take to ensure effective communication with the patient?

SINUSITIS

Overview

- *Sinusitis* is the inflammation of the *paranasal sinuses*, or the mucus-lined, air-filled pockets in the head.
- The sinuses become inflamed when viruses, bacteria, and fungi get trapped within them.
- Sinusitis can be acute or chronic.

COMPLICATIONS

Complications of sinusitis arise from the proximity of the infection to areas such as the eyes, facial bones, and brain. Complications include brain abscess, mastoiditis, orbital abscess or cellulitis, and osteomyelitis.

Signs and Symptoms

- Congestion
- Cough
- Facial pain or pressure
- Fever
- Halitosis
- Postnasal drip
- Runny nose
- Sore throat

Diagnosis

Labs
- CBC with differential to assess basophils

Diagnostic Testing
- CT/radiographs
- Cultures of nasal drainage
- Sinus and facial x-rays

Treatment

- Antibiotics, if bacterial (see Table A.1)
- Antifungals, if fungal (see Table A.1)
- Antihistamines, if allergy
- Humidifier
- Nasal saline washes/saline drops
- Warm compresses

Nursing Interventions

- Administer medications as ordered.
- Assess pain levels.
- Decrease stimulation.
- Educate on preventive measures.
- Encourage fluid intake to thin nasal secretions.
- Implement relaxation techniques.
- Encourage hot showers or use of steam inhaler.

Patient Education

- Avoid known allergens.
- Drink 2 to 3 L of fluids, particularly water, each day to thin nasal secretions.
- Elevate head when lying down to alleviate congestion.
- Take medications as prescribed.
- Use proper hand hygiene.

LARYNGEAL CANCER

Overview

- *Laryngeal cancer* is cancer of the *larynx*, or "voice box." The larynx is divided into the supraglottis, the glottis, and the subglottis.
- Use of tobacco products and excessive alcohol consumption increase risk.

Signs and Symptoms

- Change in voice or hoarseness
- Dysphagia
- Ear pain
- Lump in neck or throat
- Numbness of mouth, lips, or face
- Pain when swallowing
- Sore throat that does not resolve

Diagnosis

Labs
- Tumor marker

Diagnostic Testing
- Barium swallow study
- Bone scan
- CT scan
- Endoscopy
- Laryngoscopy
- MRI
- PET scan

Treatment

- Chemotherapy
- Immunotherapy
- Radiation therapy
- Surgery

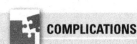 **COMPLICATIONS**

Complications of laryngeal cancer include airway obstruction, disfigurement of face or neck, permanent damage to larynx resulting in loss of voice, metastasis, and need for long-term tube feeding due to the inability to safely swallow.

Nursing Interventions

- Assess and maintain airway patency.
- Administer medications as ordered.
- Encourage patient to cough, turn head, and deep breathe every 2 to 4 hours.
- Elevate the head of the bed to at least 30 degrees.
- Suction as necessary.

Patient Education

- Avoid smoking and alcohol consumption.
- Keep all follow-up appointments.

DYSPHAGIA

Overview

- *Dysphagia* is difficulty swallowing.
- There are different degrees of dysphagia. Some people cannot swallow liquids, some cannot swallow solids, and some cannot swallow at all.
- Causes can be idiopathic or neurologic (e.g., stroke, MS, brain trauma, brain tumor).

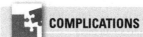

COMPLICATIONS

The most common side effect of dysphagia is aspiration, which can lead to aspiration pneumonia.

Signs and Symptoms

- Congestion after eating or drinking
- Coughing/gagging during or after swallowing
- Excess saliva/drooling
- Frequent heartburn
- Odynophagia
- Pocketing of food
- Sensation of food stuck in throat
- Unexplained weight loss

Diagnosis

Labs
There are no labs specific to diagnosing dysphagia.

Diagnostic Testing
- Barium swallow study
- Barium x-ray
- Endoscopy
- Manometry
- FEES

Treatment

- Diet changes
- Esophageal dilation
- Feeding tube
- Oral medications to reduce acid
- Speech therapy
- Surgery

(continued)

Nursing Interventions

- Administer tube feeding when appropriate and ordered.
- Assess for pocketing of food.
- Feed patient small bites, allowing for breaks between bites.
- If dysphagia is caused by stroke, place food in the back of the mouth on the unaffected side.
- Sit the patient upright at a 90-degree angle during meals.
- Suction as needed.
- Thicken liquids as prescribed by speech therapist, using additives if indicated. Some patients may need varying levels of thickening with nectar, honey, or pudding.
- When administering medications, crush pills (if appropriate for type of medication) and place in applesauce or gelatin.

Patient Education

- Avoid foods, beverages, and substances that exacerbate heartburn, such as tobacco, alcohol, and caffeine.
- Avoid foods that are difficult to swallow.
- Cut food into small bites.
- Eat small, frequent meals.

> **POP QUIZ 4.4**
>
> The nurse has admitted a patient to the floor, and the patient asks for something to drink. Upon drinking, the patient holds the fluid in their mouth, drooling a bit. What are the appropriate nursing interventions?

ORAL CANCER

Overview

- Oral, or oropharyngeal, cancer comprises all cancers of the mouth and pharynx.
- Oral cancer can affect the tongue, soft and hard palate, throat, sinuses, cheeks, and lips.
- Causes include age older than 40 years, HPV, UV sunlight, and alcohol and tobacco use.
- If not detected early, it can metastasize.

> **COMPLICATIONS**
>
> Complications of oral cancers include airway obstruction, disfigurement of face or neck, dysphagia, and mucositis.

Signs and Symptoms

- Chronic sore throat
- Dysphagia
- Dysarthria
- Ear pain
- Hoarseness
- Numbness in oral cavity
- Sensation that object is stuck in throat
- Ulceration or growth in mouth or throat that does not go away
- White or red patch in mouth

Diagnosis

Labs

- Tumor marker

Diagnostic Testing

- Biopsy
- Dental examination

Treatment

- Chemotherapy
- Radiation therapy
- Surgery
- Targeted therapy

Nursing Interventions

- Administer medications as prescribed.
- Allow adequate time to communicate.
- Assess and maintain airway patency.
- Encourage patient to cough, turn head, and deep breathe every 2 to 4 hours.
- Provide emotional support.

Patient Education

- Begin a smoking cessation program as needed.
- Brush teeth twice daily, and floss teeth daily.
- Limit alcohol consumption.
- Eat a nutritious diet.
- Maintain yearly dental examinations.

Appendix 4.1 Eyes, Ears, Nose, and Throat Medications

Indications	Mechanism of Action	Contraindications, Precautions, and Adverse Effects
Miotics/cholinergics (pilocarpine HCl)		
• Used to decrease IOP	• Directly stimulate cholinergic receptors • Increase outflow of aqueous humor in open-angle glaucoma • Open the angle of the anterior chamber of the eye and allow aqueous humor to exit in closed-angle glaucoma	• Oral route is contraindicated in closed-angle glaucoma and uncontrolled asthma. • Use caution in patients with cardiac disease. • Medication may cause dimmed vision, especially at night.
Prostaglandin analogs (latanoprost)		
• Used to decrease IOP with open-angle glaucoma	• Selective agonist at a FP receptor • Increase the outflow of aqueous humor, which reduces IOP	• Medication may cause dizziness, headache, or arthralgia. • Medication is contraindicated in closed-angle glaucoma.

RESOURCES

Gawlik, K. S., Melnyk, B. M., & Teall, A. M. (2020). *Evidence-based physical examination best practices for health & well-being assessment.* Springer Publishing Company.

Harding, M., Kwong, J., Roberts, D., Hagler, D., & Reinisch, C. (2020). *Lewis's medical-surgical nursing: Assessment and management of clinical problems* (11th ed.). Elsevier.

Herndon, J. R. (2019, February 1). *Indocyanine green angiography.* https://maculardegeneration.net/indocyanine-green-angiography

Hinkle, J. L., & Cheever, K. H. (2018). *Brunner & Suddarth's textbook of medical-surgical nursing* (14th ed.). Wolters Kluwer Health/Lippincott Williams & Wilkins.

National Institute of Dental and Craniofacial Research. (2018). *Oral cancer*. U.S. Department of Health and Human Services, National Institute of Dental and Craniofacial Research. https://www.nidcr.nih.gov/health-info/oral-cancer

Prescribers' Digital Reference. (n.d.). *Humalin R* [Drug information]. https://www.pdr.net/drug-summary/Amoxicillin-Tablets-amoxicillin-2350

Prescribers' Digital Reference. (n.d.). *Augmentin* [Drug information]. https://www.pdr.net/drug-information/augmentin-xr?druglabelid=2206

Prescribers' Digital Reference. (n.d.). *Sproranox* [Drug information]. https://www.pdr.net/drug-summary/Sporanox-Capsules-itraconazole-930

Prescribers' Digital Reference. (n.d.). *Prednisone* [Drug information]. https://www.pdr.net/drug-summary/Prednisone-Tablets-prednisone-3516.6194

Tkacs, N. C., Linda, L. H., & Randall, L. J. (2020). In C. T. Nancy, L. H. Linda, & L. J. Randall (Eds.), *Advanced physiology and pathophysiology: Essentials for clinical practice*. Springer Publishing Company.

5

FLUID/ELECTROLYTE/ CELLULAR REGULATON

ACID–BASE IMBALANCE

Overview

- The concentration of acids and bases in the body must be regulated so that the pH is maintained between 7.35 and 7.45.
- This dynamic is known as *acid–base balance*.
- Whenever there is an imbalance, the body attempts to implement compensatory mechanisms to restore the acid–base balance in the blood.
- Normal values:
  - pH: 7.35 to 7.45
  - $PaCO_2$: 35 to 45 mmHg
  - HCO_3^-: 22 to 26 mEq/L
- There are four acid–base imbalance states:
  - Respiratory acidosis is caused by a buildup of CO_2 as a result of poor lung function or breathing. $PaCO_2$ will be elevated.
  - Respiratory alkalosis is characterized by low CO_2 levels because of rapid breathing (hyperventilation). $PaCO_2$ will be normal or decreased.
  - Metabolic acidosis is caused by overproduction of acid or excessive loss of HCO_3^-.
  - Metabolic alkalosis results from excess HCO_3^- or loss of acid from the blood.

NURSING PEARL

The metabolic states of metabolic acidosis are due to issues with the kidneys.

COMPLICATIONS

Complications related to the acid–base balance include a pH lower than 7.35 (considered acidic and leads to a state of acidosis) and a pH above 7.45 (considered alkaline and leads to a state of alkalosis).

Signs and Symptoms

- Metabolic acidosis:
  - Confusion
  - Fatigue
  - Rapid breathing
- Respiratory acidosis:
  - Confusion
  - Fatigue
  - Headache
  - Shortness of breath
- Respiratory and metabolic alkalosis:
  - Irritability
  - Muscle twitching and cramps
  - Nausea and vomiting
  - Paresthesia
  - Tremors

Diagnosis

Labs
- ABGs: will be altered based on acidosis/alkalosis and correction by lungs or kidneys
- CMP: may reflect electrolyte abnormalities
- UA
- Urine pH: may be low in metabolic acidosis

Diagnostic Testing
There are no diagnostic tests specific to diagnosing acid–base imbalance.

Treatment
- Underlying cause must be treated to reverse acid–base imbalances.

Nursing Interventions
- Administer medications as ordered.
- Assess breathing.
- Assess level of orientation (if confusion is present) and reorient as necessary.
- Provide oxygen and reassurance for a patient who is hyperventilating.

POP QUIZ 5.1

An older adult patient presents with shortness of breath, confusion, and cyanosis. The patient has a history of COPD, leukemia, and GERD. ABG reveals pH: 7.38; $PaCO_2$: 47; PaO_2: 85%; HCO_3: 25; SaO_2: 90%. What is the most likely diagnosis?

Patient Education
- Electrolyte imbalances can lead to acid–base imbalances. Take electrolyte supplements, such as potassium, as instructed.
- Report any abnormal signs and symptoms to provider, especially confusion.

ELECTROLYTE IMBALANCE

- Electrolyte imbalance occurs when the body's concentrations of electrolytes become either too high or too low.
- Figure 5.1 shows the normal distributions of electrolytes in the plasma, intracellular space, and extracellular spaces.

COMPLICATIONS

Complications of electrolyte imbalances include headache, nausea, vomiting, muscle cramps, cerebral edema, heart arrythmias, and death.

SODIUM

Overview
- *Hyponatremia*, a low level of sodium in the blood, occurs when the body loses too much water or sodium electrolytes. Additionally, hyponatremia can be caused by excessive water gain, which dilutes sodium electrolytes.
- *Hypernatremia*, excess sodium in the blood, occurs when the body does not take in enough water, has excess water loss, and/or has a sodium gain.
- A normal sodium level is 135 to 145 mEq/L.

Signs and Symptoms
- Hyponatremia:
  - Confusion
  - Dizziness
  - Headache
  - Lethargy

COMPLICATIONS

Complications of hyponatremia include headache, nausea, vomiting, muscle cramps, cerebral edema, and death.

(continued)

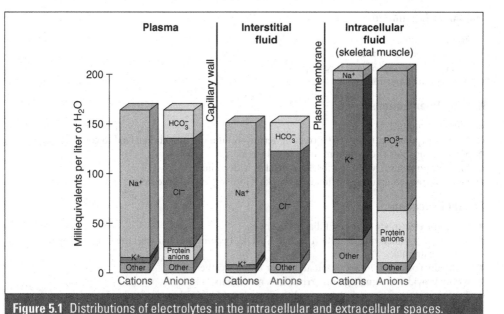

Figure 5.1 Distributions of electrolytes in the intracellular and extracellular spaces.

Source: Tkacs, N., Herrmann, L. L., and Johnson, R. (2020). *Advanced physiology and pathophysiology: essentials for clinical practice.* Springer Publishing Company.

Signs and Symptoms *(continued)*

- Hypernatremia:
  - Coma
  - Confusion
  - Hyperreflexia
  - Seizures

Diagnosis

Labs

- BMP for sodium level:
  - Elevated in hypernatremia
  - Low in hyponatremia
- Urine sodium:
  - Random urine sodium: 20 mEq/d
  - 24-hour urine sodium test range: 40 to 220 mEq/L

Diagnostic Testing

There are no diagnostic tests specific to diagnosing sodium levels.

Treatment

- Treatment for underlying cause
- Hyponatremia:
  - Modified medications for sodium imbalance cause or exacerbation
  - Decreased water intake
  - IV sodium (Appendix 5.1 at the end of this chapter)

(continued)

Treatment *(continued)*

- Hypernatremia:
  - Increased water intake
  - IV D$_5$W. or 0.45% NaCl (see Appendix 5.1)
  - Sodium restriction

Nursing Interventions

- Closely monitor I/O.
- Correct hyponatremia slowly. Correcting serum sodium too quickly can lead to cerebral edema.
- Monitor for signs and symptoms of cerebral edema.
- Monitor potassium, which is closely correlated with sodium.
- Perform frequent neurologic function checks if infusing hypertonic saline.

Patient Education

- Consume electrolyte solution if diarrhea occurs.
- If there is an underlying condition such as SIADH, become familiar with the signs and symptoms of hyponatremia.
- Maintain a balanced intake of salt and water in hot weather.
- Notify provider if vomiting or diarrhea lasts more than 48 hours.
- Take medications for underlying conditions, such as SIADH, that may lead to hyponatremia.

POTASSIUM

Overview

- Potassium is important for nerve impulses and muscle contraction, especially in the heart. It is also vital in bone health and in regulating blood pressure.
- Hypokalemia can be caused by excess excretion of or inadequate intake of potassium.
- A normal potassium level is 3.5 to 5.0 mmol/L.

COMPLICATIONS

Hyperkalemia can cause potentially lethal cardiac arrythmias.

Signs and Symptoms

- Hypokalemia:
  - Constipation
  - Dysrhythmias
  - Fatigue
  - Muscle cramps
  - Palpitations
  - Weakness
- Hyperkalemia:
  - Chest pain
  - Dysrhythmias
  - Muscle weakness
  - Nausea
  - Numbness
  - Palpitations
  - Shortness of breath
  - Tingling

Diagnosis

Labs

- Serum potassium:
  - Elevated in hyperkalemia
  - Decreased in hypokalemia
- Urine potassium:
  - Random urine potassium: 20 mEq/L
  - 24-hour urine potassium test range: 25 to 125 mEq/L

Diagnostic Testing

There are no diagnostic tests specific to diagnosing potassium levels.

Treatment

- Treatment for underlying cause
- Hypokalemia:
  - IV potassium administered slowly (not exceeding 10 mEq/hr) (see Appendix 5.1)
  - Potassium supplements
  - Potassium-rich diet
- Hyperkalemia:
  - Diuretics for urine output to measure 0.5 mL/kg/hr to ensure renal efficiency
  - Low-potassium diet
  - Potassium binders

Nursing Interventions

- Administer medications as ordered.
- If patient requires insulin to lower potassium, monitor the patient's blood glucose closely.
- Monitor lab values, especially sodium, which is closely correlated with potassium.
- Monitor patient on continuous telemetry if there is significant derangement of potassium.

NURSING PEARL

Sodium and potassium often conversely affect one another. When sodium increases, potassium often decreases, and vice versa. Close monitoring of one is required if the other is high or low.

Patient Education

- Adhere to hemodialysis schedule, if applicable.
- Avoid salt alternatives with elevated potassium.
- Notify provider of vomiting or diarrhea that lasts more than 48 hours.
- Take medications as instructed.

CALCIUM

Overview

- Calcium is vital in transmitting nerve impulses and regulating muscle contraction and relaxation, especially in the heart.
- *Hypocalcemia*, or serum calcium levels that are lower than normal, can be the result of primary hypoparathyroidism or surgical hypoparathyroidism.
- A normal serum calcium level is 8.5 to 10.5 mg/dL.

COMPLICATIONS

Hypercalcemia is typically due to an overactive parathyroid gland and can cause kidney stones, weak bones (osteoporosis), and cardiac arrythmias. It can also alter brain function.

Signs and Symptoms

- Hypocalcemia:
  - Arrythmias
  - Mood changes
  - Paresthesia
  - Seizures
  - Tetany
- Hypercalcemia:
  - Bone pain
  - Confusion
  - Digestive issues: constipation, vomiting, nausea, poor appetite
  - Excessive thirst
  - Frequent urination
  - Lethargy

Diagnosis

Labs

- Serum calcium:
  - Elevated in hypercalcemia
  - Decreased in hypocalcemia
- Serum PTH:
  - Normal value 10 to 55 pg/mL
  - Elevated if calcium level is low
- Serum vitamin D: normal level is 20 to 50 ng/mL; needed to absorb calcium
- Urine calcium: 24-hour urine test to show level of calcium excreted in urine

Diagnostic Testing

- X-ray

Treatment

- Treatment for underlying cause
- Hypocalcemia:
  - Calcium supplements
  - IV calcium
  - Vitamin D therapy: increases calcium absorption
- Hypercalcemia:
  - Medications to lower calcium (corticosteroids, bisphosphonates, calcitonin, diuretics) (see Appendix 5.1)
  - Surgery

Nursing Interventions

- Administer medications as ordered.
- Assess patient for Chvostek's and Trousseau's signs.
- Monitor patient on continuous telemetry if there is significant calcium derangement.
- Closely monitor patients who have had surgical removal of the parathyroid for hypocalcemia.
- Monitor patients with metastatic bone lesions closely for development of hypercalcemia.

 ALERT!

Calcium is a vital electrolyte in regulating muscle contractility. Both hypocalcemia and hypercalcemia can cause life-threatening cardiac arrythmias. A patient with serum calcium derangement should be placed on telemetry.

Patient Education

- Notify provider if taking long-term antacids, as these may decrease calcium absorption.
- Take medications as instructed.
- With hypercalcemia, avoid over-the-counter antacids that contain calcium.

MAGNESIUM

Overview

- Magnesium is an activator of many intracellular enzyme systems. It is important for carbohydrate and protein metabolism.
- Hypomagnesemia is usually linked to hypocalcemia and hypokalemia. It may occur with alcohol withdrawal or administration of tube and parenteral feedings.
- Hypermagnesemia is most often caused by renal failure, but can also be caused by adrenocortical insufficiency, DKA, and hypothermia.
- A normal magnesium level is 1.5 to 2.5 mEq/L.

 COMPLICATIONS

A malnourished patient who is started on enteral or parenteral nutrition is at risk for hypomagnesemia as a result of refeeding syndrome. Careful reintroduction of carbohydrates and close monitoring of electrolytes is imperative during early reintroduction of nutrition.

Signs and Symptoms

- Hypomagnesemia:
  - Ataxia
  - Dizziness
  - Hallucinations and psychoses
  - Mood disturbances (apathy, depression, agitation)
  - Positive Chvostek's and Trousseau's signs
- Hypermagnesemia:
  - Cardiac arrest
  - Dysarthria
  - Facial flushing
  - Lethargy
  - Loss of deep tendon reflexes
  - Nausea and vomiting

 NURSING PEARL

Chvostek's and Trousseau's signs are both symptoms of hypocalcemia and hypomagnesemia. Chvostek's sign is contraction of facial muscles that occurs when lightly tapping over the facial nerve anterior to the ear. Trousseau's sign is indicated by flexion of the wrist and fingers when the upper arm is compressed. This test is often done using a blood pressure cuff to compress the upper arm.

Diagnosis

Labs
Serum magnesium:
- Elevated in hypermagnesemia
- Decreased in hypomagnesemia

Diagnostic Testing
There are no diagnostic tests specific to diagnosing magnesium levels.

Treatment

- Treatment for underlying cause
- Hypomagnesemia: magnesium-rich foods, such as whole grains, nuts, legumes, seafood, and green, leafy vegetables
- Hypermagnesemia:
  - 0.45% NaCl (see Appendix 5.1)
  - Loop diuretics
  - IV calcium gluconate

Nursing Interventions

- Administer medications as ordered.
- If significant derangement in magnesium is present, place patient on seizure precautions.
- Monitor for diarrhea, which can be a side effect of oral magnesium.
- Monitor lab values.

Patient Education

- Follow hemodialysis schedule, if applicable.
- Limit alcohol intake.
- Notify provider of diarrhea or vomiting lasting longer than 48 hours.
- Take medications as instructed.

 POP QUIZ 5.2

A patient is admitted under a nurse's care and is placed on telemetry. What lab value is suspected to be low if torsade de pointes is noted on the telemetry strip?

PHOSPHORUS

Overview

- Phosphorus is an important component of body tissues. It is also important to the function of muscles and RBCs and the formation of ATP.
- Phosphorus is inversely related to calcium.
- Hypophosphatemia is a low concentration of serum inorganic phosphorus. It can occur in the presence of normal total body phosphorus levels.
- Hyperphosphatemia is usually caused by renal failure.
- A normal phosphate level is 2.5 to 4.5 mg/dL.

 COMPLICATIONS

Chronic hypophosphatemia can lead to bone pain and fractures. Critically low phosphorus can lead to coma and death.

Signs and Symptoms

- Hypophosphatemia:
  - Confusion
  - Fatigue
  - Irritability
  - Numbness
  - Paresthesia
  - Seizures
  - Weakness
- Hyperphosphatemia:
  - Can be asymptomatic unless calcium binds with phosphorus to create signs of hypocalcemia
  - Hyperreflexia
  - Muscle cramping
  - Numbness and tingling in extremities and around mouth
  - Seizures
  - Tetany

Diagnosis

Labs
Serum phosphorus levels:
- Elevated in hyperphosphatemia
- Decreased in hypophosphatemia

Diagnostic Testing
There are no diagnostic tests specific to diagnosing phosphorus levels.

 NURSING PEARL

Glucose or insulin administration will cause a slight decrease in the serum phosphorus level. The nurse should be mindful when reviewing laboratory results.

Treatment

- Treatment for underlying cause
- Hypophosphatemia:
  - IV phosphorus
  - Phosphorus supplements
- Hyperphosphatemia:
  - Dialysis
  - Phosphate-binding antacids
  - Restricting dietary phosphorus
  - Vitamin D preparations

Nursing Interventions

- Administer medications as ordered.
- If significant phosphorus derangement is present, the patient may need to be monitored on continuous telemetry.
- Monitor electrolytes, as increased phosphorous leads to a decrease in calcium.
- Monitor for phosphate derangement in patients with hyperparathyroidism.

Patient Education

- Adhere to dialysis schedule.
- Take medications as instructed and avoid over-the-counter medications as instructed.
- Restrict intake of foods and fluids containing phosphorus.
- With hyperphosphatemia, take oral phosphate-binding agents as directed by provider.

 POP QUIZ 5.3

The nurse is assessing a patient who has been agitated, aggressive, and confused. The nurse taps lightly over the patient's facial nerve, and the patient's facial muscles twitch. The nurse suspects that the patient is experiencing a deficit of which electrolyte? What intervention will the nurse expect to perform?

FLUID IMBALANCES

Hypervolemia

- Volume fluid excess, or *hypervolemia*, is an isotonic expansion of the ECF caused by the abnormal retention of sodium and water.
- It is always secondary to an increase in total body sodium levels, which increases total body water.
- Contributing factors are HF, renal failure, and cirrhosis of the liver.

 COMPLICATIONS

Hypervolemia can be caused by HF. However, hypervolemia caused by other illnesses such as kidney failure can also lead to HF.

Signs and Symptoms

- Distended neck veins
- Edema
- Lung crackles

Diagnosis

Labs

- BMP to assess electrolytes, which may be low due to dilution of serum
- BNP to determine level of HF
- BUN:
  - Normal levels: 6 to 24 mg/L
  - Decreased in hypervolemia

(continued)

Labs (continued)

- Hematocrit:
  - Decreased in hypervolemia
  - Normal values for men: 41% to 50%
  - Normal values for women: 36% to 38%
- Urine sodium: less than 20 mEq/L

Diagnostic Testing

- Chest x-ray

Treatment

- Diuretics
- Hemodialysis
- Sodium-restricted diet

Nursing Interventions

- Assess edema.
- Assess respiratory status.
- Measure daily standing weights.
- Measure intake and output at regular intervals.

Patient Education

- Follow a sodium-restricted diet.
- Limit fluid intake.
- Monitor for weight gain and edema.
- Report signs of respiratory distress to provider.

POP QUIZ 5.4

While measuring a patient's morning daily weight, the nurse notices that the patient has gained 10 lb since yesterday. The nurse also notices that the patient is having a hard time breathing. When the patient is assessed, the nurse hears increased crackles in all lung fields. After ensuring airway patency, what should the nurse do next?

HYPOVOLEMIA

Overview

- *Hypovolemia*, or fluid volume deficit, occurs when extracellular volume exceeds fluid intake volume.
- When water and electrolytes are lost in the same proportion as they exist in normal body fluids, the result is hypovolemia.
- Abnormal fluid losses through illness or hemorrhage lead can lead to hypovolemia.
- Hypovolemic shock is the most common form of shock and is exemplified by decreased intravascular volume.
  - Subsequent to the decrease in intravascular volume is decreased venous return of blood to the heart and decreased ventricular filling.
  - Decreased ventricular filling leads to decreased stroke volume and cardiac output.
  - When cardiac output decreases, blood pressure decreases, and the body's tissues cannot be adequately perfused.

COMPLICATIONS

Complications of illnesses causing extreme volume losses such as DI, intractable nausea and vomiting, and adrenal insufficiency can lead to hypovolemia.

Signs and Symptoms

- Hypovolemia:
  - Acute weight loss
  - Cool, clammy skin
  - Decreased skin turgor

(continued)

Signs and Symptoms *(continued)*

- Flattened neck veins
- Muscle cramps
- Weakness
- Hypovolemic shock:
  - Cool, clammy skin
  - Decreased or no urine output
  - Decreased skin turgor
  - Flattened neck veins
  - Rapid breathing
  - Sweating

Diagnosis

Labs

- BUN: elevated in hypovolemia
- CMP to assess kidney function and electrolytes
- Hematocrit: may be elevated due to concentrated serum volume
- Urine osmolality
- Urine specific gravity: may be elevated due to urine concentration

Diagnostic Testing

There are no diagnostic tests specific to diagnosing hypovolemia.

Treatment

- Increased oral intake of fluid if tolerated
- IV lactated Ringer's or 0.9% NaCl (see Table A.3)
- Oral isotonic electrolyte solution, once stable

Nursing Interventions

- Measure intake and output at regular intervals.
- Measure daily weights with a consistent method or scale.
- Monitor skin color and turgor.

Patient Education

- Replace fluids and electrolytes as soon as possible after abnormal fluid loss.
- Report acute weight loss.
- Take medications, as needed, to treat underlying cause.

Appendix 5.1 Medications to Correct Fluid and Electrolyte Imbalances		
Indications	**Mechanism of Action**	**Contraindications, Precautions, and Adverse Effects**
Bisphosphonates (pamidronate, zoledronic acid)		
• Used to treat hypercalcemia	• Bone uptake of excess calcium • Interfere with osteoclasts	• Medication can cause hypovolemia. • Use with caution in electrolyte imbalances. • Use with caution in diabetes, hypertension, osteoporosis, and renal failure.

(continued)

Appendix 5.1 Medications to Correct Fluid and Electrolyte Imbalances *(continued)*

Indications	Mechanism of Action	Contraindications, Precautions, and Adverse Effects
Calcitonin		
• Used to lower hypercalcemia	• Calcitonin receptor agonist	• If administered nasally, medication is contraindicated in patients with nasal trauma. • Use caution in patients with fish sensitivity.
Crystalloids (0.9% sodium chloride)		
• Fluid and electrolyte replacement • Helpful in hypovolemic shock	• Isotonic • Remain in the extracellular compartment when administered • Help restore blood volume and support peripheral perfusion	• Medication can cause pulmonary edema. • Monitor for hypernatremia.
Diuretics (bumetanide, furosemide)		
• Used to treat hyperkalemia • Used to treat hypercalcemia	• Enhance renal potassium excretion	• Medication can cause hypotension. • Use with caution in patients with electrolyte imbalances. • Medication can impair glucose tolerance and cause hyperglycemia. • Medication can cause dehydration.
Potassium binders (calcium polystyrene, sodium polystyrene, sodium zirconium cyclosilicate)		
• Used to treat hyperkalemia	• Insoluble resin binds to potassium in gastrointestinal tract • Excess potassium excreted in feces	• Medication is contraindicated in colitis and inflammatory bowel diseases. • Use with caution in patients with hypocalcemia and hypomagnesemia.
Sodium bicarbonate		
• Used to increase plasma bicarbonate levels • Raise pH • Combat acidosis	• After administration, disassociates into sodium and bicarbonate. • Bicarbonate anions consume more hydrogen and convert to carbonic acid. • Carbonic acid breaks down into water and carbon dioxide for excretion from the lungs.	• Medication may cause metabolic alkalosis, muscle pain, headache, and restlessness. • Medication is contraindicated in metabolic and respiratory alkalosis. • Rapid administration may lead to pulmonary edema.

RESOURCES

American Heart Association. (2020). *Advanced cardiovascular life support provider manual*. American Heart Association.

Hinkle, J. L., & Cheever, K. H. (2018). *Brunner & Suddarth's textbook of medical-surgical nursing* (14th ed.). Wolters Kluwer Health/Lippincott Williams & Wilkins.

Prescribers' Digital Reference. (n.d.[a]). *Bumetanide* [Drug information]. https://www.pdr.net/drug-summary/Bumetanide-Injection-bumetanide-1535.1100

Prescribers' Digital Reference. (n.d.[b]). *Calcitonin-salmon* [Drug information]. https://www.pdr.net/drug-summary/Fortical-calcitonin-salmon--rDNA-origin--1939.1801#14

Prescribers' Digital Reference. (n.d.[c]). *Prednisone* [Drug information]. https://www.pdr.net/drug-summary/Prednisone-Tablets-prednisone-3516.6194#14

Prescribers' Digital Reference. (n.d.[d]). *Sodium polystyrene sulfonate* [Drug information]. https://www.pdr.net/drug-summary/Kayexalate-sodium-polystyrene-sulfonate-2925

Prescribers' Digital Reference. (n.d.[e]). *Sodium chloride* [Drug information]. https://www.pdr.net/drug-summary/Kayexalate-sodium-polystyrene-sulfonate-2925

Prescribers' Digital Reference. (n.d.[f]). *Zoledronic acid* [Drug information]. https://www.pdr.net/drug-summary/Reclast-zoledronic-acid-437.5883#14

Tkacs, N. C., Herrmann, L. L., & Johnson, R. L. (Eds.). (2020). *Advanced physiology and pathophysiology: Essentials for clinical practice*. Springer Publishing Company.

6

GASTROINTESTINAL SYSTEM

APPENDICITIS

Overview

- *Appendicitis* is an inflammation of the appendix, the tube-like protrusion that extends out from the cecum area of the colon. It is often precipitated by obstruction of the appendiceal lumen.
- It is one of the most common causes of the acute abdomen and one of the most frequent indications for an emergency abdominal surgical procedure.
- Causes of appendicitis include infection, malignancy, obstruction by a foreign body or fecalith, or stricture.

Signs and Symptoms

- Anorexia
- Blumberg sign (rebound tenderness)
- Generalized or periumbilical abdominal pain initially possible
  - Pain usually starts in the periumbilical area and moves to the right lower abdomen.
  - As inflammation worsens, pain typically increases and can become severe.
  - Pain may be worse when patient coughs, walks, or makes any sudden movements.
- Fever: low grade initially but may worsen as illness progresses
- Localized RLQ pain (late sign)
- Nausea
- Vomiting
- Loss of appetite
- Abdominal bloating
- Constipation or diarrhea
- Obturator sign: pain with internal rotation of flexed right thigh
- Psoas sign (iliopsoas test): pain with right thigh extension
- Positive Rovsing's sign: RLQ pain when pressure is applied to the LLQ
- Tachycardia

Diagnosis

Labs

- BMP to assess electrolytes if the patient has been anorexic or vomiting
- CBC to assess for elevated WBC

NURSING PEARL

A *fecalith* is a hard mass of feces. It can cause obstruction in the appendix or diverticula or partial bowel obstruction in the colon. In rare instances, large fecaliths have caused complete bowel obstruction.

COMPLICATIONS

Untreated appendicitis can be fatal. Gangrene can develop as the inflamed tissue dies, resulting in perforation, peritonitis, sepsis, and death.

NURSING PEARL

The PQRST mnemonic is a helpful tool to use to perform a thorough pain assessment:

  P (provokes): What provokes the pain? What makes it better or worse?
  Q (quality): What does the pain feel like?
  R (radiation): Where is the pain located? Does it radiate?
  S (severity): How do you rate your pain on a 1–10 scale?
  T (time): How long have you had the pain? Does it come and go?

Diagnostic Testing

- CT scan (abdomen, pelvis) if further imaging is needed
- Ultrasound to assess a nonperforated appendix

Treatment

- Antibiotics: The first few doses will be given by IV in the hospital; then the severity of the infection or the presences of an abscess will determine the course of antibiotic treatment
  - Treatment is typically 3 to 5 days but sometimes may be 2 to 4 weeks or more if the infection was severe.
  - Antibiotics are usually given by mouth as long as patient tolerates it well.
  - In some cases, the surgeon may have the patient take antibiotics prior to surgery to control the infection first (if the appendix has not ruptured) or to see if the appendicitis resolves with antibiotics alone (in mild appendicitis).
  - Antibiotics that may be prescribed (see Table A.1) include the following:
    - Ampicillin
    - Cefotetan
    - Piperacillin
- Surgical removal of the appendix: It is usually laparoscopic, but open surgery may be needed if the appendix has ruptured and infection has spread beyond the appendix or if there is an abscess.
  - An open surgery may be necessary to clean out the abdominal cavity.
  - Some patients may not need surgery and may be managed with antibiotics alone.

Nursing Interventions

- Administer antibiotics, if ordered.
- Assess pain and manage as necessary. Administer pain medications PRN, as ordered.
- Assess incision(s) for surgical complications such as dehiscence or infection.
- Encourage activity as tolerated in the postoperative period.
- Ensure patient has patent IV access.
- Provide IV hydration both prior to and after surgery as patient may be dehydrated and malnourished.
- Encourage IS use after surgery to help with deep breathing.
- Ensure NPO status is maintained if ordered or preparing for surgery.
- Instruct the patient to splint abdomen while coughing to minimize pain.
- Monitor vital signs closely.
- Perform a focused abdominal assessment.
- Place the patient in a position of comfort, often in a semi-Fowler's position, supine with hips and knees flexed.
- Prepare patient for transfer to the OR for surgical intervention, including witnessing surgical consents and performing any preoperative bathing with chlorhexidine.

Patient Education

- After general anesthesia or while taking pain medication, do not operate machinery, drive, or drink alcohol until approved by surgeon.
- Complete coughing and deep-breathing exercises to prevent pneumonia.
- Complete course of antibiotics as prescribed.
- Gradually increase activity level to help recovery, starting with light activities around the house and walking.
- Monitor incision site for any signs of infection, such as fever, redness, swelling, drainage, or increased pain, and report these to the provider.

 POP QUIZ 6.1

A patient with appendicitis is admitted to the medical-surgical floor for antibiotics and IV fluids in preparation for an appendectomy the following day. Despite pain medication, the patient continues to have severe pain. Which position should the nurse place the patient in to help reduce pain?

(continued)

Patient Education *(continued)*

- Know that normal activity can usually resume within a week, but avoid strenuous activity and heavy lifting until cleared by the surgeon.
- Schedule a follow-up appointment with the surgeon to assess postsurgery recovery.
- Take laxatives and stool softeners PRN, maintain hydration, and maintain activity as tolerated to prevent constipation from pain medications and immobility.
- Take pain medications only as needed. Do not share narcotic pain medications.

CELIAC DISEASE

Overview

- *Celiac disease* is a chronic digestive and autoimmune disorder in which the immune system damages the small intestine after the ingestion of gluten.
- This small bowel disorder is characterized by mucosal inflammation, villous atrophy, and crypt hyperplasia, which occur after exposure to dietary gluten.
- *Gluten* is a protein found in grains such as barley, rye, and wheat.
- Celiac disease is genetic. First-degree family members of a person with celiac disease have up to a 40% chance of developing celiac disease.

Signs and Symptoms

- Abdominal pain and distention
- Bloating
- Constipation
- Diarrhea
- Flatulence
- Foul-smelling stools
- Greasy stools
- Nausea
- Nutritional deficiencies
- Vomiting

 COMPLICATIONS

Untreated celiac disease can lead to malnutrition, anemia, and weight loss. In children, malnutrition can cause slow growth and short stature. Malabsorption of calcium and vitamin D can also lead to bone weakening and loss of bone density.

 NURSING PEARL

Celiac disease was once referred to as celiac sprue. This term is outdated; however, nurses should be familiar with the term. Celiac sprue and celiac disease are the same illness. If a patient has refractory celiac disease, the small intestine will not heal, and the patient will need to see a specialist. Refractory celiac disease can be serious, and there is currently no proven treatment.

Diagnosis

Labs

- Tissue transglutaminase IgA antibody to confirm celiac: positive in 98% of patients on a gluten-containing diet
- Total serum IgA level: to exclude selective IgA deficiency
- Positive test results: refer to gastroenterologist for tissue biopsy to confirm diagnosis
  - Individuals with a high probability of celiac disease should have serologic testing and small bowel biopsy.

Diagnostic Testing

- Biopsy from intestinal tissue
- CT scan to assess for small bowel wall thickening, dilation, or vascular abnormalities
- Endoscopy to examine intestinal tissue

Treatment

- A strict gluten-free diet must be followed by the patient. Foods that must be avoided include barley, bulgur, durum, farina, graham flour, malt, rye, semolina, spelt, triticale, wheat, modified food starch, and some preservatives.
- Other items that may contain gluten and should be avoided by the patient include some prescription and OTC medications, vitamin supplements, herbal and nutritional supplements, some cosmetics, some toothpastes and mouthwashes, and envelope adhesive.
- If anemia or nutritional deficiencies are present, it may be recommended that the patient take supplements, including copper, folate, iron, zinc, and vitamins B12, D, and K.
- If the digestive tract has difficulty absorbing vitamins, it may be recommended for the patient to get supplements by injection.
- Medications prescribed to control intestinal inflammation include the following:
  - NSAIDs
  - Steroids: short term while the intestine heals
- Clinical trials should be considered for prevention, detection, treatment, and management of celiac disease.
- Genetic testing is recommended for family members of those diagnosed with celiac disease.

Nursing Interventions

- Ensure that the patient is on a gluten-free diet.
- Ensure that gluten is listed under the patient's allergies.
- Provide education on a gluten-free diet.
- If inpatient, have dietitian meet with patient for nutrition counseling.

Patient Education

- Check all food labels for the presence of gluten.
- Check products such as lip balm and OTC medications for the presence of gluten.
- Seek out support groups or other emotional support in the community.
- See a dietitian or nutritionist for diet education.
- Be aware of the following nutrition information:
  - Soybean or tapioca flours, rice, corn, buckwheat, and potatoes are safe.
  - It is important to read labels on prepared foods and condiments carefully, paying particular attention to additives that may contain gluten.
  - Distilled alcoholic beverages, wine, and most vinegars are gluten free. However, beer and malt vinegar should be avoided because they are often made from gluten-containing grains and are not distilled.
  - Dairy products may not be well tolerated initially, since celiac disease may be accompanied by secondary lactose intolerance. Lactose-containing products should initially be avoided if symptoms appear to be worsened by them.
  - Oats should be introduced into the diet with caution. Oat consumption should be limited to 50 to 60 g/d (approximately 2 ounces) in mild disease or disease in remission after a stringent gluten-free diet. Oats should be avoided altogether in severe disease.

 POP QUIZ 6.2

A patient is newly diagnosed with celiac disease. The patient is preparing to be discharged from the hospital and asks the nurse if there are any dietary restrictions. How should the nurse respond?

CHOLECYSTITIS

Overview

- *Cholecystitis* is acute or chronic inflammation of the gallbladder.

(continued)

Overview *(continued)*

- It is commonly associated with gallstones (cholelithiasis) but can also occur in the absence of stones (acalculous).
- Symptoms often are precipitated by a large or high-fat meal.
- Secondary bacterial infection occurs in about 50% of cases.

Signs and Symptoms

- Abdominal muscle rigidity
- Abdominal tenderness
- Fever
- Muscle guarding and rebound pain
- Nausea
- Positive Murphy's sign: deep pain on inspiration while fingers are placed under the right rib cage
- Jaundice (if common bile duct obstructed by gallstones)
- RUQ tenderness to palpation
- Steady, severe abdominal pain that may also appear in epigastrium or right hypochondrium
- Tachycardia
- Relief of symptoms after vomiting

COMPLICATIONS

Cholecystitis can lead to gallbladder gangrene and bile duct injury, which can affect the liver. If the gallbladder is not removed and the patient has recurrent episodes of cholecystitis, it can lead to chronic long-term cholecystitis. This can damage the walls of the gallbladder, and over time the gallbladder will be less able to store and release bile. The patient will eventually require a cholecystectomy.

NURSING PEARL

The phrenic nerve passes near the gallbladder and into the shoulder. Gallbladder inflammation can irritate this nerve, causing referred pain in the back and shoulder, often on the right side.

Diagnosis

Labs

- Amylase/lipase assays to assess for pancreatitis: amylase is elevated in cholecystitis (normal amylase range is 40–140 U/L; normal lipase range is 0–160 U/L)
- Serum bilirubin: may be elevated
- BMP to assess electrolytes, especially with anorexia or intractable vomiting
- CBC: WBCs often elevated
- Hepatic function panel: increased serum ALT, AST, LDH, and alkaline phosphatase levels

Diagnostic Testing

- Abdominal ultrasound is the gold standard diagnostic test.
- Plain x-ray films may show radiopaque gallstones.
- Endoscopic retrograde cholangial-pancreatography is used to diagnose diseases of the gallbladder, bile system, pancreas, and liver.

Treatment

- Manage pain as needed with pain medications (Appendix 6.1 at the end of this chapter) until gallbladder inflammation resolves.
  - Meperidine
  - Hydrocodone/acetaminophen
  - Oxycodone/acetaminophen
- Administer antibiotics to prevent or treat infection.
  - Ampicillin (see Table A.1)
  - Cephalosporin-based therapies such as cefazolin or cefotetan (see Table A.1)
  - Ciprofloxacin (see Table A.1)
  - Metronidazole
  - Piperacillin (see Table A.1)

(continued)

Treatment *(continued)*

- Administer anticholinergic medications such as dicyclomine to reduce bile duct spasms.
- Perform lithotripsy using ultrasound waves to break up gallstones.
- NGT for gastric decompression may be needed.
- Patient may be NPO to provide gallbladder rest and before surgery if indicated.
- Administer IV fluids: usually crystalloid therapies to treat hemodynamic instability.
- Implement low-fat diet.
- Administer medications to dissolve gallstones.
- Consult GI or hepatobiliary specialist to determine if laparoscopic cholecystectomy is necessary.

Nursing Interventions

- Maintain patient's NPO status prior to surgery.
- Advance patient's diet as tolerated after surgery.
- Assess and manage ABC.
- Administer IV fluids as ordered.
- Assess and manage pain as needed.
- Manage nausea as needed.
- Monitor vital signs and assess for any postoperative signs or symptoms of infection.
- Monitor intake and output (including appearance of stool) before and after surgery
- Assess bowel sounds as ordered.
- Encourage ambulation as tolerated in the postoperative period.
- Monitor drainage from drains or tubes, if present.
- Monitor for jaundice.
- Monitor surgical incisions for complications such as dehiscence or infection.

Patient Education

- Implement diet modifications:
  - Decrease fat intake.
  - Increase fiber intake.
  - Maintain adequate hydration.
- If medications to dissolve gallstones are prescribed, take them for 6 to 12 months or as prescribed.
- Exercise regularly.
- Take medications as prescribed.
- Take pain medications as needed.

 POP QUIZ 6.3

A patient comes into the hospital after having had a cholecystectomy 1 week earlier. The patient states that they have been eating a high-fat diet over the last week. What education would the nurse provide to the patient?

CLOSTRIDIUM DIFFICILE

Overview

- *Clostridioides difficile* is a spore-forming, toxin-producing, gram-positive anaerobic bacterium. It colonizes the human intestinal tract and causes antibiotic-associated colitis after the normal gut flora has been disrupted.
- One of the most common HAIs, *C. difficile* infection may cause significant morbidity and mortality.
- *C. difficile* spores can live on surfaces and soil for months or even years.

 COMPLICATIONS

Clostridioides difficile infection that is severe and sudden, an uncommon condition, may also cause intestinal inflammation leading to enlargement of the colon (also called toxic megacolon) and sepsis. Sepsis is a life-threatening condition that occurs when the body's response to an infection damages its own tissues. Patients with these conditions are admitted to the ICU.

Signs and Symptoms

- Abdominal distention and cramping
- Lower abdominal pain
- Fever
- Nausea
- Blood in the stool
- Dehydration
- Profuse, watery diarrhea

Diagnosis

Labs

- CBC to assess for leukocytosis
- BMP
- *C. difficile* stool sample

Diagnostic Testing

- Abdominal x-ray
- CT scan

Treatment

- Antibiotics such as vancomycin (see Table A.1)
- IV hydration
- Supportive care
- Fecal transplant (stool from a donor placed into the gut of the patient to introduce healthy bacteria)

Nursing Interventions

- Administer medications as ordered.
- Maintain contact isolation precautions, including use of gowns and gloves and washing hands with soap and water.
  - Wipe down all surfaces where spores may be present.
- Monitor I/O closely to assess fluid balance.
- Assist with perineal hygiene to prevent skin breakdown.
- If skin breakdown is present, provide skin barrier cream.

Patient Education

- Do not take antidiarrheal medications because the toxins produced can cause serious colon damage.
- Do not take antibiotics that are not prescribed.
- Finish prescribed antibiotic course after discharge to prevent drug-resistant infections.
- Perform frequent hand hygiene with soap and water.
- Wash frequently touched surfaces in the home.

ALERT!

A rare but serious complication of *C. difficile* infection colitis is toxic megacolon. Toxic megacolon occurs when the colon rapidly swells, causing obstruction. Symptoms can rapidly progress to systemic symptoms such as fever, tachycardia, hypotension, abdominal distention, inability to pass gas or stool, and shock. Toxic megacolon is a medical emergency.

COLORECTAL CANCER

Overview

- *Colorectal cancer* is caused by a malignant tumor in the large intestine (colon) or rectum.
- Colon cancer is the third most common cancer in the United States.
- Tumors in the sigmoid and descending colon often grow circumferentially.

COMPLICATIONS

Complications of colorectal cancer include bowel obstruction, perforation, peritonitis, and sepsis. If the tumor invades the surrounding blood vessels, the patient is at a risk for hemorrhage.

(continued)

Overview *(continued)*

- Tumors in the ascending colon are often large at diagnosis and can sometimes be palpated.
- Colorectal cancer usually progresses slowly and has a better prognosis if diagnosed before nodal involvement occurs.
  - The most common indicator of outcome following resection of colon cancer is the pathologic stage.

Signs and Symptoms

- Anemia
- Black, tarry stools
- Blood in the stool
- Melena
- Hematochezia
- Rectal bleeding
- Change in bowel habits
- Constipation
- Diarrhea
- Abdominal distention
- Nausea
- Vomiting
- Dull abdominal pain
- Fatigue
- Unintentional weight loss
- Rectal or abdominal mass

Diagnosis

Labs

- CBC to assess for anemia
- CEA
- Iron studies to assess for causes of anemia, if present
- Fecal immunochemical test to assess for hidden blood in the stool, which can be an early sign of cancer
- Fecal occult blood test
- Stool DNA test to look for abnormal DNA associated with colon cancer: positive result usually requires colonoscopy

Diagnostic Testing

- CT scan of the chest, abdomen, and pelvis
- Colonoscopy with biopsy, if lesions are noted
- Digital rectal examination to assess for rectal or perianal lesions
- MRI
- Rectal ultrasound

Treatment

- Endoscopic resection is a reasonable option for selected early-stage colon cancers arising in a polyp, as long as they meet certain criteria for favorable risk.
- Surgical resection is the only curative modality for localized colon cancer.

 NURSING PEARL

Signs and symptoms of colorectal cancer depend on the location of the malignancy, and there are often no symptoms.

- Early-stage right-sided tumors often do not cause symptoms because stool is liquid when it enters the colon.
- Symptoms often do not develop until the disease has progressed to later stages.
- Patients with colorectal cancer may present in one of three ways:
  - Suspicious symptoms and/or signs
  - Asymptomatic with disease discovered by routine screening
  - Emergency admission with an intestinal obstruction, perforation, or, rarely, an acute GI bleed.

 ALERT!

Depending on location of the tumor, disease burden, and level of resection, the patient may need a permanent colostomy.

(continued)

Treatment *(continued)*

- Patients with potentially resectable disease should undergo resection, rather than upfront chemotherapy or chemoradiotherapy, if they are surgical candidates.
  - Following potentially curative resection, postoperative (adjuvant) chemotherapy eradicates micrometastases, reduces the likelihood of disease recurrence, and increases cure rates.
- Most patients who present with metastatic disease are not surgical candidates, and palliative chemotherapy is generally recommended.
- Surgical procedures include the following:
  - Hemicolectomy for advanced disease
  - Local resection of small lesions
  - Total colectomy for advanced disease not able to be resected by hemicolectomy

Nursing Interventions

- Administer medications as ordered.
- Advance diet as tolerated by patient.
- Monitor surgical incisions for complications such as dehiscence or infection (redness, swelling, skin warm to the touch, drainage from the incision site).
- Monitor for signs and symptoms of peritonitis, including fever, abdominal pain that is worse with movement, hypotension, and abdominal tenderness.
- Monitor fluid and electrolyte balance.
- Assist with ostomy care (if applicable); teach patient how to change bag appliance, monitor output of stool, assess stoma site, and provide care of surrounding skin.
- Provide emotional support to the patient and family.
- Monitor ostomy output if colostomy is present.

Patient Education

- Comply with prescribed diet, which varies based on surgical site and on whether an ostomy is present.
- Notify provider of acute changes such as new blood in stool or inability to have a bowel movement.
- Learn how to care for new ostomy: how to change ostomy bag, monitor output of stool, assess stoma site, and care for surrounding skin.
- Learn what a healthy stoma looks like (beefy red) and when to report concerns to provider, such as a dusky blue stoma.
- Learn how to order ostomy supplies as needed.
- Consult support groups and additional cancer resources such as the American Cancer Society or the Colon Cancer Alliance.

DIVERTICULITIS

Overview

- Diverticulosis is a condition in which small pouches or sacs form and push outward through weak areas in the muscle wall of the colon.
- Diverticulitis occurs when one or a few of the pouches become inflamed.
- Patients may have diverticulosis (the presence of diverticula) and be asymptomatic.

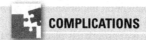 **COMPLICATIONS**

Inflammation of the diverticular sac occurs when undigested food and bacteria become trapped inside the sac. This can lead to abscess, peritonitis, perforation, obstruction, or hemorrhage.

Signs and Symptoms

- Diarrhea
- Anorexia

(continued)

Signs and Symptoms *(continued)*

- Nausea/vomiting
- Diminished or absent bowel sounds
- Changes in bowel habits (constipation or loose stools)
- Fever
- Inability to have a bowel movement
- Leukocytosis
- LLQ abdominal pain and cramping
- Rigid abdomen

Diagnosis

Labs

- CBC to assess for leukocytosis
- BMP to assess electrolyte imbalance
- Elevated ESR
- Fecal occult blood test
- CRP
- Lactate level
- Stool culture

Diagnostic Testing

- CT scan of the abdomen to evaluate potential abscess
- Abdominal ultrasound
- Barium enema
- Plain abdominal films to look for free air (pneumoperitoneum)
- Colonoscopy

Treatment

- NPO for complete bowel rest or clear liquids for milder cases
- Pain management with acetaminophen or NSAIDs
- Antibiotics if infection is suspected (IV progressing to oral as indicated):
    - Metronidazole
    - Amoxicillin
- Anticholinergics such as hyoscyamine to reduce spasms
- IV hydration
- High-fiber diet after the acute period
- Possible colonic resection in severe cases
    - Surgery indicated for severe infection or peritonitis in 20% to 30% of patients
- Temporary colostomy

Nursing Interventions

- Educate patient on importance of high-fiber diet.
- Monitor vital signs.
- Ensure IV is appropriately placed and patent.
- Administer IV hydration as ordered.
- Monitor for signs and symptoms of diverticular perforation, including blood in the stool and peritonitis.
- Monitor stool output.
- Monitor surgical incisions, if present, for complications such as dehiscence or infection.
- Provide ostomy care and teaching if applicable.
- Monitor for pain and manage as needed.

Patient Education

- Consume high-fiber diet with adequate fruits and vegetables and whole grains.
- Consult with dietitian or nutritionist if necessary.
- Maintain hydration to decrease constipation.
- Know signs and symptoms of infection and when to notify provider.
- Notify provider for blood in stool.
- Seek urgent evaluation for uncontrolled pain.
- Take laxatives and stool softeners if prescribed.
- Take medications, such as antibiotics, as prescribed.

ESOPHAGEAL CANCER

Overview

- Esophageal cancer is caused by a malignant tumor occurring in the esophagus.
- SCC and adenocarcinoma account for more than 95% of esophageal malignant tumors.

Signs and Symptoms

- Dysphagia
- Weight loss
- Hoarseness
- Cough
- Difficulty swallowing
- Feeling of fullness
- Hiccups
- Regurgitation
- Substernal pain

Diagnosis

Labs
- CBC with differential
- CMP

Diagnostic Testing
- CT scan of the head, neck, and chest
- Endoscopic ultrasound with biopsy
- Chest x-ray
- PET scan to assess stage of disease

Treatment

- Early-stage cancers can be treated with endoscopic procedures such as radiofrequency ablation or endoscopic mucosal resection.
    - Frequent follow-up endoscopies are important after treatment to continue to assess for precancerous cells.
- Esophagectomy may be indicated in healthy individuals to remove cancer that is in early stage (T1).
    - Chemoradiation may be indicated after surgery if there are signs that not all cancer was removed.

COMPLICATIONS

Complications from esophagectomy occur in approximately 40% of patients. The morbidity associated with the surgery consists mostly of respiratory, cardiac, and septic complications. Septic complications include wound infection, anastomotic leak (breakdown of the new connection between the stomach and esophagus), and pneumonia. Anastomotic leaks and stricture may require dilatation. Leaks may be treated with endoscopic placement of self-expanding, removable plastic stents.

NURSING PEARL

When discovered early, the goal of treatment is curative. When the disease is discovered in later stages, the goal of treatment is palliative. The prognosis and treatment depend on the stage of the cancer (whether it affects part of the esophagus, involves the whole esophagus, or has metastasized); whether the tumor can be completely surgically removed; and the patient's overall health.

(continued)

Treatment (continued)

- For slightly more advanced cancer, such as stage T2, chemoradiation may be recommended prior to surgery.
  - Surgery alone may be an option for smaller tumors.
  - If the cancer is located near the stomach, only chemotherapy may be given prior to surgery.
  - If there is any remaining cancer after chemoradiation and surgery, immunotherapy may be recommended.
  - If the cancer is in the upper part of the esophagus, chemoradiation may be recommended instead of surgery. For some patients, this may cure the cancer.
- Stage II cancer has grown into the main muscle layer of the esophagus or into the connective tissue on the outside of the esophagus. Stage III cancer has grown through the wall of the esophagus to the outside layer and grown into nearby organs, tissues, or lymph nodes.
  - For patients who are healthy enough, treatment is usually chemoradiation followed by surgery.
  - If there is any remaining cancer after chemoradiation and surgery, immunotherapy may be recommended.
- Stage IV cancer has spread to distant lymph nodes or other distant organs.
  - This stage is not usually curable, so surgery is not the best option unless it is palliative to relieve symptoms.
  - Chemotherapy along with targeted therapy or immunotherapy may be given to help patients feel better or live longer.
  - Intention for this stage is palliative, not curative.
- Esophageal dilation and or stenting may be done to keep the esophagus open to allow food and liquids to pass through to the stomach.

Nursing Interventions

- Advance diet as tolerated.
- Consider dietitian/nutritionist consult prior to patient discharge to assess for nutrition resources and provide education for discharge.
- Consult with speech pathology to assess for dysphagia/safe swallowing.
- Monitor BMI, calorie counts, and albumin levels to ensure patient is well nourished.
- Maintain adequate nutrition through enteral or parenteral feedings, as ordered.
- Assess and maintain drain care (nasogastric, nasoduodenal, nasojejunal, G-tube, G/J tube).
- Monitor telemetry:
  - Tumor burden putting pressure on great vessels can lead to arrythmias.
- Place the patient in semi-Fowler's or low Fowler's position to reduce gastric reflux.

Patient Education

- Consider a smoking cessation program, if applicable.
- Reduce or eliminate alcohol consumption.
- Take medications as prescribed, especially antacid medications.
- See a dietitian/nutritionist for follow-up to maintain adequate nutrition.
- If necessary, maintain safe swallowing: Elevate HOB 45 to 90 degrees when eating, take small sips, and eat meals with supervision or assistance as needed.
- Visit speech therapist as referred.

GASTRITIS

Overview

- *Gastritis* refers to acute or chronic irritation and inflammation of the stomach lining.
- It is usually caused by infectious agents (most commonly *Helicobacter pylori*), excessive alcohol intake, or certain medications (e.g., chronic NSAID use) or is immune mediated; however, the cause is frequently unknown.

Signs and Symptoms

- Abdominal pain
- Early satiety
- Epigastric pain
- Indigestion
- Nausea
- Vomiting
- Burning sensation in the stomach
- Anorexia
- Blood in emesis or stool

Diagnosis

Labs
There are no labs specific to diagnosing gastritis. However, the following may be helpful in diagnosis:
- CBC
- CMP
- Fecal occult blood test
- Guaiac test of gastric contents
- H. pylori
- Immunologic markers

Diagnostic Testing
- Endoscopy
- Gastric biopsy and histology
- Abdominal CT
- Upper GI series

 COMPLICATIONS

Left untreated, gastritis may lead to stomach ulcers and hemorrhage. Rarely, some forms of chronic gastritis may increase the risk of stomach cancer, especially if there is extensive thinning of the stomach lining and changes in the lining's cells.

 NURSING PEARL

Helicobacter pylori is a common infectious organism that causes gastritis. Chronic *H. pylori* infection can lead to gastritis and ulcers and eventually progress to gastric cancers. *Helicobacter pylori* treatment involves a combination therapy of antibiotics and a proton pump inhibitor to treat the infection. Frequently, the patient is asked to follow up after the medication course is completed to ensure eradication of the bacteria.

Treatment

- Gastric/bowel rest
- Medications (see Appendix 6.1) to reduce acid secretion such as omeprazole or lansoprazole
- Antibiotics such as metronidazole or amoxicillin (see Appendix 6.1)
- Treatment of underlying causes such as autoimmune disorders or other types of chronic gastritis, such as lymphocytic gastritis or radiation gastritis

Nursing Interventions

- Perform focused GI assessment.
- Assess and manage pain.
- Monitor intake and output.
- Administer medications and crystalloid IV fluids as ordered.
- Administer PRN medications such as antiemetics, as ordered.
- Encourage PO intake of bland foods.

Patient Education

- Avoid foods that trigger symptoms, such as spicy or acidic foods.
- Complete full course of antibiotics, if ordered.
- Avoid alcohol consumption and stop smoking, if applicable.
- Avoid taking NSAIDs, if indicated.
- Follow up with provider for increased pain or deceased ability to eat.
- Monitor for signs of GI bleeding, including dark, tarry stools.
- Take medications as prescribed.

GASTROINTESTINAL BLEEDING

Overview

- GI bleeding can be chronic and occur from inflammation such as gastritis, or it can be acute and caused by rupture or erosion into a blood vessel.
- GI bleeds occur in both the upper and the lower GI tract. Upper GI bleeding is the most common.
- Symptoms and presentation vary based on location.
- Upper GI hemorrhage is often caused by:
  - Peptic ulcer disease
  - Esophageal varices
  - Postsurgical bleeds
  - Mallory-Weiss tears
  - Stress ulcers
  - Cancer
  - GI tumors
  - Gastritis
  - Duodenitis
  - Esophagitis
- Lower GI hemorrhage is caused by:
  - Infectious or ischemic colitis
  - UC
  - Crohn's disease
  - Angiodysplasia
  - Intestinal polyps
  - IBS
  - Hemorrhoids
  - Colon cancer
  - Anal fissures
  - Postsurgical bleeding

Signs and Symptoms

- Abdominal pain
- Black, tarry stools
- Blood in the stool or vomit
- Coffee ground emesis
- Unexplained anemia
- Upper GI hemorrhage presenting with any of the following:
  - Abdominal tenderness
  - Decreased pulse pressure
  - Epigastric pain
  - Hematemesis (bright red or coffee ground)
  - Hyperactive bowel sounds
  - Hypotension
  - Melena
  - Nausea and vomiting
  - Orthostatic hypotension
  - Pale skin and mucous membranes
  - Presyncope/syncope
- Lower GI hemorrhage presenting with any of the following:
  - Abdominal cramping or discomfort

 COMPLICATIONS

Acute GI hemorrhage is a GI bleed that results in rapid blood loss. This hemodynamic instability decreases blood flow to the organs, causing tissue hypoxia, which can result in organ failure, seizures, coma, and death. Timely identification and treatment of acute GI hemorrhage is essential to preventing these complications and improving patient outcomes.

 ALERT!

Past medical history relevant to bleeding sources include:

- Alcohol misuse
- Diverticulitis
- *H. pylori* infection
- Hemorrhoids
- Inflammatory bowel disease
- Portal hypertension
- Tobacco use
- Gastric varices
- Ulcers
- NSAID misuse or overdose
- Recent anticoagulation or antiplatelet therapy

(continued)

Signs and Symptoms *(continued)*

- Diarrhea
- Hematochezia, often bright or dark red; may pass clots with stool
- Hypotension
- Orthostatic hypotension
- Pale skin and mucous membranes
- Presyncope/syncope

Diagnosis

Labs
- CBC to assess hemoglobin and hematocrit and need for possible transfusion
- CMP
- Coagulation panel to assess for bleeding times
- Guaiac test of gastric and stool contents
- *H. pylori* blood sample
- Stool sample
- Type and screen

Diagnostic Testing
- Colonoscopy
- EGD
- *H. pylori* via biopsy
- Imaging:
  - CT scan of chest, abdomen, and pelvis
  - Doppler ultrasound of portal veins
  - X-ray of chest and abdomen

Treatment

- Blood transfusion (PRBC, FFP, and platelets) as indicated if large-volume hemorrhage occurs
  - Massive transfusion protocol may be necessary depending on patient condition.
- Cauterization of bleeding vessels
- Holding of anticoagulant medications if indicated
- TIPS procedure if cause of bleeding is variceal
- Balloon tamponade: Sengstaken–Blakemore or Minnesota tube
- Medications (see Appendix 6.1):
  - Vasopressors
  - Isotonic fluid resuscitation
  - H2 antagonist or PPI
  - Somatostatin
- Nasogastric decompression (if appropriate based on location)
- Surgical intervention:
  - Endoscopic banding or cautery procedures
  - Endoscopic clipping or sewing of vessel
  - Exploratory laparotomy
  - Partial gastrectomy

 ALERT!

An acute rupture of esophageal varices results in sudden-onset projectile hematemesis, which can be bright red or coffee ground in appearance. This is an emergency. The nurse should act quickly to notify the provider and GI team. A Sengstaken–Blakemore tube is often inserted to tamponade variceal hemorrhage. If insertion is delayed, rapid acute hemorrhage may result in death.

Nursing Interventions

- Administer oxygen as needed.
- Assess ABC often.

(continued)

Nursing Interventions *(continued)*

- Administer blood products as ordered.
  - Monitor for blood transfusion reaction.
- Administer medications as ordered.
- Keep the patient NPO until source of bleeding is identified and controlled.
- Maintain two large-bore IVs in case of need for rapid transfusion.
- Maintain patency of NG tube, if ordered.
- Monitor for signs and symptoms of bleeding.
- Monitor hemodynamics and vital signs.
- Monitor for signs of aspiration and changes in respiratory status.
- Monitor serial CBCs to assess for a change in blood counts.
- Monitor volume and characteristics of stool and emesis output.
- Prepare to transfer to OR or IR as indicated for surgical intervention.

Patient Education

- Begin a smoking cessation program, if necessary.
- Eliminate use of NSAIDs, as these are gastric irritants.
- Follow up with gastroenterologist for management of varices.
- Follow up with hepatologist for management of cirrhosis.
- Monitor for signs and symptoms of bleeding (e.g., frank blood or black tarry stools, nosebleeds) and notify provider if present.
- Self-assess for any changes or signs of worsening anemia:
  - Pallor, dizziness, fatigue, lightheadedness, palpitations, SOB
- Stop any anticoagulants as indicated by provider.
- Take medications as prescribed.
- Reduce or eliminate alcohol consumption.

GASTROESOPHAGEAL REFLUX DISEASE

Overview

- The passage of gastric contents into the esophagus is a normal physiologic process that may occur in all patients but does not cause symptoms, injury, or complications.
- Gastroesophageal reflux becomes a disease when it causes macroscopic damage to the esophagus or when symptoms appear.
- GERD is the result of an incompetent lower esophageal sphincter and/or delayed gastric emptying.

 COMPLICATIONS

If GERD is left untreated, esophagitis can cause hemorrhage, ulcers, and chronic scarring. This scarring can cause narrowing of the esophagus, eventually interfering with the ability to swallow. One major complication that occurs in about 10% to 15% of people with chronic or longstanding GERD is Barrett's esophagus.

Signs and Symptoms

- Belching
- Burning epigastric pain
- Chest pain
- Chronic cough
- Dysphagia
- Feeling of reflux when lying down
- Heartburn
- Hoarseness

(continued)

Signs and Symptoms *(continued)*

- Hypersecretion of saliva
- Increased pain after eating
- Nausea
- Regurgitation

Diagnosis

Labs
There are no labs specific to diagnosing GERD, but the following are helpful in the initial workup:
- CBC
- CMP

Diagnostic Testing
- Barium swallow exam
- ED to rule out cancer, Barrett's esophagus, and peptic ulcer disease
- Esophageal pH testing

Treatment

- Antacid medication to relieve symptoms of GERD:
  - Aluminum hydroxide
  - Calcium carbonate
  - Magnesium trisilicate
- H2 receptor antagonists
  - Can be given in high doses at night or divided into twice a day dosing
- PPIs if H2 blockers are ineffective
- Surface agents and alginates, such as sucralfate
- Lifestyle modifications, such as:
  - Eating smaller, more frequent meals
  - Sleeping with HOB elevated to relieve symptoms (more common at night and when in recombinant positions)
- GI or surgical consult as needed
- For varices:
  - Liquid adhesive injection into the vein
  - Medications to control portal hypertension
  - TIPS procedure to reduce portal hypertension
  - Variceal banding

Nursing Interventions

- Encourage compliance with lifestyle modifications.
- Position the patient in semi-Fowler's or Fowler's position to reduce reflux.
- Provide education about the causes and symptoms of GERD.

Patient Education

- Avoid eating a large meal late at night and then lying down.
- Avoid tobacco and alcohol (both reduce lower esophageal sphincter pressure; smoking also diminishes salivation).
- Comply with medication regimen.
- Eliminate dietary triggers such as caffeine, chocolate, spicy or high-fat foods, carbonated beverages, and peppermint.
- Exercise daily.
- Plan for regular endoscopies if provider is concerned about Barrett's esophagus.

(continued)

Patient Education *(continued)*

- Promote salivation by using oral lozenges or chewing gum to neutralize refluxed acid and increase the rate of esophageal clearance.
- Use abdominal breathing exercises to strengthen the anti-reflux barrier of the lower esophageal sphincter.

GASTROPARESIS

Overview

- *Gastroparesis* is delayed gastric emptying without evidence of obstruction. This disorder slows or stops the movement of food from the stomach to the small intestine.
- Uncontrolled diabetes is the most common cause of gastroparesis.

Signs And Symptoms

- Abdominal distention
- Bloating
- Early satiety
- Halitosis
- Nausea
- Vomiting
- Weight loss

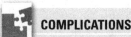

COMPLICATIONS

In the majority of patients with insulin-dependent diabetes, gastroparesis is often overlooked and underdiagnosed, especially in its early stages. Approximately 5% to 10% of patients with insulin-dependent diabetes may progress to severe symptomatic gastroparesis. The characteristics of poor glucose control and acid reflux are often the only signatures of delayed gastric emptying. The typical picture seen in the diabetic gastroparetic stomach is low blood glucose levels at bedtime with very high blood glucose levels by the next morning.

Diagnosis

Labs
- BMP to assess electrolytes and serum glucose

Diagnostic Testing
- Abdominal ultrasound
- CT scan
- Endoscopy
- Gastric emptying study
- Upper GI series

Treatment

- Assess for dehydration and malnutrition.
- Use gastric stimulator.
- Place jejunostomy tube for patients who cannot tolerate oral nutrition or have severe gastric emptying and are severely malnourished.
- Administer medications (see Appendix 6.1):
  - Metoclopramide: increases contraction of stomach wall to help with gastric emptying (also helps with nausea and vomiting)
  - Ondansetron: helps with nausea
- Implement parenteral nutrition for severe gastroparesis when other treatments are ineffective.

Nursing Interventions

- Administer medications as ordered.
- Maintain patency of jejunostomy tube or other feeding tube if indicated.

(continued)

Nursing Interventions *(continued)*

- Measure gastric residuals.
- Monitor glycemic control.
- Monitor labs.
- Monitor vital signs.

Patient Education

- Abstain from alcohol.
- Abstain from smoking.
- Follow dietary instructions.
  - Eat foods low in fat and fiber.
  - Eat five or six small, nutritious meals a day instead of two or three large meals.
  - Eat soft, well-cooked foods.
  - Avoid carbonated, or fizzy, beverages.
  - Drink plenty of water or liquids that contain glucose and electrolytes, such as:
    - ○ Low-fat broths or clear soups
    - ○ Naturally sweetened, low-fiber fruit and vegetable juices
    - ○ Sports drinks
    - ○ Oral rehydration solutions
  - Do gentle physical activity after a meal, such as taking a walk.
  - Avoid lying down for 2 hours after a meal.
  - Take a multivitamin each day.
- Follow up with endocrinologist for management of diabetes.
- Follow up with gastroenterologist for management of gastroparesis.
- Maintain euglycemia.
- Take medications as prescribed.

HEPATITIS

Overview

- *Hepatitis* is inflammation of the liver with resultant liver dysfunction.
- It can be acute or chronic:
  - Acute liver failure involves hepatic injury of less than 26 weeks without prior history of liver disease, encephalopathy, and coagulopathy, with an INR of ≥1.5. It is a process of hepatocellular necrosis (Table 6.1).
  - Chronic liver failure, or end-stage liver disease, involves irreversible cirrhosis by progressive fibrosis, nodular regeneration after necrosis, and chronic inflammation.
- Hepatitis can be caused by a multitude of factors, including bacteria, viruses, trauma, toxins, and immune disorders.
- Types of hepatitis are shown in Table 6.2.

 ALERT!

Adults should not take more than 4,000 mg of single-ingredient acetaminophen per day. Patients older than 65 years should take no more than 3,000 mg/d. A dose of 7,000 mg or more can lead to severe liver damage and possible liver failure, requiring a liver transplant. If the nurse suspects acetaminophen overdose, the nurse should talk with the patient about how often and what dose they ingest, including combination medications that contain acetaminophen.

Table 6.1 Causes and Symptoms of Acute and Chronic Liver Failure

	Acute Liver Failure	Chronic Liver Failure
Etiology	• Acetaminophen toxicity • Autoimmune condition • Graft-versus-host disease following bone marrow transplantation • Hepatotoxic drugs • Reye's syndrome • Veno-occlusive disease • Viral infections (herpes, hepatitis A and B) • Wilson's disease	• Alcoholism • Autoimmune hepatitis • Hepatic vein thrombosis • Nonalcoholic fatty liver • Right-sided HF • Toxins • Viral hepatitis • Wilson's disease
Signs and Symptoms	• Coagulopathy • Fever • Flu-like symptoms • Hepatic encephalopathy with rapid progression to coma • Hepatorenal syndrome • Hyperdynamic circulation • Hyperventilation respiratory alkalosis • Hypoglycemia • Intracranial hypertension • Systolic ejection murmur	• Altered mental status • Anemia • Ascites • Asterixis • Clay colored stools • Fatigue • Hepatic bruit • Hyperdynamic circulation • Insomnia • Jaundice • Muscle wasting • Musty breath • Poor dentition • Splenomegaly • Systolic ejection murmur

Table 6.2 Types of Hepatitis

Type	Hepatitis A (HAV)	Hepatitis B (HBV)	Hepatitis C (HCV)	Hepatitis D (HDV)	Hepatitis E (HEV)
Method of Transmission	Fecal-oral (contaminated food or water)	Blood and other bodily fluids	Blood	Blood and other bodily fluids	Fecal-oral (contaminated food or water)
Labs	Anti-HAV specific antibody, DNA	HBV surface protein, anti-HBV specific antibody	PCR of viral RNA, anti-HCV antibody	Anti-HBV specific antibody	Anti-HEV specific antibody, PCR of viral RNA
Chronic Hepatitis	No	Yes, 10% chance	Yes, >50% chance	Yes, <5% coinfections; >80% superinfections	No

Signs and Symptoms

- Abdominal pain in the RUQ
- Altered mental state
- Anemia
- Anorexia

(continued)

Signs and Symptoms *(continued)*

- Ascites
- Asterixis
- Ecchymosis
- Edema
- Encephalopathy
- Enlarged, nodular liver
- Esophageal or gastric varices
- Fatigue
- Itching
- Jaundice
- Low-grade fever
- Nausea
- Orange- or brown-colored urine
- Peripheral edema
- Poor appetite
- Pruritis
- Thrombocytopenia
- Unintentional weight loss
- Vomiting

Diagnosis

Labs

- Ammonia: high levels associated with alcoholic hepatitis (common with hepatic encephalopathy)
- Albumin levels: drop with liver damage (normal range 3.5–5 g/dL)
- ALT and AST: high levels mean the liver is leaking enzymes
    - Normal range of AST: 0 to 140 U/L
    - Normal range of ALT: 7 to 56 U/L
- Bilirubin:
    - A normal, functioning liver removes bilirubin from the blood; when the liver is damaged, bilirubin is elevated. Most patients become jaundiced.
    - Normal range is 0.1 to 1.0 mg/dL.
- BMP: usually hyponatremia and hypokalemia in cirrhosis patients
- CBC to assess for anemia and thrombocytopenia
- Coagulation panel
- Creatinine: elevated in late stages of cirrhosis (increase in serum creatinine ≥0.3 mg/dL within 48 hours, or 50% or 1.5-fold from baseline in less than 7 days)
- Hepatitis panel:
    - HAV: IgM HAV antibody
    - HBV: surface antigen or HBV antibody
    - HCV: anti-HCV or HCV viral load
- Hepatic function panel to measure liver involvement associated with viral or alcoholic hepatitis
- Herpes simplex virus
- Toxicology screen to assess for drug use

Diagnostic Testing

- Abdominal CT scan
- Abdominal ultrasound
- Liver biopsy
- MRI

 COMPLICATIONS

Hepatic failure may result in protein and nutritional deficiencies as well as significant fluid shifts. Hemorrhage may occur secondary to portal hypertension with resultant esophageal varices. The decreased ability of clotting factors also contributes to an increased risk for bleeding. Severe systemic effects of hepatic failure include sepsis, renal failure, respiratory failure, encephalopathy, hepatic coma, brainstem herniation, and death.

 NURSING PEARL

Cirrhosis represents a late stage of progressive hepatic fibrosis. The liver is permanently damaged, and the only treatment option may be a liver transplantation.

 NURSING PEARL

The most common cause of acute hepatic failure is acetaminophen overdose. The most common cause of chronic liver failure is alcohol toxicity.

Treatment

- Administer vitamin K for prolonged PT.
- Administer lactulose 30 mL orally or rectally for elevated ammonia levels.
- Administer antiviral drugs.
- Avoid alcohol or other drugs detoxified by the liver.
- Identify and reverse cause of acute hepatic failure.
- Administer immunosuppressants.
- Increase fluids.
- Perform liver resection.
- Perform liver transplantation.
- Administer medications (see Appendix 61.).
  - N-acetylcysteine and activated charcoal for acetaminophen overdose; most effective when given within 8 hours of ingesting acetaminophen
- Perform TIPS procedure.
- Treat hepatitis C (see Appendix 6.1).
- Treat cirrhosis:
  - Fluid restriction
  - Treatment/management of hepatic encephalopathy if present (monitor ammonia levels and manage with lactulose and/or rifampin; see Appendix 6.1)
  - Management of coagulopathies or uncontrolled bleeding
  - Antibiotics as indicated for secondary infections
  - Treatment/management of hepatorenal syndrome if present (may require dialysis)
  - Low-sodium, high-protein diet
  - Potassium-sparing diuretics to reduce ascites and edema
  - Removal of excess fluid (with diuretics and/or paracentesis for ascites)
  - Prophylactic antibiotics to prevent SBP
  - GI/surgery consultation for procedures including an endoscopy, a TIPS procedure, liver resection, and/or liver transplantation

 NURSING PEARL

A TIPS procedure connects the portal vein to the hepatic vein via a shunt placed in the liver. This shunt helps to decrease portal hypertension and allow for the delivery of venous return back to the heart. Without this shunt, patients with portal hypertension are at risk for worsening ascites and edema, esophageal varices, portal gastropathy, and hydrothorax.

Nursing Interventions

- Administer medications as ordered.
- Assess ABC.
- Assess abdomen frequently for changes.
- Assess neurologic status for evidence of worsening disease.
- Assess vital signs and hemodynamic stability.
- Assist with perineal hygiene/toileting with lactulose doses.
- Closely monitor I/O, especially for patients receiving diuretics and/or lactulose.
- Draw and monitor serial labs as ordered.
- Encourage activity as tolerated.
- If patient has hepatic encephalopathy:
  - Provide frequent reorientation.
  - Maintain patient safety.
  - Assess neurologic status for evidence of worsening hepatic encephalopathy.
- Maintain appropriate sleep/wake cycles.
- Monitor and record bowel movement frequency, consistency, and volume.
- Monitor for signs and symptoms of bleeding.
- Monitor labs.
- Perform interventions for postoperative liver transplant:
  - Administer hemodynamic support with albumin, fluids, or vasopressors.
  - Assess and monitor all lines, drains, and tubes.

(continued)

Nursing Interventions *(continued)*

- Monitor vital signs.
- Draw and monitor serial labs, tacrolimus levels, and blood glucose.
- Encourage advanced diet as tolerated once extubated.
- Encourage working with PT and OT to regain functional ability postsurgery.

Patient Education

- Abstain from alcohol.
- Be mindful of safe acetaminophen dosage and other analgesics.
- Call provider for any signs of change in mental status or confusion.
- Call provider with any new or worrisome bleeding, including increased bruising.
- Follow up with alcohol and tobacco cessation or mental health resources as indicated.
- Maintain fluid restriction, if prescribed.
- Maintain low-sodium, high-protein diet if prescribed.
- Monitor for changes in behavior and orientation.
- Monitor for worsening symptoms of disease.
- Strictly adhere to follow-up office visits and testing.
- Take medications as prescribed.
  - If continuing lactulose at home, be aware that diarrhea is an expected effect of the medication.
  - Learn about lactulose dosing and how to titrate doses appropriately.
  - If liver transplant has been received, take antirejection and immunosuppressive medications as prescribed.

INFLAMMATORY BOWEL DISEASE

Overview

- Inflammatory bowel disease is an umbrella term describing disorders that involve chronic inflammation of the digestive tract: Crohn's disease and UC.
- Crohn's disease usually affects the end of the small intestines and the beginning of the colon but can occur anywhere in the GI tract; UC affects only the colon.

 COMPLICATIONS

A common complication of inflammatory bowel disease is toxic megacolon, which is a total or segmental nonobstructive colonic dilation that occurs in the context of systemic toxicity. As a result, the colon stops working and in severe cases may rupture. Antibiotics and steroids are the typical treatment for this diagnosis. In severe cases septic shock may be present, and the patient will be admitted to the ICU.

Signs and Symptoms

- Abdominal pain
- Anorexia
- Anxiety/stress
- Blood in the stool
- Diarrhea or constipation
- Weight loss

Diagnosis

Labs

- CBC to assess for anemia
- BMP to assess electrolytes in setting of diarrhea
- CRP and ESR to assess inflammation
- Fecal occult blood test
- Stool culture

Diagnostic Testing

- Abdominal CT
- Barium x-ray
- Biopsy
- Colonoscopy
- Fecal calprotectin to measure inflammation levels in the intestines; may eliminate more invasive tests
- Upper endoscopy

Treatment

- Anxiety medication or antidepressant
- Colostomy or ileostomy
- Dietary modifications, such as:
  - Eat a low-fiber diet. Limit foods such as seeds, nuts, beans, fruit, and bran.
  - Avoid caffeine.
  - Drink plenty of water to stay hydrated.
  - Elimination diet to establish which foods are triggers.
- Immunosuppressant medications
- Medications to control intestinal inflammation, such as:
  - NSAIDs
  - Steroids (for short-term use)
- Pain medications
- Surgery for fistula repair, if applicable

Nursing Interventions

- Administer IV fluids, such as crystalloids, to maintain hydration status.
- Administer medications as ordered.
- Assist patient to maintain adequate hydration.
- Assist patient with perineal hygiene and incontinence episodes as needed.
- Instruct patient on prescribed diet modifications to reduce symptom severity.
- Maintain patency of NG tube, if applicable.
- Monitor bowel sounds.
- Monitor intake/output, including stool characteristics.
- Monitor for signs and symptoms of bleeding.
- Monitor vital signs.
- Provide analgesics and antiemetics as needed.
- Provide ostomy care, if needed.

Patient Education

- Avoid large quantities of fluids with meals to minimize abdominal distention.
- Avoid smoking and alcohol consumption.
- Care for ostomy, if applicable.
- Exercise regularly.
- Follow dietary recommendations.
- Follow up with gastroenterologist.
- Identify and avoid foods and stressful situations that may trigger symptoms.
- Maintain adequate hydration and fiber intake to manage constipation.
- Monitor for signs and symptoms of worsening disease.
- Take medications as prescribed.

INTESTINAL OBSTRUCTION

Overview

- A bowel obstruction is a blockage of the lumen of the intestine that impedes the passage of gas and contents through the bowel.
- Bowel obstructions can occur in either the small or the large intestine and can be classified as either of the following:
  - A mechanical obstruction results from something outside or within the intestine that causes a blockage. These include obstructions such as adhesions, strictures, volvulus, impaction, intussusception, and tumors.
  - A nonmechanical obstruction develops when the muscular activity of the intestine decreases. Functional causes include paralytic ileus, inflammatory disease, or prior intestinal surgeries that alter regular bowel function.
- Obstructions can cause partial or complete intestinal blockage.
- Signs and symptoms may vary depending upon the location of the obstruction.
- *Ileus* is the inability to tolerate oral intake due to a lack of gastrointestinal motility without obstruction.
  - Common causes of ileus include surgery, medication, peritonitis, and trauma.

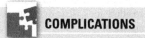

COMPLICATIONS

An untreated, intestinal obstruction can cause serious, life-threatening complications, including:

- **Tissue death.** Intestinal obstruction can cut off the blood supply to part of the intestine. Lack of blood causes the intestinal wall to die. Tissue death can result in a perforation in the intestinal wall, which can lead to infection.
- **Infection.** Peritonitis is a life-threatening condition that requires immediate medical and often surgical attention.

Signs and Symptoms

- Abdominal pain, tenderness, and distention
- Anorexia
- Bilious or feculent vomiting
- Constipation
- Dehydration
- High-pitched "tinkling" bowels sounds
- Intermittent feculent vomiting
- Inability to pass stool or gas

Diagnosis

Labs
- BMP
- CBC to check for leukocytosis
- Serum lactate: levels may be elevated in dehydration or decreased tissue perfusion
- BUN and creatinine: levels may be elevated with dehydration

Diagnostic Testing
- Abdominal CT scan
- Abdominal ultrasound
- Abdominal x-ray

Treatment

- Bowel rest (NPO)
- Conservative management with observation
  - If no improvement or deterioration, surgical intervention may be needed.
- Electrolyte replacement

(continued)

Treatment *(continued)*

- IV hydration
- Management of underlying condition
- NG tube to allow for gastric decompression
- Pain management

Nursing Interventions

- Administer medications as prescribed to manage nausea and vomiting.
- Assess and manage pain.
- Assess for signs and symptoms of infection or acute abdomen.
- Assist with oral care if patient is NPO.
- Ensure large-bore IV is placed and patent.
- Insert/manage NG tube as ordered.
- Monitor I/O, including characteristics of stool.
- Monitor lab values.
- Perform focused abdominal assessment to monitor for bowel sounds and assess gastric distention.
- Prepare patient for transfer to OR as indicated.

Patient Education

- Ambulate as tolerated to encourage bowel motility.
- Monitor and track bowel movements.
- Follow up with appropriate provider based on cause of obstruction.
- Maintain oral hygiene if oral intake is temporarily not permitted.
- Monitor for symptoms or worsening condition and follow up as needed.
- Take medications only as prescribed, including stool softeners as needed.
- Advance diet:
  - Take NPO until obstruction is resolved.
  - When able to eat, begin with clear liquids and advance diet as tolerated or per provider instructions.

MALABSORPTION SYNDROME

Overview

- Malabsorption syndrome is characterized by the inability of the small intestine to absorb nutrients.
- There are many causes of malabsorption syndrome, including:
  - Biliary atresia
  - Medications that injure the lining of the intestine
  - Damage to the intestine from infection, inflammation, trauma, or surgery
  - Diseases of the gallbladder, liver, or pancreas
  - Lactase deficiency or lactose intolerance
  - Parasitic diseases
  - Prolonged use of antibiotics
  - Radiation therapy

 COMPLICATIONS

Hypoalbuminemia is a common finding among hospitalized individuals. The presence of a decreased serum albumin is related to increased patient morbidity and mortality. Management of hypoalbuminemia is contingent on treatment of the underlying disease.

Signs and Symptoms

- Decreased PO intake
- Dehydration

(continued)

Signs and Symptoms *(continued)*

- Edema
- Electrolyte abnormalities:
  - Hypokalemia:
    - Muscle twitching or cramps
    - Palpitations or dysrhythmia
    - Hypomagnesemia:
    - Anorexia
    - Fatigue
    - Nausea and vomiting
    - Weakness
    - Tetany
  - Hypocalcemia:
    - Cramps and spasms
    - Circumoral numbness
    - Chvostek's sign
    - Carpopedal spasm (Trousseau's sign)
    - Paresthesia
    - Seizures
    - Tetany
- Hair loss
- Hypoglycemia:
  - Anxiety
  - Hunger
  - Irritability
  - Palpitations
  - Sweating
- Infections
- Mood changes:
  - Apathy
  - Anxiety
  - Depression
  - Self-neglect
- Nutritional deficiencies
- Pressure ulcers
- Slow wound healing
- Weight loss

Diagnosis

Labs

- BMP to assess electrolytes in setting of diarrhea or severe emesis
- CBC to assess for anemia and leukocytosis
- CRP and ESR to assess inflammation
- Serum albumin: hypoalbuminemia possible in malabsorption
- Calcium; phosphorous; magnesium; vitamins D, B1, and B12; and folic acid levels
- Renal and liver function tests to evaluate proteins, electrolytes, and organ function
- Serum osmolality to measure dehydration, electrolytes, and glucose levels

Diagnostic Testing

- Diagnosis by clinical presentation, BMI, and associated laboratory findings
- CT scan
- EKG to assess for electrolyte abnormalities that may be present
- Stool tests to measure fat levels(fat usually present in stool with malabsorption syndrome)
- Thorough history and physical exam to assess for malabsorption

Treatment

- Nutritional supplementation, including necessary vitamins and protein if not contraindicated
- Appetite stimulants in certain patients, such as those with malignancies and those receiving chemotherapy (see Appendix 6.1)
- Electrolyte replacement based on CMP results
- PO intake as tolerated
- Enteral nutrition via temporary (or permanent) tube feeding: nasogastric, orogastric, gastrostomy, or jejunostomy
  - Parenteral nutrition (IV), if patient unable to tolerate enteral feeds (such as TPN)
- IV fluid resuscitation
- Medication management dependent on condition for patients with malnourishment

Nursing Interventions

- Administer medications as ordered.
- Assess vital signs for early indications of change in status (deterioration).
- Draw and monitor serial labs as ordered.
- Minimize interruptions in enteral and parenteral nutrition.
- Monitor blood glucose when initiating TPN.
- Monitor for signs of malnutrition, including routine skin assessment for wounds.
- Monitor for signs of respiratory distress or aspiration following.
- Monitor I/O and nutritional intake.
- Monitor securement and site marking for nasogastric or other gastric tubes.
- Provide protein supplementation as indicated.

Patient Education

- Choose calorie-, nutrient-, and protein-dense foods to receive adequate daily nutrition.
- Consider working with a dietitian or nutritionist to receive additional nutritional education and establish optimal lifestyle habits.
- Reduce or stop alcohol consumption.
- Take medications as ordered.
- Take nutritional supplements as recommended by your provider.

PANCREATITIS

Overview

- *Pancreatitis* is an inflammatory condition of the pancreas caused by leakage of pancreatic enzymes into the surrounding tissues, resulting in an autodigestive state of the pancreas.
- Patients can develop multisystem organ failure secondary to inflammatory chemicals secreted throughout the body.
- Pancreatitis can be classified as either of the following:
  - *Acute pancreatitis* is the result of pancreatic injury, commonly caused by gallstones.
  - *Chronic pancreatitis* occurs when permanent damage is sustained to the structure and endocrine and exocrine functions of the pancreatitis.
- Causes of pancreatitis include heavy alcohol use, trauma, infection, hypercalcemia, hyperlipidemia, medications (e.g., sulfonamides, thiazides, furosemide, estrogen, azathioprine), and obstruction of the bile ducts.

 COMPLICATIONS

Local complications include fluid collection, ascites, pancreatic pseudocyst, pancreatic necrosis, and infective pancreatic necrosis. These complications are twice as frequent in patients with alcoholic and biliary pancreatitis. Pancreatic necrosis is a significant complication of acute pancreatitis and may result in mortality rates as high as 15%. In necrotizing pancreatitis, there is obstruction of the pancreatic microcirculation. Treatment of infected pancreatic necrosis depends on the pattern and anatomic location. Treatment options include surgical debridement of necrotic tissue (reduces mortality rates when done early in the course of pancreatitis) or percutaneous drainage.

Signs and Symptoms

- Abdominal distention
  - Upper abdomen may be tender to palpation
- Abrupt onset of steady, severe epigastric pain (relieved by sitting and leaning forward)
- Anorexia
- Anxiety
- Dehydration
- Diaphoresis
- Hemorrhagic signs:
  - Grey Turner's sign: flank discoloration
  - Cullen's sign: umbilical discoloration
- Hypoactive or absent bowel sounds
- Low-grade fever
- Nausea
- Mild jaundice
- Pallor, cool skin
- Radiating back or shoulder pain
- Tachycardia
- Vomiting

Diagnosis

Labs

- BUN and coagulation values: may be elevated
- CBC to assess for leukocytosis, hyperglycemia, and hypocalcemia
- CRP: may be elevated in pancreatic necrosis
- Hepatic function panel: may be elevated in acute biliary pancreatitis if stones are present
- Serum LDH: may be elevated
- Serum lipase/amylase levels:
  - Typically three times normal level during acute pancreatitis episode
  - May only be slightly elevated with chronic pancreatitis
- ALT/AST: may be elevated if gallstones are present

Diagnostic Testing

- Chest, abdomen, and pelvis CT scan
- ERCP if biliary tract occlusion suspected
- MRI
- Abdominal ultrasound to assess gallbladder
- X-ray

Treatment

- Electrolyte replacement
- Enzymes to improve digestion in chronic pancreatitis, such as:
  - Pancrelipase: given for symptoms of malabsorption
- ERCP to assess pancreatic and bile ducts
- IV hydration to prevent dehydration
- NPO status initially to provide bowel rest
- Pain management
- Surgery if indicated to relieve pressure/blockage in pancreatic duct.

Nursing Interventions

- Administer analgesics and antiemetics as ordered.
- Administer medications as ordered.
- Assess for signs of retroperitoneal bleeding.
- Assess respiratory status for early signs of atelectasis or effusions.

(continued)

Nursing Interventions *(continued)*

- Provide blood pressure support as needed; in severe pancreatitis blood pressure may drop.
- Draw and monitor serial labs as ordered.
- Monitor for signs of hyperglycemia as needed; they may develop due to pancreatic islet cell damage.
- Monitor I/O (monitor urine output for signs of hypoperfusion as well as adequate resuscitation).
- Monitor stool for signs of fat malabsorption (yellow, floating, or greasy stools and diarrhea).
- Monitor vital signs frequently.
- Monitor securement and site marking for NGT if indicated:
  - May be used for gastric decompression, to remove gastric fluids, and/or to remove air to let the pancreas rest and heal
  - May be used for enteral nutrition
- Once patient is pain free and has bowel sounds, start clear diet or enteral feeding below the duodenum.

Patient Education

- Discuss a low-fat diet with a dietitian.
- Eliminate alcohol consumption. If diagnosis is alcoholic pancreatitis, consider treatment and addiction resources.
- Follow recommended dietary changes.
- Take medications as advised (see Appendix 6.1).
  - Take pancreatic enzymes to help with digestion.
  - Take vitamin supplements for malabsorption.

PEPTIC ULCER DISEASE

Overview

- Peptic ulcers are defects in the gastric or duodenal mucosa that extend through the muscularis mucosae. Ulcers develop and persist due to the acid-peptic activity in gastric juice.
- Peptic ulcer disease is associated with two major factors: *H. pylori* infection and the consumption of NSAIDs. Family history can also be a factor.
- There are two types of ulcers:
  - Duodenal ulcers:
    - Pain occurs when the stomach is empty.
    - Pain is typically relieved with food or antacids.
  - Gastric ulcers:
    - Pain occurs with eating.
    - Patients tend to have weight loss.

Signs and Symptoms

- Acid brash
- Acid reflux
- Anorexia
- Burning abdominal pain
- Dizziness
- Epigastric pain
- Feeling of abdominal fullness
- Hematemesis
- Hematochezia

COMPLICATIONS

There are four major complications of peptic ulcer disease: bleeding, perforation, penetration, and obstruction. Hemorrhage is the most frequent complication, and its incidence is increasing in comparison to perforation and stenosis. Therapeutic endoscopy is considered the treatment of choice for bleeding ulcers, reducing the need for emergent surgical procedures to 10% to 20% of cases.

NURSING PEARL

Peptic ulcer disease can occur in patients with Zollinger–Ellison syndrome, which is a rare gastrinoma. These tumors can produce too much of a hormone called gastrin, which can lead to peptic ulcers.

(continued)

Signs and Symptoms *(continued)*

- Nausea
- Syncope
- Vomiting
- GI bleeding (in severe cases):
  - Melena
  - Hematemesis
  - Coffee ground emesis
- Signs of perforation (in severe cases):
  - Severe epigastric pain
  - Board-like, rigid abdomen
  - Quiet bowel sounds

Diagnosis

Labs
- CBC to assess for anemia
- BMP
- Coagulation panel
- *H. Pylori* (blood or stool)

Diagnostic Testing
- Biopsy to assess cause of ulcer
- Upper endoscopy
- X-ray of abdomen and chest

Treatment

- *H. pylori* treatment: combination therapy of antibiotics and a proton pump inhibitor
  - PPI: may include omeprazole or lansoprazole
  - Antibiotics such as metronidazole or amoxicillin
- Diet modifications:
  - Elimination of dietary triggers such as caffeine, chocolate, spicy or high-fat foods, carbonated beverages, and peppermint
- Lifestyle modifications to heal and prevent:
  - Balanced diet
  - Regular exercise
  - Successful coping with stress
  - Avoidance of smoking
  - Limiting of alcohol intake
  - Sufficient sleep
- Medications such as proton pump inhibitors or histamine blockers
- Medications such as sucralfate or bismuth subsalicylate (see Appendix 6.1) to cover the ulcer and create a protective layer to prevent further damage

Nursing Interventions

- Administer medications as ordered.
- Assess for pallor and fatigue.
- Encourage compliance with ordered diet.
- Encourage smoking cessation.
- Monitor vital signs.
- Monitor for GI bleeding.
- Monitor for signs and symptoms of acute abdomen.
- Prep patient for scope as indicated.

Patient Education

- Avoid medications that can trigger symptoms, including aspirin, ibuprofen, and naproxen.
- Begin a smoking cessation program, if appropriate.
- Discuss modifying use of NSAIDs with provider.
- Follow up with gastroenterologist.
- Consume high-fiber diet consisting of adequate fruits, vegetables, and whole grains.
- Consider referral to dietician or nutritionist if necessary.
- Reduce alcohol consumption.
- Take medications as prescribed.

Appendix 6.1 Gastrointestinal Medications

Indications	Mechanism of Action	Contraindications, Precautions, and Adverse Effects
Antidiarrheals (loperamide)		
• Treatment of diarrhea	• Interfere with peristalsis by direct action on the circular and longitudinal muscles of the intestinal wall to slow motility	• Contraindications include dysentery, fever, gastroenteritis, infection, pseudomembranous colitis, cardiac arrhythmia, constipation, toxic megacolon, UC, and AIDS. • Use caution in hepatic disease. • Adverse effects include ileus, toxic megacolon, angioedema, lethal arrhythmias and cardiac arrest, constipation, rash, respiratory depression, and QT prolongation.
Antidote, other (activated charcoal)		
• Emergency use following toxic ingestion/poisoning	• Absorbs ingested toxin, preventing it from being systemically absorbed in the stomach	• Use caution in intestinal bleeding, blockage or perforation, decreased LOC, dehydration, slow digestion, and recent surgery. • Adverse effects include diarrhea, black stools, or vomiting.
Antiemetic, serotonin/5HT3 antagonist (ondansetron)		
• Treatment of nausea and vomiting	• Blocks the serotonin 5-HT3 receptors at the peripheral vagal nerve terminals in the intestines, blocking signal transmission to the CNS to antagonize the effect of serotonin and decrease the presence of nausea and vomiting	• Use caution with hepatic disease, PKU, GI obstruction or ileus, any cardiac arrhythmia, electrolyte imbalance, malnutrition, MI, and thyroid disease. • Monitor for QT prolongation and resultant arrythmias including torsades de pointes. • Adverse effects include bradycardia, bronchospasm, hepatic failure, arrhythmia, angioedema, laryngeal edema, laryngospasm, constipation, urinary retention, hypokalemia, and hypotension.

(continued)

Appendix 6.1 Gastrointestinal Medications *(continued)*

Indications	Mechanism of Action	Contraindications, Precautions, and Adverse Effects

Antiemetic, other, antipsychotic, phenothiazine (prochlorperazine maleate)

Indications	Mechanism of Action	Contraindications, Precautions, and Adverse Effects
• Treatment of nausea and vomiting, including postoperative and postoperative prophylaxis • Management of the manifestations of psychotic disorders such as schizophrenia • Short-term management of nonpsychotic anxiety • Acute treatment of migraines • Treatment of pregnancy-induced nausea and vomiting	• Prochlorperazine blocks postsynaptic dopamine receptors in the mesolimbic system and increases dopamine turnover by blockade of the dopamine D2 somatodendritic autoreceptor. • The decrease in dopamine neurotransmission has been found to correlate with the antipsychotic effects. • Possesses moderate anticholinergic and alpha-adrenergic receptor blocking effects. Blockade of alpha 1 adrenergic receptors produces sedation; muscle relaxation; and cardiovascular effects such as hypotension, reflex tachycardia, and minor changes in ECG patterns. • Exerts an antiemetic effect through a depressant action on the chemoreceptor trigger zone. • Blocks H1-receptors, causing anticholinergic actions to result in reduced CNS stimulation of nausea and motion sickness	• Possible risk factors for leukopenia/neutropenia include preexisting low WBC count and history of drug-induced leukopenia/neutropenia. • Drug should not be administered at doses of more than 20 mg/d in adults or for longer than 12 weeks when used in the treatment of nonpsychotic anxiety, because use of prochlorperazine at higher doses or for longer intervals may cause tardive dyskinesia that may become irreversible. • Drug can cause motor and sensory instability, which may lead to falls with the potential for fractures and other injuries. • Contraindicated in patients in comatose states or in the presence of large amounts of CNS depressants (e.g., alcohol, barbiturates, narcotics). • Avoid use, if possible, in patients with other forms of CNS depression. • May potentiate hypotension caused by hypovolemia, the presence of antihypertensive drugs, or a dehydrated state. • Should be used cautiously in patients with significant cardiac disease or pulmonary disease. Phenothiazines may induce angina, tachycardia, and/or orthostatic hypotension. Sudden, unexpected deaths have been reported in some patients, appearing to result from asphyxia or cardiac arrest. QT prolongation may occur. • Hypotension, syncope, cardiac arrhythmias, and respiratory arrest may be associated with aggressive dose titration. • This is hepatically metabolized. Hepatic disease could compromise prochlorperazine's metabolism, leading to excessive concentrations.

(continued)

Appendix 6.1 Gastrointestinal Medications *(continued)*

Indications	Mechanism of Action	Contraindications, Precautions, and Adverse Effects

Antiemetic, other, antipsychotic, phenothiazine (prochlorperazine maleate) (continued)

- Drug can lower the seizure threshold and should be used with caution in patients with a seizure disorder.
- Because of mild anticholinergic activity, patients with glaucoma, urinary retention, and benign prostatic hypertrophy can experience exacerbation of symptoms.
- Use with caution in patients with GI obstruction or ileus as it can mask their symptoms such as vomiting.
- Drug has been reported to disrupt the body's ability to reduce core body temperature, presumably through effects in the hypothalamus, and they predispose patients to hyperthermia. Patients receiving prochlorperazine should be advised of conditions that contribute to an elevation in core body temperature (e.g., strenuous exercise, ambient temperature increase, dehydration).
- Drug may cause hyperprolactinemia; the elevation in prolactin persists during chronic administration. Elevated prolactin levels may induce infertility or cause other endocrine abnormalities such as sexual dysfunction, gynecomastia, or menstrual irregularities.
- Patient should use drug during pregnancy only if the potential benefit justifies the potential risk to the fetus.
- Monitor for oversedation.
- Monitor IV side for extravasation and tissue necrosis.

(continued)

Appendix 6.1 Gastrointestinal Medications *(continued)*

Indications	Mechanism of Action	Contraindications, Precautions, and Adverse Effects

Antiemetic, antihistamine, anticholinergic, phenothiazine (promethazine)

- Prevention of motion sickness
- Treatment of nausea and vomiting, including postoperative and postoperative prophylaxis
- Treatment of allergic reactions to blood or plasma
- For preoperative and postoperative sedation as an adjunct to analgesics

- Antagonist of H1-receptors (although classified as a phenothiazine)
- Does not prevent the release of histamine, but competes with free histamine for binding at H1-receptor sites
- Histamine receptors in the GI tract, uterus, large blood vessels, and bronchial muscle are blocked.
- The relief of motion sickness and nausea and vomiting appear to be related to central anticholinergic actions and may implicate activity on the medullary chemoreceptor trigger zone.
- Other CNS receptor sites can also be affected, since promethazine is believed to indirectly reduce stimuli to the brain stem reticular system.
- Sedation is significant at concentrations achieved from therapeutic dosages.
- Mild antitussive activity has been attributed to promethazine, but this effect probably results from anticholinergic and sedative actions.

- Drug is contraindicated in patients who have experienced agranulocytosis, blood dyscrasias, bone marrow suppression, or jaundice due to phenothiazine therapy.
- Promethazine is also contraindicated in patients who are in a coma.
- The use of promethazine via intraarterial administration or subcutaneous administration is contraindicated due to risk of severe tissue necrosis, gangrene, or other tissue damage.
- Proper intravenous administration is well generally tolerated; however, due to the increased risk of severe tissue necrosis and injury, the preferred route of administration is deep intramuscular injection.
- Phenothiazine derivatives lower the seizure threshold through their effect on GABA; therefore, promethazine should be avoided, if possible, in patients with a seizure disorder or those receiving anticonvulsants. Extreme caution should be used when combining phenothiazine agents with other agents that can lower the seizure threshold, such as opioids or local anesthetics.
- It should be avoided in those who have experienced a worsening in respiratory status due to H1-antagonist therapy. The anticholinergic activity of H1-antagonists, such as promethazine, may result in thickened bronchial secretions in the respiratory tract, thereby aggravating acute asthmatic attack or COPD.

(continued)

Appendix 6.1 Gastrointestinal Medications *(continued)*

Indications	Mechanism of Action	Contraindications, Precautions, and Adverse Effects

Antiemetic, antihistamine, anticholinergic, phenothiazine (promethazine) (continued)

- The metabolism of promethazine may be reduced in the presence of hepatic disease, hepatic encephalopathy, or liver impairment. Those with significant hepatic disease receiving H1-antagonists should be monitored for liver function and side effects; dosage adjustments may be required in some patients.
- Contraindicated for use in children younger than 2 years due to the risk for fatal respiratory depression. Seizures and/or paradoxical CNS stimulation may also occur in this age group.
- No adequate studies in pregnant people are available; promethazine should be considered during pregnancy only when the benefits of therapy outweigh the risks to the fetus.
- Should be avoided, if possible, in patients with open-angle or closed-angle glaucoma; an H1-antagonist with fewer anticholinergic effects should be substituted. An increase in IOP may occur from the anticholinergic actions of the drug, precipitating an acute attack of glaucoma.
- Drug has substantial anticholinergic effects, and a worsening of symptoms may be seen in patients with bladder obstruction, GI obstruction or ileus, benign prostatic hypertrophy, or urinary retention.
- Use with caution in patients with conditions that may increase the risk of QT prolongation, including congenital long QT syndrome, bradycardia, AV block, HF, stress-related cardiomyopathy, MI, stroke, hypomagnesemia, hypokalemia, and hypocalcemia.

(continued)

Appendix 6.1 Gastrointestinal Medications *(continued)*

Indications	Mechanism of Action	Contraindications, Precautions, and Adverse Effects
Antiemetic, prokinetic agent (metoclopramide)		
• Treatment of nausea and vomiting	• Inhibits dopamine receptors in the chemoreceptor trigger zone and decreases the sensitivity of the visceral afferent nerves that transmit from the GI system to the vomiting center in the chemoreceptor trigger zone	• Medication is contraindicated in patients with paraben and procainamide hypersensitivity. • Use caution in GI bleed, obstruction or perforation, Parkinson's disease, seizures or tardive dyskinesia, cardiac disease, HF, hypertension hepatic disease, renal failure, breast cancer, and malignant hyperthermia. • Adverse effects include seizure, suicidal ideation, tardive dyskinesia, arrhythmia, hepatotoxicity, angioedema, serotonin syndrome, depression, confusion, and hepatic and renal disease.
Antivirals: NS5A protein inhibitor antiviral in combination with NS5B polymerase inhibitor antivirals for hepatitis C		
• Hepatitis C	• Inhibit HCV protein replication	• Contraindications include pregnancy and breastfeeding. • Adverse effects include angioedema, hepatic failure, hepatitis B exacerbation, dyspnea, depression and SI, hyperbilirubinemia.
Appetite stimulants (megestrol acetate)		
• Treatment of anorexia, cancer, or malnutrition	• Induce endometrial secretory changes, increase body temperature, and inhibit pituitary function	• Medication is contraindicated in pregnancy. • Use caution in hepatic or renal disease, thromboembolic disease, breast cancer, or dysfunctional uterine bleeding. • Adverse effects include diarrhea, flatulence, dyspepsia, hypersalivation, diaphoresis, dizziness, and malaise.

(continued)

Appendix 6.1 Gastrointestinal Medications *(continued)*

Indications	Mechanism of Action	Contraindications, Precautions, and Adverse Effects
Gallstone dissolution agents, bile acid agent (ursodiol)		
• Treatment of cholelithiasis via the dissolution of radiolucent cholesterol gallstones. • For gallstone dissolution via use of ursodiol alone • Treatment of primary biliary cirrhosis • For gallstone prophylaxis during rapid weight loss • Treatment of NASH • Treatment of cholestasis	• Decrease the cholesterol content of bile and associated gallstones by reducing the hepatic synthesis and secretion of cholesterol and fractional reabsorption of cholesterol by the intestine • Improve hepatic flow, decrease bile viscosity, reduce portal inflammation • Interfere with the intrahepatic circulation of bile acids by inhibiting reupdate of endogenous bile acids in the terminal ileum	• Contraindicated in patients with biliary obstruction, biliary tract disease, biliary-GI fistula, bleeding, cholangitis, encephalopathy, esophageal varices, jaundice, pancreatitis. • Monitor LFTs and bilirubin. • Use caution in pregnant and breastfeeding patients.
Hepatic encephalopathy, antibiotic (rifampin)		
• Treatment of hepatic encephalopathy	• A broad-spectrum antibiotic with activity against both gram-positive and gram-negative bacteria, especially anaerobic enteric bacteria. It binds to the beta-subunit of DNA-dependent RNA polymerase, inhibiting RNA synthesis, thus lowering ammonia levels.	• Drug may cause bacteria resistance or *C. diff* infection • Drug may cause low plasma levels and altered metabolism of other drugs
H2 receptor antagonists (e.g., famotidine)		
• Esophagitis • Gastric ulcer prophylaxis • GERD	• Inhibit binding of histamine to H2 receptors on gastric cells decreasing gastric acid secretions	• Use caution in gastric cancer, GI bleed, infection, hepatic disease, QT prolongation, renal impairment, PKU, vitamin B12 deficiency, and smoking. • Adverse effects include seizures, angioedema, arrhythmia, agranulocytosis, pancytopenia, rhabdomyolysis, constipation, liver impairment, renal impairment, delirium, confusion, and hallucinations.

(continued)

Indications	Mechanism of Action	Contraindications, Precautions, and Adverse Effects
Laxatives, stimulants (senna glycoside, bisacodyl)		
• Treatment of constipation	• Directly stimulate peristaltic movement of the intestine via local mucosal irritation, thus increasing motility and reducing colonic water absorption • Can alter permeability of cell walls in the colon because it increases cyclic 3',5'-adenosine monophosphate, which also regulates active ion secretion. The result is increased fluid accumulation in the colon and a laxative action. • More recent studies suggest that bisacodyl promotes evacuation of the colon by altering intestinal fluid and electrolyte absorption.	• Avoid with GI obstruction, rectal bleeding, GI disease, inflammatory bowel disease, and signs of appendicitis. • Drug is contraindicated for use of more than a week. • Avoid stimulant laxatives when possible during pregnancy because some may induce premature labor. • Drugs may cause flatulence, bloating, and abdominal pain in debilitated or older patients.
Laxatives, osmotic (e.g., polyethylene glycol, magnesium citrate, magnesium hydroxide)		
• Treatment of constipation • Hepatic encephalopathy	• Increase osmotic pressure, which causes fluid accumulation that breaks down stool • Ionize ammonia in the colon to the ammonium ion, preventing ammonia diffusion into the bloodstream to lower serum ammonia levels by 25%–50%	• Use caution in renal disease. • Use caution in patients with abdominal pain, GI bleeding, GI obstruction, GI perforation, ileus, toxic megacolon, and vomiting. • Monitor for hypernatremia, hypokalemia, and metabolic acidosis.
Laxatives, softener (docusate sodium)		
• Treatment of constipation	• An anionic surfactant • Decreases surface tension to allow water and lipids to penetrate the stool, hydrating it and allowing it to be passed.	• Use caution in patients with abdominal pain of unknown origin, GI bleeding, GI obstruction, GI perforation, ileus, toxic megacolon, and vomiting. • Concurrent use of docusate sodium with mineral oil to relieve constipation is not recommended because docusate sodium can increase the systemic absorption of mineral oil. Inflammation of the intestinal mucosa, liver, spleen, and lymph nodes may occur due to a foreign body reaction. • Adverse reactions include diarrhea.

(continued)

Appendix 6.1 Gastrointestinal Medications *(continued)*

Indications	Mechanism of Action	Contraindications, Precautions, and Adverse Effects
Mucolytics, systemic antidotes (acetylcysteine)		
• Antidote for acetaminophen	• Bind to oxygen free radicals to excrete them out of the body without causing cellular and organ damage	• Use cautiously in patients with history of asthma or bronchospasm. • Use cautiously in patients with esophageal ulcers, as it may induce vomiting and potentiates risk for GI bleed. • Adverse effects include flushing, rash, itching, nausea, and vomiting.
Opioid pain medication (meperidine)		
• Treatment of severe pain for which alternative treatments are inadequate • For treatment of shaking chills induced by intravenous infusions of amphotericin B or for postoperative shivering.	• Stimulant effect by inhibition of dopamine transporter (DAT) and norepinephrine transporter (NET) • Binds with mu kappa opioid receptors	• Contraindicated in patients with known or suspected GI obstruction, including paralytic ileus. Due to the effects of opioid agonists on the GI tract, meperidine should be used cautiously in patients with GI disease, such as UC. Patients with UC or other inflammatory bowel disease may be more sensitive to constipation caused by opioid agonists. Opioid agonists may obscure the diagnosis or clinical course in patients with acute abdomen. • Monitor patients with biliary tract disease, including acute pancreatitis, for worsening symptoms. Drug may cause spasm of sphincter of Oddi, and patients may have increased serum amylase concentrations. • Drug is contraindicated in patients with asthma or significant respiratory depression. • Monitor patients closely for respiratory depression, profound sedation, coma, and death. • Drug is contraindicated in patients who are receiving MAOIs or in those who have received MAOI therapy within the past 14 days. Therapeutic doses of meperidine have occasionally precipitated unpredictable, severe, and fatal reactions in patients who received MAOIs. • There is abuse potential with this medication; use caution with patients who have a substance use history.

(continued)

Appendix 6.1 Gastrointestinal Medications *(continued)*

Indications	Mechanism of Action	Contraindications, Precautions, and Adverse Effects
Opioid pain medication (meperidine) (continued)		
		• Use with caution in patients with CNS depression, toxic psychosis, head trauma, and intracranial mass/pressure. • Drug may increase the frequency of seizures in patients with a seizure history. • Use caution in patients with renal impairment and hepatic disease. • Drug may cause bradycardia or vasovagal syncope; use caution in patients with cardiac history. • Abrupt discontinuation of this medication may lead to withdrawal symptoms. • Use caution in patients with adrenal insufficiency, hypothyroidism, or myxedema. • Drug is contraindicated in pregnant and breastfeeding people.
Pancreatic enzymes (pancrelipase)		
• Management of exocrine pancreatic insufficiency	• Release lipase, amylase, and protease in high levels to assist with the hydrolysis of fats and breakdown of starches into sugars and proteins into peptides	• Use caution in patients with porcine protein hypersensitivity, gout, renal impairment, and hyperuricemia. • Adverse effects include abdominal pain, elevated hepatic enzymes, hyperuricemia, and nausea and vomiting.
Proton pump inhibitors (e.g., pantoprazole, omeprazole)		
• GERD • Empirically used for upper GI bleeds • Gastric and duodenal ulcers • Peptic ulcer prophylaxis • Eradication of *H. pylori* in combination with antibiotics	• Suppress gastric acid secretion by inhibiting hydrogen-potassium gastric ATPase enzyme pump on the parietal cells	• Contraindications include interstitial nephritis. • Use caution in hepatic disease, gastric cancer, colitis, diarrhea, vitamin B12 and zinc deficiency, bone fractures, osteopenia/osteoporosis, hypomagnesemia, prolonged QT interval, and lupus. • Adverse reactions include GI bleeding, seizures, MI, arrhythmias, elevated hepatic enzymes, interstitial nephritis, anemias, headache, nausea, and abdominal pain.

(continued)

Appendix 6.1 Gastrointestinal Medications *(continued)*

Indications	Mechanism of Action	Contraindications, Precautions, and Adverse Effects

Somatostatin and analogs (e.g., octreotide)

• Dumping syndrome • Enterocutaneous fistula • Upper GI hemorrhage • Variceal hemorrhage	• Binds to somatostatin receptors • Leads to smooth muscle contraction in blood vessels • Decreases GI blood flow and variceal pressure • Increases splanchnic arteriolar resistance • Inhibits secretion of hormones involved in vasodilation	• Monitor for QT interval prolongation • Use caution in patients with biliary disease as cholelithiasis may occur. • Use caution in pancreatitis, hepatic or renal disease, diabetes mellitus, biliary obstruction, goiter, hypothyroidism, vitamin deficiency, alcoholism, and cardiac arrhythmia and disease. • Adverse effects include bradycardia and arrhythmia, GI bleeding or obstruction, hyperglycemia, constipation, goiter, edema, jaundice, ascites, nausea, abdominal pain, and rash.

Peptic ulcer and GERD agents, other (sucralfate or bismuth subsalicylate)

• Treatment of duodenal ulcer not related to NSAID use • Treatment of gastric ulcer not related to NSAID use • For NSAID-induced ulcer prophylaxis • Stress-induced gastritis prophylaxis • Treatment of aphthous ulcer or palliative treatment of stomatitis • Alternative treatment of proctitis due to UC	• Cover the ulcer and create a protective layer to prevent further damage	• Use cautiously in patients with DM as it may cause hyperglycemia. • Use caution in patients with dysphagia or gag reflex depression as this drug may cause respiratory complications. • Use caution in patients receiving dialysis, with renal failure/ impairment, because it contains small amounts of aluminum that are cleared by the kidneys • Use caution in pregnant and breastfeeding patients.

RESOURCES

Columbia Surgery. (2013). *What you need to know about pancreatic enzymes.* https://columbiasurgery.org/news/2013/12/20/what-you-need-know-about-pancreatic-enzymes#:~:text=There%20are%20six%20FDA%20approved,Ultresa%2C%20Viokace%2C%20and%20Pertzye.

Harding, M., Kwong, J., Roberts, D., Hagler, D., & Reinisch, C. (2020). *Lewis medical-surgical nursing* (11th ed.). Elsevier.

John Hopkins Medicine. (n.d.). *Acute pancreatitis.* https://www.hopkinsmedicine.org/gastroenterology_hepatology/_pdfs/pancreas_biliary_tract/acute_pancreatitis.pdf

Longe, J. L (Ed.). (2018). *The Gale encyclopedia of nursing and allied health* (4th ed.). Gale. https://link.gale.com/apps/pub/07UZ/GVRL?u=kcls_main&sid=GVRL

Mayo Clinic. (n.d.). *Intestinal obstructions.* causes/syc-20351460#:~:text=Intestinal%20obstruction%20can%20cut%20off,Infection

Medscape. (n.d.). *Esophageal cancer treatment and management.* https://emedicine.medscape.com/article/277930-treatment#d11

Prescriber's Digital Reference. (n.d.[a]). *Amitriptyline-Hydrochloride.* https://www.pdr.net/drug-summary/ Amitriptyline-Hydrochloride-amitriptyline-hydrochloride-1001#11
Prescriber's Digital Reference. (n.d.[b]). *Actigall.* https://www.pdr.net/drug-summary/Actigall-ursodiol-1231
Prescriber's Digital Reference. (n.d.[c]). *Carafate.* https://www.pdr.net/drug-summary/Carafate-Suspension-sucralfate-2243#10
Prescriber's Digital Reference. (n.d.[d]). *Ledipasvir/Sofosbuvir.* https://www.pdr.net/drug-summary/ Harvoni-ledipasvir-sofosbuvir-3630#11
Prescriber's Digital Reference. (n.d.[e]). *Loperamide hydrochloride.* Retrieved from https://www.pdr.net/ drug-summary/Loperamide-Hydrochloride-Capsules-loperamide-hydrochloride-2664#15
Prescriber's Digital Reference. (n.d.[f]). *Pantoprazole sodium.* Retrieved from https://www.pdr.net/drug-summary/ Protonix-I-V--pa ntoprazole-sodium-2096.5821
Prescriber's Digital Reference. (n.d.[g]). *Promethazine.* https://www.pdr.net/drug-summary/ Promethazine-Hydrochloride-Injection-promethazine-hydrochloride-3471.1583#11
Prescriber's Digital Reference. (n.d.[h]). *Ondansetron.* https://www.pdr.net/drug-summary/ Ondansetron-ondansetron-hydrochloride-3428.2904
Prescriber's Digital Reference. (n.d.[i]). *Meperidine.* https://www.pdr.net/drug-summary/Meperidine-Hydrochlorid e-Oral-Solution-and-Tablets-meperidine-hydrochloride-1164#15
Prescriber's Digital Reference. (n.d.[j]). *Metoclopramide.* https://www.pdr.net/drug-summary/Reglan-Tablet s-metoclopramide-956.5843#15
Prescriber's Digital Reference. (n.d.[k]). *Metronidazole.* https://www.pdr.net/drug-summary/Flagyl-Tablet s-metronidazole-2892
Prescriber's Digital Reference. (n.d.[l]). *Urso Forte.* https://www.pdr.net/drug-summary/Urso-250-Urso-Fort e-ursodiol-2807#14
Pub Med/NIH. *Complications of peptic ulcer disease.* https://pubmed.ncbi.nlm.nih.gov/22095016/
Pub Med/NCBI. *Lifestyle and peptic ulcer disease.* https://pubmed.ncbi.nlm.nih.gov/29745325/#:~:text=Pylori%20 infection%2C%20having%20a%20balanced,prevention%20and%20healing%20of%20PUD
Rare Diseases. *Gastroparesis.* https://rarediseases.org/rare-diseases/gastroparesis/
Up-to-Date: *Esophageal Cancer.* https://www.uptodate.com/contents/clinical-manifestation s-diagnosis-and-staging-of-esophageal-cancer?search=esophageal%20 cancer&source=search_result&selectedTitle=1~150&usage_type=default&display_rank=1
Up-To-Date. *Management of celiac disease in adults.* https://www.uptodate.com/ contents/management-of-celiac-disease-in-adults?search=celiac%20disease%20 treatment&source=search_result&selectedTitle=1~150&usage_type=default&display_rank=1#H7
Up-To-Date. *Clinical manifestations, diagnosis, and staging of esophageal cancer.* Retrieved from https://www.uptodate.com/contents/clinical-manifestation s-diagnosis-and-staging-of-esophageal-cancer?search=esophageal%20 cancer&source=search_result&selectedTitle=1~150&usage_type=default&display_rank=1
Up-To-Date. *Overview of the management of primary colon cancer.* https://www.uptodate.com/ contents/overview-of-the-management-of-primary-colon-cancer?search=colorectal%20 cancer&source=search_result&selectedTitle=1~150&usage_type=default&display_rank=1#H40

HEMATOLOGICAL SYSTEM

ANEMIA

Overview

- Anemia indicates a reduction in the number or volume of RBCs, or a reduction in circulating hemoglobin and hematocrit.
- Anemia reduces the amount of available oxygen in the blood, potentially leading to hypoxia.
- Three main factors lead to anemia (Table 7.1):
  - Blood loss
  - Decreased production of RBCs
  - Destruction of RBCs
- *Aplastic anemia* is a rare form of pancytopenia (decrease of all blood cell types):
  - Can be caused by drugs, infections, radiation, or toxins
  - Ranges from slow onset to rapid onset
- *Autoimmune hemolytic anemia* is a rare condition in which the immune system makes antibodies that attack RBCs:
  - Antibody reactions (leukemia, medications)
  - Infectious reactions (cytomegalovirus, hepatitis, HIV)
  - Physical destruction (hemodialysis)
- *G6PD deficiency* is a hereditary condition (X-linked recessive mutation) in which RBCs are hemolyzed due to the enzyme G6PD defect. Causes include:
  - Certain foods, such as fava beans
  - Infections
  - Stress

> **COMPLICATIONS**
>
> Severe untreated anemia can affect age groups differently. In younger populations, impaired neurologic development may occur. In pregnant patients, severe anemia can lead to early labor and premature birth. Complications of severe anemia, such as multiorgan failure or death, are most common in older adults due to preexisting comorbidities in this population.

(continued)

Table 7.1 Conditions That Cause Anemia

Blood Loss	Increased RBC Destruction	Reduced RBC Production
<ul><li>Acute</li><li>Chronic</li><li>May be related to:<ul><li>Coagulopathies</li><li>Frequent phlebotomy</li><li>Surgery</li><li>Trauma</li></ul></li></ul>	<ul><li>Damage by artificial valves</li><li>Immune destruction (e.g., hemolytic transfusion reaction)</li><li>Inherited disorders (e.g., G6PD, sickle cell anemia)</li><li>RBC membrane defects</li><li>Splenic destruction</li><li>Thalassemia</li></ul>	<ul><li>Aplastic anemia</li><li>Bone marrow malignancies</li><li>Chemotherapy or radiation</li><li>Chronic inflammatory conditions</li><li>CKD</li><li>Nutritional deficiencies:<ul><li>Vitamin B12</li><li>Folate</li><li>Iron</li></ul></li><li>Stem cell transplant</li></ul>

Overview *(continued)*

- Iron-deficiency anemia occurs when ferritin, hemoglobin, hematocrit, and serum iron blood levels are low. Causes include:
  - Blood loss
  - Malabsorption
  - Poor dietary intake
- *Sickle cell anemia* is a common inherited form of anemia. Hallmark findings include crescent- or sickle-shaped RBCs; this decreases oxygen-carrying capacity and can obstruct blood flow to other areas of the body.
  - Timely recognition and intervention are key to preventing severe complications.
- *Thalassemia* is a genetically inherited disorder (autosomal recessive trait) resulting in abnormal hemoglobin production and microcytic, hypochromic anemia.
  - Alpha thalassemia occurs when a gene or genes related to the alpha globin proteins are missing or mutated.
  - Beta thalassemia occurs when similar gene defects affect the production of the beta globin protein.
  - Both conditions include thalassemia major and minor.
- Vitamin B12 (cobalamin) and folic acid deficiencies cause megaloblastic anemia because cobalamin and folic acid are necessary for producing healthy RBCs. Causes include:
  - Alcohol misuse
  - Certain drugs (metformin, proton pump inhibitors)
  - Gastric issues
  - Impaired DNA synthesis
  - Pernicious anemia caused by absence of intrinsic factor required for absorption of vitamin B12 in the GI tract

Signs and Symptoms

- Mild anemia may be asymptomatic.
- Severe anemia symptoms may include any of the following:
  - Altered mental status
  - Bone marrow hyperplasia (thalassemia)
  - Brittle nails
  - Chest pain
  - Decreased exertional tolerance
  - Delayed growth
  - Dizziness
  - Dyspnea, especially on exertion
  - Fatigue, weakness, and lethargy
  - Hair loss
  - Headache
  - Hypotension
  - Jaundice

 NURSING PEARL

Sickle-shaped RBCs have a much shorter life span than disc-shaped RBCs. This shortened life span contributes to anemia, as blood cells are broken down faster than they are replaced.

 ALERT!

Patients with sickle cell anemia can suffer from severe pain due to vaso-occlusive crisis. Contributing factors to vaso-occlusive crisis include:

- Changes in body temperature
- Dehydration
- Hypoxia

In addition to acute pain episodes, patients with sickle cell disease may also develop chronic pain due to joint damage and chronic inflammation.

 ALERT!

Sickle cell crisis may be triggered by infection, hypoxia, acidosis, and dehydration, among other stressors. Sickle cell crises may present in any of three categories (Table 7.2). Identification of the appropriate phase of crisis can help guide treatment.

(continued)

Table 7.2 Manifestations of Sickle Cell Crisis

Hematologic aplastic crisis	• Exacerbation of anemia with significant drop in hemoglobin • Symptomatic anemia
Infectious crisis	• Elevated risk of secondary infections (e.g., pneumonia, bloodstream infections, meningitis, osteomyelitis) • Sickle cell occlusions in the spleen reducing immunologic function
Vaso-occlusive crisis	• Microvascular occlusions caused by sickled RBCs • Severe pain possible in abdomen, chest, bones, and joints • Tissue and organ ischemia

Signs and Symptoms *(continued)*

- Koilonychia (spooning nails)
- Pallor
- Petechiae
- Pica
- Splenomegaly or hepatomegaly
- Tachycardia

Diagnosis

Labs

- Vitamin B12 less than 180 ng/L
- Bilirubin greater than 1.2 mg/dL in hemolytic anemia
- Blood films/smears showing abnormally sized RBCs
- CBC
- Hematocrit less than 38% in men and less than 35% in women
- Hemoglobin less than 13 g/dL in men and less than 12 g/dL in women
- Coombs test: may be positive
- Folate less than 2.7 ng/mL
- Homocysteine level
- High performance liquid chromatography (sickle cell)
- Iron/ferritin less than 30 ng/mL
- Methylmalonic acid level (for vitamin B12 deficiency)
- Reticulocyte count: varies by type of anemia
- Serum iron: may vary by type of anemia
- Schilling test (pernicious anemia)
- Stool: guaiac test may be positive
- Total iron-binding capacity

Diagnostic Testing

- Chest x-ray
- CT scan
- Pelvic ultrasound
- Upper GI endoscopy (if suspected GI hemorrhage)

Treatment

- Treatment is dependent on etiology.
- Aplastic anemia may require bone marrow transplant.
- Vitamin B12, iron, or folate deficiency may require PO or IV replacement of these nutrients (Appendix 7.1, located at the end of this chapter) and blood transfusion.

(continued)

Treatment *(continued)*

- Chronic anemia treatment is based on the following:
  - Renal failure: erythropoietin (see Appendix 7.1)
  - Autoimmune or rheumatologic condition: management of causative disease
- Treatment of RBC destruction (hemolytic anemia) includes the following:
  - Sickle cell: blood transfusions, exchange transfusions, antibiotics, opioids, hydroxyurea (see Appendix 7.1), IV hydration, oxygen therapy, stem cell/bone marrow transplants
  - Medication mediated: discontinuation of medication immediately (if possible)
  - DIC: antifibrinolytic agents (see Appendix 7.1)
  - Faulty mechanical values: valve replacement treatment
  - If persistent despite treatment: splenectomy
- Treatment of thalassemia includes the following:
  - Bone marrow transplant to help treat the disease in certain patients, especially children
  - Chelation therapy to remove excess iron from the body
  - Mild to moderate cases: no treatment
  - RBC transfusions or splenectomy in severe cases

Nursing Interventions

- Assess ABC.
- Assess for signs of hemorrhage and occult bleeding.
- Assess for signs of infection.
- Assess for signs of respiratory distress or hypoperfusion.
- Assess for worsening signs of fatigue, weakness, and lethargy.
- Draw and monitor serial CBCs to assess RBC, hemoglobin, and hematocrit.
- Elevate extremities to prevent swelling.
- Initiate fall precautions if patient is experiencing weakness.
- Monitor electrolyte and blood levels following transfusion of blood products.
- Monitor perfusion and oxygenation.
- Position patient with HOB at 30 degrees or higher to improve oxygenation and perfusion.
- Prepare patient for administration of blood transfusion for severe anemia.
- Promote appropriate diet choices for deficiency anemias.
- Provide therapeutic communication and support: discuss condition specific to anemia diagnosis and assess for willingness to accept blood transfusions.

Patient Education

- After discharge, avoid extreme temperatures and changes in altitude that could cause a vaso-occlusive crisis in sickle cell anemia.
- Avoid offending drug or drug class if hemolytic anemia is a result of medication therapy.
- Avoid smoking due to nicotine's ability to attach to hemoglobin and cause decreased oxygen delivery.
- Follow up regularly with hematologist (in sickle cell anemia, PKU, and G6PD deficiency) for monitoring.
- Seek genetic counseling in thalassemia, if desired.
- If a splenectomy was performed, follow infection prevention techniques:
  - Hand washing
  - Staying up to date on vaccinations
  - Taking prophylactic antibiotics as prescribed
- Increase iron-rich foods in the diet for iron-deficiency anemia:
  - Dark green, leafy vegetables
  - Dried fruit
  - Iron-fortified cereals, breads, and pastas
  - Legumes

(continued)

Patient Education *(continued)*

- ● Red meat, pork, or poultry
- ● Seafood
- Incorporate vitamin C–containing foods to enhance iron absorption for iron-deficiency anemia:
  - ● Broccoli
  - ● Grapefruit
  - ● Kiwi
  - ● Green, leafy vegetables
  - ● Melons and oranges
- With thalassemia, avoid excessive iron in the diet.
- Recognize that black, tarry stools and constipation may occur with iron replacement therapy.
- Recognize that fortified foods are necessary to treat vitamin B12 deficiency.
- Self-monitor for symptoms of worsening anemia.
- Take medications and iron or vitamin supplements as indicated by the provider.

POP QUIZ 7.1

A patient has a new diagnosis of iron-deficiency anemia and asks the nurse what foods to eat to help manage the condition. How does the nurse reply?

DISSEMINATED INTRAVASCULAR COAGULATION

Overview

- DIC is a rare and life-threatening abnormal activity of the coagulation cascade that causes extensive inappropriate clotting; then, as the clotting factors are exhausted, uncontrolled bleeding occurs.
- DIC can occur as the result of many conditions, including:
  - ● Blood transfusion reactions
  - ● Cancer such as leukemia or metastatic carcinoma
  - ● Cardiac arrest
  - ● Cirrhosis
  - ● Fat embolism
  - ● Heat stroke
  - ● Infections such as gram-negative or gram-positive septicemia; viral, fungal, or rickettsial infections; or protozoal infections (falciparum malaria).
  - ● Intraoperative cardiopulmonary bypass
  - ● Large hemangioma
  - ● Obstetric complications such as abruptio placentae, amniotic fluid embolism, or retention of a dead fetus
  - ● Purpura fulminans (a severe, rapidly fatal form of nonthrombocytopenic purpura)
  - ● Severe venous thrombus
  - ● Tissue necrosis from extensive burns or trauma, brain tissue destruction, transplant rejection, or hepatic necrosis

COMPLICATIONS

Complications of DIC are MI, PE, multiorgan failure, and death. The mortality rate is higher than 80%.

Signs and Symptoms

- Abnormal bleeding such as:
  - ● Bleeding from IV sites
  - ● Bruising without injury
  - ● Cutaneous oozing

(continued)

Signs and Symptoms (continued)

- GI bleeding
- Hematoma
- Hematuria
- Melena
- Petechiae
- Other symptoms that may be present:
  - Dyspnea
  - Nausea and vomiting
  - Oliguria
  - Severe muscle, back, and abdominal pain

Diagnosis

Labs

- CBC
  - Platelet count: rapidly decreases in DIC, usually to <100,000
  - Hgb: will be decreased
- CMP
  - BUN > 25 mg/dL
  - Serum creatinine > 1.3 mg/dL
- Coagulation panel
  - PT > 15 seconds
  - PTT > 60 seconds
- D-dimer
- Fibrin degradation products > 100 mcg/mL
- Fibrinogen levels < 150 mg/dL
- Type and screen
- Urine output < 30 mL/hr

Diagnostic Testing

- There are no tests specific to diagnosing DIC, but the following may be used to find the underlying cause and determine treatment:
  - Chest x-ray
  - CT scan
  - Ultrasound

Treatment

- Electrolyte replacement
- Exogenous clotting factors
- Heparin to prevent further clotting
- IV hydration
- Specialist consultation (e.g., OB/GYN, oncology, surgery) as required
- Supplemental oxygen
- Supportive care until underlying cause identified and treated
- TXA (see Appendix 7.1)
- Transfer to higher level of care if mechanical ventilation, sedation, and vasopressors needed
- Transfusion of blood, FFP, platelets, or packed RBCs to support hemostasis
- Treatment of underlying cause

Nursing Interventions

- Administer IV hydration as ordered.
- Administer blood products as ordered and monitor of signs and symptoms of transfusion reaction.

(continued)

Nursing Interventions *(continued)*

- Administer medications as ordered.
- Administer supplemental oxygen to maintain $SpO_2 > 94\%$.
- Apply pressure to sites of bleeding.
- Draw labs such as coagulopathies, CBC, fibrinogen, and electrolytes, and notify provider for critical results.
- Encourage bedrest to decrease chance of bleeding.
- Establish at least two large-bore peripheral IVs.
- Expedite transfer to critical care unit if indicated.
- Monitor intake and output.
- Monitor for signs of ischemia.
- Monitor for signs and symptoms of bleeding, including bleeding from IV sites, oral bleeding, hematuria, and rectal bleeding.
- Monitor vital signs closely.
- Perform head-to-toe assessment and immediately address any uncontrolled bleeding.
- Place patient on continuous cardiac monitoring with continuous pulse oximetry.
- Avoid scrubbing bleeding areas to prevent clots from dislodging.

Patient Education

- Follow up with appropriate specialists (e.g., hematology/oncology), if needed.
- Monitor for signs and symptoms of bleeding.
  - Be aware of increased risk for bleeding with certain medical conditions, such as liver disease and certain hematologic disorders/cancers.
  - Watch for signs and symptoms of occult bleeding:
    - Dark, tarry stools
    - Coffee-ground emesis
- Seek emergency medical care for difficulty breathing or chest pain.
- Seek emergency medical care if prolonged and uncontrolled bleeding occurs.
- Take medications as prescribed.
- Take precautions to avoid falls and injuries

POP QUIZ 7.2

A patient with end-stage liver failure has been admitted for peritonitis. The patient calls the nurse into the room and reports chest pain and difficulty breathing. The nurse checks the patient's vital signs; the heart rate is 134 and the SpO_2 is 88%. The patient is at risk for DIC due to liver failure. What acute event may this patient be experiencing?

HEMOPHILIA

Overview

- *Hemophilia* is a hereditary clotting disorder carried on the X chromosome that results from a lack of specific clotting factors.
- There are two types of hemophilia:
  - *Hemophilia A*, also called classic hemophilia, is caused by an insufficient amount of clotting factor VIII (seen in 80% of hemophilia cases).
  - *Hemophilia B*, also referred to as Christmas disease, is caused by an insufficient amount of clotting factor IX (seen in roughly 15% of hemophilia cases).
- Patients may experience unexplained bleeding, which varies based on whether the hemophilia is mild, moderate, or severe.
  - Mild hemophilia:
    - Bleeding does not occur spontaneously or after minor trauma.
    - Major trauma or surgery typically causes prolonged bleeding.

(continued)

Overview *(continued)*

- Moderate hemophilia:
  - ○ Spontaneous occasional bleeding occurs.
  - ○ Major trauma or surgery causes excessive bleeding.
- Severe hemophilia:
  - ○ Bleeding occurs spontaneously.
  - ○ Bleeding may be severe even with minor trauma, leading to subcutaneous and deep intramuscular hematomas.

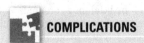

COMPLICATIONS

Complications of hemophilia include GI bleeding, persistent bleeding from minor trauma, uncontrolled bleeding after dental extractions, and splenic rupture with impact injury.

Signs and Symptoms

- Bleeding gums
- Excessive bleeding after injections, such as vaccinations
- Frequent or hard-to-control epistaxis
- Hemarthrosis, most commonly affecting the knees, elbows, and ankles
- Hematochezia
- Hematuria

Diagnosis

Labs

- Antigens for von Willebrand's disease: may be drawn if the patient has no known family history of hemophilia to rule out other causes of bleeding
- CBC: normal PLT level
- Coagulation panel:
  - Normal PT
  - Prolonged PTT
- Factor assays to identify factor VIII or factor IX (factor deficiency determines the severity of the illness):
  - Mild hemophilia: factor levels 5% to 40% of normal
  - Moderate hemophilia: factor levels 1% to 5% of normal
  - Severe hemophilia: factor levels <1% of normal
- Fibrin levels

Diagnostic Testing

There are no tests specific to diagnosing hemophilia.

Treatment

- Aminocaproic acid to inhibit fibrinolysis (often used for oral bleeding)
- Cryoprecipitate AHF to raise clotting factor levels above 25%
- Desmopressin to increase factor VIII
- FFP administration
- Hemostatics
- Recombinant factor VIIa (see Appendix 7.1)

Nursing Interventions

- Administer clotting factors as ordered.
- Administer medications as ordered.
- Administer blood products as ordered and monitor for signs and symptoms of transfusion reaction
- Administer supplemental oxygen to maintain SpO_2 > 94%
- Assess for signs and symptoms of bleeding.
- Assess function of musculoskeletal joints.

(continued)

Nursing Interventions *(continued)*

- Control any active bleeding.
- Encourage rest after episodes of bleeding.
- Establish IV access.
- If bleeding into joint occurs, immediately elevate affected joint.
- Manage pain with analgesics.
- Monitor vital signs frequently.
- Perform head-to-toe assessment with focused cardiovascular and musculoskeletal evaluation. Alert provider to any signs and symptoms of active bleeding or bruises.
- Prevent injury and trauma.

Patient Education

- Apply firm, direct pressure to any bleeding.
- Do not take aspirin-containing medications because they decrease platelet adherence and may worsen bleeding.
- Exercise to help protect your joints.
- Follow up with a provider at a hemophilia treatment center.
- Get tested regularly for bloodborne infections.
- Receive vaccinations to eliminate the likelihood of infection with preventable illnesses.
- Report any prolonged/uncontrolled bleeding, tarry stools, or coffee-ground emesis to provider.

LEUKEMIA

Overview

- *Leukemia* is cancer of the body's blood-forming tissues, including the bone marrow and the lymphatic system.
- Leukemia is classified as either acute or chronic.
  - *Acute leukemia* is uncontrolled proliferation of immature WBCs; it must be treated quickly and aggressively.
  - Chronic leukemia occurs when too many or too few cells are produced. This process is much slower, and treatment is not as aggressive.
- Leukemia is secondarily classified by the cell type from which it arises.
  - Lymphocytic leukemia arises from lymphatic tissue.
  - Myelogenous leukemia arises from myeloid cells, the precursor to blood cells.
- The most common types of leukemia include the following:
  - *Acute lymphocytic leukemia* is the most common type of leukemia in young children. It can also affect adults. The hallmark of the disease is pancytopenia with circulating blasts.
  - *Acute myelogenous leukemia* is the most common type of acute leukemia in adults.
  - *Chronic lymphocytic leukemia* is the most common chronic adult leukemia. Many patients feel well for years before needing treatment. The hallmark of the disease is lymphocytosis.
  - Chronic myelogenous leukemia mainly affects adults. The patient may have no symptoms for months or years before the cells begin to proliferate quickly. The Philadelphia chromosome is seen in leukemic cells.
- Less common forms of leukemia include hairy cell leukemia, myelodysplastic syndromes, and myeloproliferative disorders.

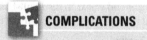

COMPLICATIONS

Complications of leukemia include anemia, bleeding, and increased risk of infections.

Signs and Symptoms

- Anorexia
- Bone pain or tenderness

(continued)

Signs and Symptoms *(continued)*

- Chills
- Diaphoresis
- Easy bleeding or bruising
- Fatigue
- Fever
- Frequent or severe infections
- Generalized lymphadenopathy
- Hepatomegaly
- Pallor
- Petechiae
- Recurrent epistaxis
- Splenomegaly
- Swollen lymph nodes
- Weight loss
- Weakness

Diagnosis

Labs

- CBC
  - Hemoglobin decreased (anemia)
  - Neutrophils decreased (neutropenia)
  - Platelets decreased (thrombocytopenia)
  - WBC abnormal: will indicate acute versus chronic disease
- Elevated ESR
- Peripheral blood smear to distinguish acute and chronic leukemia
- Uric acid measurement to detect hyperuricemia

Diagnostic Testing

- Bone marrow biopsy
- Lumbar puncture to detect meningeal involvement

Treatment

- Antibiotics if infection occurs
- Blood transfusions to prevent anemia
- Bone marrow transplant if appropriate
- Chemotherapy
- Expert consultation to oncology/hematology for ongoing care
- Fluid resuscitation if indicated and ordered by provider
- Initiation of allopurinol to reduce tumor lysis syndrome in high-risk patients
- Stem cell transplant
- Symptom relief
- Antibiotics, antifungals, and antivirals to control infection as needed

Nursing Interventions

- Administer blood products as ordered.
- Administer medications as ordered.
- Assess closely for potential infection.

 NURSING PEARL

Neutropenic precautions are put in place to protect severely immunocompromised patients from infection and include:

- All visitors and healthcare staff must don gowns, gloves, and masks before taking care of the patient.
- Visitors or staff who exhibit signs of illness are not permitted to enter the patient's room.
- No foods such as sushi, rare meats, or soft cheeses are allowed in the room. All fruits and vegetables should be thoroughly washed before the patient eats them.
- No live plants or flowers are allowed in the room.
- Single-use equipment should be used with the patient and should not be shared with other patients (e.g., stethoscopes, thermometers).
- Patient's door must remain closed.
- Patient should be placed in a private room, preferably one with HEPA filtration.

(continued)

Nursing Interventions *(continued)*

- Avoid indwelling catheters and intramuscular injections to prevent infection.
- Encourage PO intake.
- Evaluate need for treatment education relating to procedures or chemotherapy.
  - Refer the patient to resources such as the Leukemia Society of America.
- Follow neutropenic precautions.
- For patients with terminal disease, provide supportive care directed at promoting comfort.
  - Discuss resources such as hospice, palliative care, and home care.
- Monitor labs.
- Monitor temperature for fever
- Take precautions to limit bleeding.

ALERT!

Neutropenic precautions guidelines may vary slightly across healthcare facilities. Be sure to refer to institutional guidelines.

Patient Education

- Avoid contact with people with infectious illnesses.
- Avoid spicy and hot foods if experiencing mouth pain as a side effect from treatments.
- Follow neutropenic precautions.
- Maintain oral hygiene and use a soft-bristle toothbrush to avoid gum irritation and potential bleeding.
- Monitor for signs and symptoms of bleeding and know when to report abnormal bleeding.
- Stay up to date with vaccines, as advised by the provider.
- Take medications as prescribed.
- Understand how to stop bleeding, such as by applying pressure or ice.
- Be aware of the signs and symptoms of infection.

POP QUIZ 7.3

Upon assessment of a patient with leukemia, how would the nurse expect the patient to present clinically?

LYMPHOMA

Overview

- Lymphoma describes a group of malignant neoplasms arising from abnormal lymphocytes.
- The two main types of lymphoma are:
  - Hodgkin's lymphoma is characterized by enlarged painless lymph nodes.
    - 75% of all newly diagnosed patients can be cured.
    - It can be categorized as A (those without B symptoms) or B (defined general symptoms).
    - The cause is unknown.
    - It usually presents with cervical adenopathy and spreads in predictable fashion along lymph node groups.
    - Characteristic Reed-Sternberg cells differentiate Hodgkin's lymphoma from non-Hodgkin's lymphoma.
  - Non-Hodgkin's lymphoma is often disseminated at diagnosis and has a much poorer prognosis.
    - The cause is unknown but may have viral etiology.
    - The pattern is less predictable than in Hodgkin's lymphoma.
    - It is more likely to disseminate to extranodal sites.
    - It often presents with lymphadenopathy.
    - The overall survival rate at 5 years is >60%.
    - Median survival rate is 20 years.

COMPLICATIONS

Complications of lymphoma include infections due to a weakened immune system and secondary cancers, including leukemia and solid tumors

Signs and Symptoms

- Hodgkin's lymphoma symptoms (mostly in lymphoma categorized as B):
  - Drenching and reoccurring nights sweats
  - Fatigue
  - Fever 100.4°F (38°C) or higher
  - Painless, swollen lymph nodes in neck, axilla, or inguinal area
  - Pruritis, especially after bathing or ingesting alcohol
  - Weight loss of 10% or more of baseline weight in the previous 6 months
- Non-Hodgkin's lymphoma symptoms:
  - Chest pain or pressure
  - Chills
  - Easy bruising or bleeding
  - Enlarged lymph nodes
  - Fatigue
  - Severe or frequent infections
  - Shortness of breath or cough
  - Possible B symptoms
  - Swollen abdomen
  - Weight loss

Diagnosis

Labs
- CBC
- CMP
- ESR
- LDH
- Phosphorus
- Uric acid

Diagnostic Testing
- CT scan of neck, chest, abdomen, and pelvis, or metabolic imaging with PET-CT
- Excisional biopsy
- Lymphangiography
- Ultrasound or MRI to locate and stage the disease

 NURSING PEARL

Diagnosis by biopsy of enlarged lymph nodes:
- Stage 1: disease localized to a single lymph node or group
- Stage 2: more than one lymph node group involved; confined to one side of the diaphragm
- Stage 3: Lymph nodes or spleen involved; occurs on both sides of diaphragm
- Stage 4: Liver or bone marrow involved

Treatment

- Bone marrow transplant
- Chemotherapy
- Immunotherapy
- Management of infections
- Radiation
- Stem cell transplant
- Symptom management
- Targeted drug therapy

Nursing Interventions

- Administer medications as ordered.
- Discuss with patient and family what to expect with treatments such as chemotherapy or radiation.
  - Discuss side effect management.
  - Talk about supportive care and resources.
- Encourage PO intake to maintain good nutrition.

(continued)

Nursing Interventions *(continued)*

- For patients with terminal disease, provide supportive care directed at promoting comfort.
  - Discuss resources such as hospice, palliative care, and home care.
- Manage pain.
- Monitor for signs and symptoms of infection.
- Monitor for respiratory distress.
- Provide supportive care for side effects of chemotherapy and radiation.

Patient Education

- Balance rest with activity.
- Bathe or shower regularly.
- Brush your teeth with a soft-bristle toothbrush.
- Call the provider if you have any questions or are concerned about any symptoms.
- Eat small, frequent, and nutrition-dense meals.
- Keep your follow-up appointments.
- Moisturize to prevent dry skin.
- Monitor for signs and symptoms of infection.
- Take all medicines as instructed.

POP QUIZ 7.4

A nurse is teaching a group of new nurse graduates on the medical-surgical unit about oncologic disorders. A nursing graduate says that Hodgkin's disease always presents with hallmark signs of bone pain in the ribs, spine, and pelvis. The nurse knows that additional education is needed based on this comment. What would the nurse say to the nurse graduate?

MULTIPLE MYELOMA

Overview

- *Multiple myeloma* is a malignancy that affects plasma cells.
- Plasma cell myeloma penetrates the bone marrow and destroys bone, leading to bone fractures.
- Men are 50% more likely to suffer from multiple myeloma than women.

COMPLICATIONS

Complications of multiple myeloma include anemia, bone fractures or pain, frequent infections, and reduced kidney function.

Signs and Symptoms

- Bone pain, most often in the back, hips, and skull
- Bone weakness and broken bones from only minor stress or injury
- Confusion and dizziness due to hyper viscosity of blood
- Extreme thirst, frequent urination, and loss of appetite due to hypercalcemia
- Fever
- Low urine output due to kidney damage
- Fatigue
- Unintentional weight loss
- Weakness

Diagnosis

Labs

- CBC: often presents with:
  - Anemia
  - Leukopenia
  - Thrombocytopenia
- CMP:
  - Calcium levels may be high in patients with advanced myeloma.
  - Albumin may be low.
  - Creatinine may be elevated due to impaired renal function.

(continued)

Labs (continued)

- Immunoglobulins (antibodies)
- Urine protein electrophoresis to look for myeloma protein

Diagnostic Testing
- Bone marrow biopsy
- CT scan (can also be used in CT-guided biopsy)
- MRI
- PET-CT
- X-ray (bone survey or skeletal survey)

Treatment

- Bone marrow transplant
- Car T-cell therapy
- Chemotherapy
- Radiation
- Stem cell transplant

Nursing Interventions

- Administer medications as ordered.
- Administer analgesics, PRN, as ordered.
- Assist patient to maintain adequate PO hydration and good nutrition.
- Assist patient with mobility.
- Consult with PT/OT for safe mobility measures.
- Educate patient on the use of assistive devices such as a walker or cane.
- Monitor urine output to evaluate renal function.
- Provide supportive care for side effects of chemotherapy and radiation.

Patient Education

- Avoid contact with individuals with infectious diseases.
- Avoid foods high in calcium:
  - Calcium-fortified foods
  - Dairy products (e.g., cheese, milk, yogurt)
  - Dark green, leafy vegetables
  - Figs
  - Soybeans
- Avoid high-impact exercise.
- Discuss with provider what to expect with treatments such as chemotherapy or radiation.
  - Discuss side effect management with provider.
  - Talk about supportive care and resources with provider.
- Maintain adequate hydration to dilute excess calcium.
- Monitor for signs and symptoms of bleeding.
- Monitor for signs and symptoms of infection.

 POP QUIZ 7.5

A patient on the medical-surgical unit with COPD and multiple myeloma has been admitted for hypoxia due to infection with influenza A. While the nurse is assisting the patient to the bathroom, the patient feels sudden and extreme pain in the hip when getting out of bed. What is the likely cause of this pain?

THROMBOCYTOPENIA

Overview

- Thrombocytopenia is characterized by a platelet count lower than 150,000/mL.
- Platelets are essential to help the blood clot and to facilitate wound healing.

(continued)

Overview (continued)

- Women are two to three times more likely than men to be affected.
- Acute idiopathic thrombocytopenia typically affects children, with onset after a viral infection.
- Chronic idiopathic thrombocytopenia typically affects people age 20 to 50 years old.
- Thrombocytopenia has many causes, including the following:
  - Autoimmune conditions
  - Cancer
  - Cirrhosis
  - Infections
  - Medications
  - Nutritional deficiencies
  - Pregnancy

COMPLICATIONS

Complications of thrombocytopenia include anemia, brain hemorrhage, and uncontrollable bleeding.

Signs and Symptoms

- Abnormal or uncontrolled bleeding or bruising
- Bleeding (oozing) from IV sites, small lacerations, or abrasions
- Bleeding gums
- Blood in stool, urine, or emesis
- Ecchymosis
- Epistaxis
- Fatigue
- Generalized weakness
- Malaise
- Petechiae
- Purpura

Diagnosis

Labs

- BMP
- CBC: often indicate platelet counts <50,000/mL
- Coagulation panel
- D-dimer
- ELISA test for heparin-platelet factor-4 antibodies
- Fibrinogen
- Peripheral blood smear
- Thromboelastography
- Type and screen

Diagnostic Testing

- Abdominal ultrasound to check for enlarged spleen, enlarged lymph nodes, or liver cirrhosis
- Bone marrow biopsy
- Chest x-ray
- Head CT scan (if concern for intracranial bleed)

Treatment

- Apply direct pressure to any sites of bleeding.
- Administer blood transfusion as ordered by provider.
- Implement clotting factor replacement based on CBC results and trends.
- Ensure patient has two large-bore IV access sites.
- Manage condition precipitating coagulopathies (if known).
- Perform splenectomy as appropriate and indicated.

(continued)

Treatment *(continued)*

- Administer steroids or immunoglobulins that reduce platelet destruction and stimulate platelet production.
- Administer supplemental oxygen support to maintain $SpO_2 > 94\%$.
- Treat underlying condition; treatment is dependent on condition and severity.

Nursing Interventions

- Administer blood products as ordered.
- Administer medications as ordered.
- Assess ABC frequently.
- Assess for signs and symptoms of bleeding.
- Assess vital signs frequently for signs of hemodynamic instability and shock.
- Avoid multiple or unnecessary needlesticks.
- Do not unnecessarily remove formed clots or scabs.
- Draw and monitor serial CBCs and clotting factor lab trends.
- Hold firm and constant pressure when removing lines or after needlesticks to allow time for clotting to occur.
- Monitor for hypothermia; provide warming measures as ordered by provider.
- Monitor urine and stool for blood.
- Perform daily skin assessment for new appearance of bruising, bleeding, or wounds.
- Provide wound care for bleeding or oozing wounds.
- Turn and assist patient gently to avoid bruising.

Patient Education

- Adhere to fall safety precautions to mitigate injury resulting in bleeding:
  - Consider installing handrails or ramps as needed for mobility assistance.
  - Obtain fall alert bracelet or button.
  - Remove throw rugs, power cords, and other tripping hazards.
- Avoid medications, such as NSAIDs, that increase bleeding risk.
- Follow up with scheduled outpatient appointments.
- Limit alcohol intake.
- Take medications as prescribed.
- Understand complications of increased bleeding risk (e.g., falls with impact to the head can lead to intracerebral bleeding).

 ALERT!

Patients with bleeding disorders should not participate in contact sports and activities that can cause injuries.

Appendix 7.1 Hematologic Medications		
Indications	**Mechanism of Action**	**Contraindications, Precautions, and Adverse Effects**
ADH/vasopressin and analogs (desmopressin acetate)		
• Used to control bleeding in hemophilia B and to prevent and/or control bleeding in patients with hemophilia A and inhibitors to FVII	• Increase factor VIII and von Willebrand factor • Raise endogenous VII and FVII levels in mild hemophilia A	• Contraindicated in patients with moderate to severe renal impairment because of the risk of fluid overload and electrolyte abnormalities.

(continued)

Appendix 7.1 Hematologic Medications *(continued)*

Indications	Mechanism of Action	Contraindications, Precautions, and Adverse Effects
ADH/vasopressin and analogs (desmopressin acetate) (continued)		
• Used to control bleeding in some forms of von Willebrand disease • Used to replace deficient FVII in patients with hemophilia A • Desmopressin is similar to the hormone that occurs naturally in the body. It is the synthetic form of vasopressin (ADH).	• Given by many routes (e.g., oral, injection, sublingual, intranasal, IV	• Contraindicated in patients with a history of hyponatremia. • Should not be used in patients with hypersensitivity to this medication as anaphylaxis has been reported. • Contraindicated in patients with CHF, HTN, CAD due to vasoactive effects (decrease in BP and increase in HR) and risk of fluid overload and electrolyte abnormalities. • Contraindicated for bleeding abnormalities in patients with CHF or unstable angina due to its antidiuretic effects. • Contraindicated in older adult populations due to the risk of toxic reactions. • Contraindicated in patients with a high risk of intracranial pressure or history of urinary retention.
Antimetabolites/antineoplastic agents (hydroxyurea)		
• Treatment of abnormally shaped hemoglobin in sickle cell anemia	• Increase hemoglobin F or fetal hemoglobin, which is larger and more flexible than other forms of hemoglobin • Decrease propensity of sickle cells to form clots	• Patients who are pregnant or might become pregnant should not handle the medication. • Individuals touching the medication should wear disposable gloves. • It is recommended to use effective contraception while taking hydroxyurea and to discontinue medication if planning to become pregnant in the next 3 months. • Live vaccines should not be administered while taking hydroxyurea, as they can cause life-threatening infection.
Vitamin B12 supplements (e.g., cyanocobalamin)		
• Vitamin B12 deficiency, pernicious anemia	• Assists in metabolic processes, including fat and carbohydrate metabolism and protein synthesis, cell production, and hematopoiesis	• Antianemics are contraindicated in cobalt hypersensitivity (cyanocobalamin). • Use caution in renal dysfunction, folic or iron deficiency, polycythemia vera, hypokalemia, bone marrow suppression, and uremia. • Adverse effects include pulmonary edema, HF, aluminum toxicity, thrombosis, thrombocytosis, hypokalemia, and polycythemia.

(continued)

Appendix 7.1 Hematologic Medications *(continued)*

Indications	Mechanism of Action	Contraindications, Precautions, and Adverse Effects
Blood coagulations factors (AHF recombinant)		
• Used to control bleeding in hemophilia B and to prevent and/or control bleeding in patients with hemophilia A and inhibitors to FVII • Used to control bleeding in some forms of von Willebrand disease • Replace deficient FVII in patients with hemophilia A • Made from human plasma proteins, collected from many people, and then separated into components, such as clotting factors • Clotting proteins then made into freeze-dried product, tested for viruses, and treated if necessary	• Raise endogenous FVII levels in mild hemophilia A	• Medication is contraindicated in pregnancy, as it is not known how plasma-derived factor concentrates affect the fetus. • Use caution in breastfeeding, as it is not known if plasma-derived concentrates are excreted into breast milk. • Plasma-derived concentrates are treated to prevent transmission of viruses, but there is always a risk that unknown viruses can resist these treatments and pass on to the patient receiving the treatment, although methods used to treat plasma-derived products seem to be effective in preventing infections.
Blood coagulation factors (recombinant factor VIIa)		
• Used to control bleeding in hemophilia B and to prevent and/or control bleeding in patients with hemophilia A and inhibitors to FVII • Used to control bleeding in some forms of von Willebrand disease • Replace deficient FVII in patients with hemophilia A • Genetically engineered plasma concentrate • Prepared to treat, remove, or inactivate bloodborne viruses • Recombinant factors VIII and IX do not contain any plasma or albumin, and therefore cannot spread any bloodborne viruses.	• Raise endogenous FVII levels in mild hemophilia A • Activate factor X and convert prothrombin to thrombin, which converts fibrinogen to fibrin and helps form a stable clot	• Recombinant products should be used initially and subsequently in all newly diagnosed patients who require factor replacement. • Some patients using this agent may develop an inhibitor that makes it more difficult to stop a bleeding episode because it prevents the treatment from working.
Erythropoietin stimulating agents (e.g., epoetin alfa)		
• Anemia associated with chronic renal failure, malignancy, or medication therapy in HIV-infected patients	• Stimulates erythropoiesis to produce more RBCs	• Use caution with a history of seizures. • Adverse effects include seizures, CHF, MI, stroke, and hypertension.

(continued)

Appendix 7.1 Hematologic Medications *(continued)*

Indications	Mechanism of Action	Contraindications, Precautions, and Adverse Effects

Hemostatics (e.g., emicizumab)

• Used to treat hemophilia A, to prevent bleeding episodes in patients both with and without inhibitors • Imitate the way factor VIII works	• Bring together factor IX and factor X, which allows blood to clot • Humanized monoclonal modified immunoglobulin G (IgG4) antibody that binds to factor IXa and factor X and restores the function missing in factor VIII, restoring hemostasis • Do not induce or enhance the development of direct inhibitors to factor VIII • Given subcutaneously • Multiple loading doses of subcutaneous administrations of 3 mg/kg once weekly for 4 weeks and then maintenance doses established based on individual patient	• Thromboembolism has been reported when an accumulative amount of more than 100 units/kg/24 hr has been given. • This agent has been associated with birth defects and miscarriage. • This agent affects intrinsic pathway clotting–based laboratory tests, including activated clotting time, aPTT, and all assays based on aPTT. • Effects on coagulation assay testing may persist for up to 6 months after treatment.

Iron supplements (e.g., ferrous sulfate, iron sucrose)

• IV or PO replacement for iron-deficiency anemia	• Assist body in performing essential metabolic functions to maintain homeostasis • Assist with erythropoiesis	• Iron supplements are contraindicated in dialysis, hypotension, anaphylaxis, hemochromatosis, hemoglobinopathy, hemosiderosis, MRI, hepatic or gastric disease, pregnancy, and breastfeeding. • Adverse effects include angioedema, cyanosis, wheezing, hypotension, constipation, peripheral edema, chest pain, dyspnea, tachycardia, and hypertension. • Administer on an empty stomach or with orange juice to increase absorption. • To prevent teeth staining, rinse mouth with water or brush teeth after taking liquid form. • Administer iron 2 hours before or 4 hours after calcium or antacids for optimal iron absorption. • Iron may decrease concentration of levothyroxine. Administer 4 hours after levothyroxine.

Synthetic antifibrinolytics: aminocaproic acid

• Prevent clots from breaking down, resulting in firmer clots	• Inhibit fibrinolysis • Cause enhanced hemostasis when fibrinolysis contributes to bleeding	• Drug is associated with potential risk for thrombosis.

(continued)

Appendix 7.1 Hematologic Medications *(continued)*

Indications	Mechanism of Action	Contraindications, Precautions, and Adverse Effects
Synthetic antifibrinolytics: aminocaproic acid (continued)		
• Commonly used for prevention of dental bleeding after dental surgery because it blocks a substance in the saliva that breaks down clots	• Given both orally and intravenously	• Drug is contraindicated in patients with active DIC, as there are no reported cases of intravascular clotting after treatment. • Drug is contraindicated in hematuria or upper urinary tract origin. • Medication is contraindicated in hematuria of upper urinary tract origin. This agent has been known to cause intrarenal obstruction in the form of glomerular capillary thrombosis in the renal pelvis and ureters. • Use caution in pregnancy and breastfeeding, as it is not known if it can cause fetal harm.
Synthetic antifibrinolytics (tranexamic acid)		
• DIC, bleeding after trauma, hemorrhage	• Hemostatic agents bind to the lysine binding site for fibrin on the plasmin molecule.	• Antifibrinolytic therapy is contraindicated in intracranial bleed, and thrombolytic disease. • Use caution in renal impairment, seizure disorders, and surgery. • Adverse effects include thrombosis, thromboembolism, PE, renal thrombosis, visual impairments, and seizures.
Vitamins (e.g., folic acid)		
• Prevention and treatment of megaloblastic and macrocytic anemia	• Assist with protein synthesis and RBC function • Stimulate production of RBCs, WBCs, and platelets to restore normal hematopoiesis	• Antianemics are contraindicated in pernicious, aplastic, or normocytic anemias. • Use caution in undiagnosed anemias. • Adverse effects include rash, irritability, difficulty sleeping, malaise, confusion, and fever.

RESOURCES

Harding, M., Roberts, D., Kwong, J., Hagler, D., & Reinsch, C. (2020). *Lewis's medical-surgical nursing* (11 ed.). Mosby.

Johnson, L. (2020, November 1). *Vitamin B12 deficiency—nutritional disorders.* https://www.merckmanuals.com/professional/nutritional-disorders/vitamin-deficiency,-dependency,-and-toxicity/vitamin-b12-deficiency

Lewis, S. L., Dirksen, S. R., Heitkemper, M. M., Bucher, L., & Harding, M.M. (2017). *Medical-surgical nursing: Assessment and management of clinical problems* (10th ed.). Elsevier.

Longe, J. L (Ed.). (2018). *The Gale encyclopedia of nursing and allied health* (4th ed.). Gale. https://link.gale.com/apps/pub/07UZ/GVRL?u=kcls_main&sid=GVRL

Nagalla, S. (2021, September 15). *Glucose-6-Phosphate Dehydrogenase (G6PD) Deficiency.* Medscape. https://medlineplus.gov/genetics/condition/glucose-6-phosphate-dehydrogenase-deficiency/

Prescriber's Digital Reference. (n.d.[a]). *Amicar* [Drug information]. https://www.pdr.net/drug-information/amicar?druglabelid=1954

Prescriber's Digital Reference. (n.d.[b]). *Aminocaproic acid.*[Drug information]. https://www.pdr.net/drug-summary/Aminocaproic-Acid-aminocaproic-acid-3083.3768

Prescriber's Digital Reference. (n.d.[c]). *Antihemophilic-factor* [Drug information]. https://www.pdr.net/drug-summary/Advate-antihemophilic-factor--recombinant--2258.4195

Prescriber's Digital Reference. (n.d.[d]). *Desmopressin* [Drug information]. https://www.pdr.net/drug-summary/Stimate-desmopressin-acetate-821.2393#10

Prescriber's Digital Reference. (n.d.[e]). *Emicizumab* [Drug information]. https://www.pdr.net/drug-summary/Hemlibra-emicizumab-kxwh-24162

Prescriber's Digital Reference. (n.d.[f]). *Epogen* [Drug information]. https://www.pdr.net/drug-information/epogen?druglabelid=2887

Prescriber's Digital Reference. (n.d.[g]). *Hemlibra* [Drug information]. https://www.pdr.net/drug-summary/Hemlibra-emicizumab-kxwh-24162#4

Prescriber's Digital Reference. (n.d.[h]). *Hydrea* [Drug information]. https://www.pdr.net/drug-information/hydrea?druglabelid=888https://www.pdr.net/drug-information/hydrea?druglabelid=888PDR.

Prescriber's Digital Reference. (n.d.[i]). *NovoSeven* [Drug information]. https://www.pdr.net/drug-summary/NovoSeven-RT-coagulation-factor-VIIa--recombinant--458

8

IMMUNE SYSTEM

ACQUIRED IMMUNODEFICIENCY SYNDROME AND HUMAN IMMUNODEFICIENCY VIRUS

Overview

- AIDS is characterized by progressive deterioration and weakening of the immune system.
- It is an immunodeficiency disorder in which HIV uses T_4 (CD4+) cells as a receptor and reservoir for HIV.
  - HIV is transmitted through blood, semen, vaginal secretions, and breast milk.
  - It also may be transmitted by needle sharing and unprotected anal or vaginal sex.
- AIDS is diagnosed by a CD4+count of less than 200, by severity of symptoms, and/or by the presence of opportunistic infections:
  - Fungal (e.g., candidiasis in respiratory system, *Pneumocystis jiroveci* pneumonia)
  - Viral (e.g., cytomegalovirus disease, herpes simplex with chronic ulcers)
  - Protozoal (e.g., toxoplasmosis of the brain, chronic intestinal cryptosporidiosis)
  - Bacterial (e.g., *Mycobacterium tuberculosis, Salmonella septicemia*)
- While there is currently no cure for HIV, with consistent and continued adherence to ART, HIV can be contained and managed as a chronic condition.

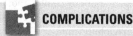

COMPLICATIONS

Complications of HIV include reduced ability to fight infections; predisposition to certain types of cancers, such as Kaposi's sarcoma and lymphoma; kidney disease; liver disease; neurologic complications; and wasting disease.

Signs and Symptoms

- Confusion
- Cough
- Dementia
- Diarrhea
- Dry skin
- Fever
- Headache
- HIV-associated encephalopathy
- Lymph node swelling
- Malaise
- Memory loss
- Nausea and vomiting
- Night sweats
- Opportunistic infections
- Pain
- Personality changes
- Poor wound healing
- Rash
- Seizures
- Shortness of breath

(continued)

Signs and Symptoms *(continued)*

- Skin lesions
- Visual changes
- Weight loss

Diagnosis

Labs

- CBC to assess for anemia, leukopenia, and thrombocytopenia
- CD4+ count: normal > 800 cells; with AIDS < 200 cells
- CD4+/CD8+ ratio
- ELISA test to detect HIV antibodies
- HIV ½ antigen/antibody combination immunoassay:
  - If positive, proceed to HIV ½ antibody differentiation immunoassay.
- Hypergammaglobulinemia
- Testing for opportunistic infections, such as tuberculosis
- Viral load: ideally zero or undetectable if medications are effective
- Western blot test

Treatment

- Combination of six main classes of HAART to inhibit HIV replication by several mechanisms:
  - NRTIs
  - NNRTIs
  - PIs
  - INSTIs
  - FIs
  - CCR5 antagonists
- Therapy for opportunistic infections (e.g., sulfamethoxazole/trimethoprim for PCP prophylaxis)
- Varying treatment of AIDS-related illnesses by type

 NURSING PEARL

As access to ART has increased, drug-resistant strains of HIV have emerged. Compliance with medication and use of PrEP in high-risk individuals can help to slow increase in drug-resistant strains.

Nursing Interventions

- Encourage activity as tolerated.
- Encourage optimal nutrition to support lean body mass.
- Encourage adequate PO hydration and IV hydration if ordered.
- Monitor oxygenation if patient is experiencing PCP; apply oxygen to maintain PaO_2 greater than 94%.
- Monitor neurologic status and provide safe environment for patient who may be confused.
- Perform skin care to reduce skin breakdown if patient is experiencing opportunistic infection.
- Restrict contact with visitors who may have transmissible infections, such as a cold or the flu.

Patient Education

- Avoid high-risk behaviors, such as sharing needles or having unprotected sex, to reduce the chance of transmission to others.
- Avoid large crowds.
- Take medications as prescribed.
- Use safe disposal of sharps and needles to prevent needlesticks.
- Watch for fevers and other signs of infection.

 POP QUIZ 8.1

A patient has recently been diagnosed with HIV and discloses intravenous drug use. What teaching is necessary for this patient?

ANAPHYLAXIS

Overview

- *Anaphylaxis* is an acute and severe allergic response between an antigen and an antibody to which the body has become hypersensitive.
- The onset is sudden and progresses rapidly.
- When the body first encounters the antigen, the immune system produces specific IgE antibodies.
- When the immune system encounters the antigen again, the IgE antibodies see the antigen as foreign and release a flood of chemical mediators.
- This release of chemical mediators can result in bronchospasm, hypotension, increased vascular permeability, and urticaria.
- Common causes of allergic reactions include environmental irritants such as pollen, food hypersensitivities such as to nuts and eggs, insect bites and stings such as with bee venom, and medications.

 COMPLICATIONS

Complications of anaphylaxis can be severe and life threatening. They include arrythmias, cardiogenic shock, kidney failure, MI, neurologic damage, respiratory failure, and death.

 ALERT!

Anaphylaxis should always be considered a life-threatening emergency. A patient who has had a mild reaction in the past can quickly progress to severe anaphylaxis if reintroduced to the same allergen. Delayed treatment of anaphylaxis can lead to death. The patient should immediately call 911 and proceed to the ED. If the patient is already in the hospital setting, the facility's anaphylaxis emergency protocol should be followed.

Signs and Symptoms

- Mild anaphylaxis occurs within 2 hours of exposure and may include the following symptoms:
  - Feeling of fullness in the throat
  - Feeling of warmth
  - Nasal congestion
  - Peripheral tingling
  - Pruritis
- Moderate anaphylaxis may occur immediately and includes the following symptoms:
  - Anxiety
  - Flushing
  - Itching
  - Warmth
- Severe anaphylaxis may also occur immediately and includes the following symptoms:
  - Anxiety
  - Chest tightness
  - Cool, clammy skin
  - Cyanosis
  - Diaphoresis
  - Difficulty swallowing or feeling of a lump in the throat
  - Dyspnea
  - Edema
  - Erythema
  - Feeling of impending doom
  - Restlessness
  - Tachypnea
  - Weakness

Diagnosis

Labs

There are no labs specific to diagnosing anaphylaxis. However, if a patient presents with respiratory distress, a full set of labs (e.g., ABG, BMP, CBC) will likely be ordered to rule out other causes.

Diagnostic Testing

- Skin testing to identify specific allergens (likely performed after acute reaction)

Treatment

- Continuous cardiac monitoring and pulse oximetry for all patients presenting with allergic reactions
- Medication administration:
  - 0.01 mg/kg of epinephrine (Appendix 8.1 at the end of this chapter) intramuscularly as soon as anaphylaxis identified; close monitoring because an additional 1 to 2 doses may be required at 5- to 15-minute intervals to control symptoms
  - Epinephrine infusion (typically a concentration of 1 mcg/mL) if symptoms are not controlled with fluids and repeated doses of IM epinephrine
  - Isotonic crystalloids as needed to support blood pressure and maintain perfusion
  - Oral or intravenous antihistamine medication, such as diphenhydramine
  - Glucocorticoids as needed to reduce inflammation and control symptoms
- Monitoring for progression of symptoms; possible additional medications if signs of worsening reaction occur, such as facial or tongue swelling, throat or chest tightness, or airway edema; immediate epinephrine injection for patients with history of severe allergic reactions or signs of anaphylaxis to prevent respiratory compromise and anaphylactic shock
- Monitoring for refractory hypotension requiring vasopressors to maintain perfusion
- Monitoring of patient's airway if anaphylactic symptoms are not immediately controlled with medications; possible intubation and mechanical ventilation, including cricothyroidotomy to permit ventilation if upper airway edema is severe
- Supplemental oxygen to maintain SpO_2 greater than 94%

Nursing Interventions

- Administer medications as ordered. IM epinephrine should be prioritized for patients experiencing signs of anaphylaxis.
- Assess ABC with priority of maintaining airway patency.
- Become familiar with institutional emergency protocols, including emergency use of epinephrine.
- Maintain IV access.
- Perform head-to-toe assessment with focused cardiovascular and respiratory assessments; alert provider immediately if respiratory distress and/or abnormal lung sounds such as stridor or wheezing are present.
- Place patient on continuous cardiac monitor with pulse oximetry, and monitor any changes.
- Reassess vital signs frequently, and monitor response to medication administration.
- Provide supplemental oxygen to maintain SpO_2 greater than 94%.

Patient Education

- Avoid allergens if possible.
- Carry two epinephrine auto-injectors at all times, and regularly check expiration dates.
- Do not consume food that contains potential allergens.
- Ensure that family and friends understand the severity of the allergy.
- Follow up with allergy specialists and learn how to use the epinephrine auto-injector.
- Teach family and friends correct use of epinephrine auto-injector.

 POP QUIZ 8.2

A patient on the medical-surgical unit with an allergy to peanuts has a visitor who brings cookies. After eating a cookie, the patient calls the nurse into the room and says their chest feels tight and they are having difficulty swallowing. The visitor notes that they baked the cookies on the same cookie sheet previously used to bake peanut butter cookies. What should the nurse prepare to do as the first-line treatment for this patient?

CANDIDIASIS

Overview

- Fungal infections are most commonly found on the skin and mucous membranes.
- The most common type of fungal infection is caused by *Candida albicans*.
- *Candida* is a common skin and mucous membrane flora. It causes infections if it grows uncontrolled in the affected area.
- Oral candidiasis is often referred to as thrush.
- Esophageal candidiasis is one of the most common opportunistic infections in patients living with HIV/AIDS.
- Invasive candidiasis can progress to candidemia, a fungal bloodstream infection.
- Candidiasis often develops in patients with other severe illnesses or compromised immune systems, so determining symptomology is difficult.

Signs and Symptoms

- Invasive candidiasis:
  - Chills
  - Fever
  - Varying symptoms based on body system affected
- Oral candidiasis:
  - Cracking or redness at corners of mouth
  - Feeling of "cotton mouth"
  - Loss of or reduction in taste
  - Odynophagia
  - Redness of mouth or throat
  - Soreness of mouth or throat
  - White patches on inside of the checks, roof of the mouth, throat, or tongue
- Vaginal candidiasis (yeast infection):
  - Abnormal vaginal discharge
  - Burning with urination
  - Painful sexual intercourse
  - Vaginal pain or itching

COMPLICATIONS

Untreated oral or vaginal thrush can lead to invasive candidiasis. Patients with compromised immune systems are also at risk for invasive candidiasis. Invasive candidiasis can lead to endocarditis, meningitis, osteomyelitis, and candidemia, which can progress to sepsis. Septic shock associated with candidemia has a very high mortality rate.

NURSING PEARL

Candida auris is a type of yeast that has developed multidrug-resistant properties and is considered a global health threat by the CDC. It has caused outbreaks in healthcare facilities.

- Some strains are resistant to all three classes of antifungals, making treatment of the fungal infection impossible.
- Strains are difficult to identify with standard laboratory equipment.
- Misidentification of the strain can lead to ineffective treatment and delays in proper antifungal management.

Diagnosis

Labs

- Blood cultures to assess for the presence of fungus in the blood
- CBC to assess for leukocytosis
- Complete set of labs for shock, if suspected
- Swabs for culture from suspected site of infection

Diagnostic Testing

- Upper endoscopy to assess site if esophageal candidiasis suspected, with possible biopsies to assess for fungal infection
- Additional diagnostic testing if sepsis suspected (e.g., CT scan, chest x-ray)

Treatment

- Clean, dry skin
- Higher level of care to support airway and perfusion: if septic shock is suspected with candidemia
- IV antifungal medications (see Appendix 8.1) for invasive candidiasis, candidemia, or oral candidiasis that is not responsive to oral or topical antifungals
- Oral, topical, and/or vaginal antifungals for oral and/or vaginal candidiasis
- Sexual abstinence or use of condoms

Nursing Interventions

- Administer medications as prescribed.
- Administer analgesics as prescribed.
- Assist patient with mouth care, including using nonirritating mouthwash and a soft toothbrush.
- Collaborate with dietician and speech therapist to provide optimal nutrition with appropriate diet order (e.g., soft diet).
- For patients with invasive candidiasis, monitor vital signs closely.
- Monitor and document color and amount of vaginal discharge.
- Provide skin hygiene.

Patient Education

- Maintain excellent oral hygiene, especially if dentures are used.
- Take antibiotics only as needed.
- Wearing cotton underwear and performing scrupulous skin/perineal hygiene may reduce the chance of vaginal candidiasis.

HEALTHCARE-ASSOCIATED INFECTIONS

Overview

- *HAIs* are infections that were not present on admission but are acquired throughout the course of a hospital stay.
- Risk factors for HAIs include:
  - Catheters (endotracheal, urinary, or vascular)
  - Improper use of antibiotics
  - Improperly or inadequately cleaned facilities
  - Injections
  - Surgery
- Common HAIs include:
  - CAUTI
  - CLABSI
  - *Clostridium difficile*
  - MRSA
  - Ventilator-associated pneumonia
  - Surgical site infections

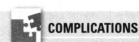 **COMPLICATIONS**

Complications from CAUTI include acute pyelonephritis, bacteremia, urosepsis, and death. Complications from CLABSI include septic shock and death. Both infections increase hospital stay.

Signs and Symptoms

- CAUTI
  - Altered mental status
  - Blood in urine
  - Chills
  - Cloudy, foul-smelling urine
  - Fever
  - Pressure or pain in lower back or stomach

Signs and Symptoms *(continued)*

- CLABSI
  - Chills
  - Erythematous central line insertion site
  - Fever
  - Pain at infection site

Diagnosis

Labs
- Blood cultures
- CBC to assess for leukocytosis
- Culture swab at site of infection
- Stool specimen testing

Diagnostic Testing
- Chest x-ray for suspected pneumonia
- CT scan or MRI if concern for abscess with surgical site infection

Treatment

- Oral antibiotics (metronidazole; see Appendix 8.1): first-line treatment for *C. difficile*
- IV antibiotics: if indicated and ordered by provider
- IV fluids: if patient is hypotensive
- Possible transfer to higher level of care: if patient develops severe systemic infection or sepsis
- Removal of infected central line, catheter, or tube

Nursing Interventions

- CAUTI prevention interventions:
  - Assess urinary output for color, consistency, and odor per institutional policy.
  - Perform peri-care every shift and after bowel movements with institutionally recommended hygiene solutions.
  - Remove or exchange urinary catheter per institutional and HOUDINI recommendations.
- CLABSI prevention:
  - Assess central line every shift.
  - Assess each port for patency every shift.
  - Change central line dressing per institutional protocol or if dirty/soiled.
  - Change IV tubing for all medications per institutional protocol.
  - Ensure dressing remains occlusive.
  - Scrub central line hubs for at least 15 seconds before using and allow to dry.
- Administer acetaminophen PRN if ordered for fever.
- Always use clean or sterile technique as appropriate to the procedure.
- Bathe patient daily with CHG baths.
- Encourage intake of probiotics or probiotic-rich foods when taking antibiotics.
- Empower patients to speak up if they see unsafe practices.
- Maintain excellent hand hygiene.
- Provide education to patients discharging with an indwelling device, such as a urinary catheter or a central line.
- Use central lines and indwelling catheters sparingly, assessing each day for necessity.

 ALERT!

Thorough hand hygiene with soap and water or an alcohol-based hand sanitizer is the easiest and most effective way to prevent HAIs. Nurses should always wash with soap and water after treating a patient who has a spore-producing bacterial illness such as *C. difficile.* Nurses should also handwash thoroughly after personal toileting, after eating, and when hands are visibly soiled. Many HAIs are preventable.

Patient Education

- If going home with a chronic indwelling urinary catheter, make sure to clean around the catheter at least daily and when soiled.
- Monitor surgical site or any indwelling device for signs and symptoms of infection.
- Practice hygienic postoperative surgical site care; keep site clean and dry.
- Shower with a chlorohexidine-based soap before surgery if instructed to do so.
- Use clean injection techniques when self-injecting.
- Wash hands often.

 NURSING PEARL

HOUDINI mnemonic for indications to maintain indwelling urinary catheter:

Hematuria
Obstruction
Urologic/abdominal/gynecologic/perineal
  surgery
Decubitus ulcer
Input and output measurement
Nursing end-of-life care
Immobility

MULTIDRUG-RESISTANT ORGANISMS

Overview

- *Multidrug resistance* develops when bacteria and other types of microorganisms evolve and become resistant to certain antibiotics, antivirals, or antifungals.
- These MDROs render many pharmacologic treatments ineffective because these antibiotics can no longer be used to control or kill the bacteria.
- MDROs have become more prevalent with the extensive use of antibiotics.
- Patients can be colonized with MDROs or have an active infection.
- Common MDROs include:
  - ESBL
  - MRSA
  - KPC
  - VRE

 COMPLICATIONS

Antibiotic-resistant infections require stronger antibiotics that can cause serious side effects, including organ failure, and can prolong recovery.

ALERT!

Patients with MDRO infections should be placed on the appropriate contact, respiratory, or airborne precautions to prevent further spread to other patients on the unit.

Signs and Symptoms

Signs and symptoms of infection vary based on the site and type of infection, but often include the following:
- Chills
- Confusion
- Fever
- Diaphoresis
- Drainage from incision or wound
- Dyspnea
- Hypotension
- Redness
- Swelling
- Tachycardia

Diagnosis

Labs
- Blood cultures
- CBC to assess leukocytosis
- Culture swab from infected site

Diagnostic Testing

- Chest x-ray
- CT scan
- MRI
- Ultrasound

Treatment

- Appropriate antimicrobial therapy based on sensitivities
- Collaboration with pharmacy to devise appropriate pharmacologic combination therapy based on cultures
- Irrigation and debridement to remove infected tissue, if applicable
- Removal of the source of infection such as catheter or central line, if possible

Nursing Interventions

- Administer medications as ordered.
- Monitor vital signs closely for signs of worsening infection.
- Practice excellent hand hygiene to prevent spreading the organism to other patients.
- Thoroughly clean or sanitize all shared equipment used by the patient.
- Wash hands before entering and leaving room.
- Wear disposable gloves and gowns to reduce transmission to other patients and reduce contact with bodily fluids.

Patient Education

- Expect a private room and a healthcare team in proper isolation protection when admitted to the hospital or when in a healthcare setting for a procedure.
- Finish all of the antimicrobial therapy prescribed as indicated, even if feeling better.
- Follow guidance, such as wearing a mask when in public spaces in the hospital.
- Once discharged from the hospital, frequently wash hands, towels, bed linens, and kitchen and bathroom countertops to prevent transmission to others.

SEPSIS

Overview

- *Sepsis* is a life-threatening systemic immune response that occurs when the body's response to infection damages its own tissues.
- It is associated with a very high mortality rate and must be treated promptly to optimize outcomes.
- If sepsis is caught early, patients have an excellent survival rate. However, if patients progress to septic shock, the mortality rate is 40%. Early detection of sepsis and immediate treatment are vital. Review sepsis protocols so implementation can begin immediately.
- Sepsis usually occurs secondary to a bacterial infection, although more rarely the source is viral or fungal.
- Patients progressing to septic shock may need a higher level of care, including vasopressors and endotracheal intubation.
- Sepsis can progress to septic shock, which can in turn progress to profound hypotension, organ failure, and death.
- Risk factors for sepsis include older age, chronic kidney or liver disease, immune compromise, diabetes, lengthy hospital stays, and the presence of invasive devices such as central lines or urinary catheters.

 COMPLICATIONS

Many patients survive sepsis without any long-term effects. However, complications from sepsis can be severe and include endocarditis leading to HF, gangrene in the extremities leading to amputation, increased risk of future infections, kidney failure, and permanent lung and neurologic damage.

Signs and Symptoms

- Change in mental status (e.g., confusion, delirium)
- Diaphoresis
- Dyspnea
- Fever or hypothermia greater than 100.4°F (38°C) or less than 96.8°F (36°C)
- Hypotension
- Known or suspected infection
- Tachycardia
- Tachypnea

Diagnosis

Labs

- ABG/VBG that may indicate acidosis, hypoxemia (PaO_2 > 300 mmHg), or hypercarbia
- Cardiac enzymes
- CMP
  - Creatinine typically increases by over 0.5 mg/dL due to renal dysfunction in sepsis.
  - Bilirubin increases (greater than 2–4 mg/dL) due to hepatic dysfunction.
  - Blood glucose will be elevated even in patients without a previous diagnosis of diabetes.
- CBC
  - Leukocytosis (WBC > 12,000 μL)
  - Leukopenia (WBC < 4,000 μL)
  - Thrombocytopenia (platelets < 80,000/mm³ in critically septic patients)
- Coagulation panel
  - INR: may be over 1.5.
  - aPTT greater than 60 seconds
- Culture of suspected infection source(s): blood, urine, wound, sputum, vascular access catheters
- D-dimer elevated in sepsis due to fibrinolysis
- Lactate acid: likely greater than 2 mmol/L if septic shock is present
- Procalcitonin: greater than 0.5 ng/mL; may indicate sepsis
- UA and urine culture

Diagnostic Testing

- CT scan or MRI to assess for source of infection if unknown
- Chest x-ray
- EKG to monitor cardiac function in severe sepsis
- Ultrasound

ALERT!

Sepsis is a life-threatening organ dysfunction caused by an infection. Septic shock is an underlying circulatory and cellular/metabolic abnormality that substantially increases mortality. Patients with septic shock can be identified with persistent hypotension requiring vasopressors to maintain MAP greater than 65 mmHg and serum lactate greater than 2 mmol/L. The mortality rate is greater than 40% if septic shock occurs. Early detection and immediate treatment is vital. Review institutional sepsis protocols so implementation can begin immediately.

NURSING PEARL

It is imperative to always draw blood cultures before starting antibiotics because it improves the chances of identifying the offending microorganism.

Treatment

- 30 mL/kg balanced crystalloid fluids within the first 3 hours for hypotensive patients or those with serum lactate level of 4 mmol/L or greater
- Blood cultures before infusing antibiotics
- Broad-spectrum antibiotics immediately (ideally within 1 hour) if high clinical suspicion for sepsis present, with transition to targeted antimicrobial therapy when appropriate
- Endotracheal intubation if respiratory status is compromised
- Monitoring of serum lactate levels (second sample if initial level >2 mmol/L)
- Preparation for transfer to ICU within 6 hours to optimize outcome
- Vasopressors for persistent hypotensive patients after fluid resuscitation with a goal of MAP (mean arterial pressure) of 65 mmHg or greater

Nursing Interventions

- Administer supplemental oxygen to maintain SpO_2 greater than 94%.
- Administer medications and IV fluids as prescribed. Aim to administer antimicrobials within the first hour of care.
- Assist to quickly obtain an EKG for interpretation by the emergency provider.
- Assist provider with central line placement if indicated; monitor site and dressing.
- Critically ill patients may require advanced airway; assist with placement of ETT (endotracheal tube) or manage noninvasive ventilation if needed.
- Establish IV access (at least two large-bore peripheral IVs initially) and draw labs as ordered.
- Monitor I/O. If ordered, place urinary catheter to obtain urine sample and monitor output.
- Perform a head-to-toe assessment and assist to identify possible sources for infection.
- Place patient on continuous pulse oximetry and cardiac monitoring and alert provider to changes in vital signs or cardiac rhythm.
- Prioritize obtaining blood cultures before administering medications.
- Reassess vital signs, including blood pressure and MAP, frequently.
- Review institutional sepsis protocols so actions can be taken quickly.

Patient Education

- Be aware that the risk of sepsis is increased with immunocompromise or a chronic health condition.
- Follow up with health care team as instructed for ongoing care and monitoring.
- If discharged home with a vascular access device (e.g., PICC, dialysis access port), adhere to instructions regarding skin care, cleansing, and dressing changes.
- Prevent infections through hand hygiene, keeping cuts and wounds clean, caring for chronic conditions such as diabetes, and discussing recommended vaccines with provider.
- Recognize the signs and symptoms of sepsis (chills, confusion, fever, increased heart rate, shortness of breath) and seek emergent care if present.
- Seek emergent care if signs of infection occur, such as fever, localized erythema, or drainage from insertion/wound sites.
- Take all medications as prescribed, ensuring that any antibiotic regimen is completed as instructed to minimize antibiotic resistance.

 POP QUIZ 8.3

The nurse is caring for a patient on the medical-surgical unit who has a UTI. The nurse notes that the patient's blood pressure is 84/52, heart rate is 112, and temperature is 104.2°F (40.1°C). The nurse notifies the provider, who orders two sets of blood cultures and broad-spectrum IV antibiotics. Which of these orders should the nurse complete first?

SYSTEMIC LUPUS ERYTHEMATOUS

Overview

- *SLE* is a chronic multisystem autoimmune disease in which the immune system attacks its own tissues, causing widespread inflammation and tissue damage in affected organs.
- Patients present with a wide range of clinical and serologic manifestations that can affect virtually any organ.
- The disease course is often marked by remissions and relapses and may vary from mild to severe.
- SLE primarily affects women of childbearing age.
- *Discoid lupus* is a mild form of SLE that primarily affects the skin. Patients with discoid lupus develop red, scaly lesions on the face, back, and upper arms, as well as hair loss.

 COMPLICATIONS

Complications of severe SLE include avascular necrosis from long-term steroid use, cataracts, complications in pregnancy, joint deformities, kidney failure, MI, skin scarring, and stroke.

Signs and Symptoms

- Anorexia
- Arthritis with synovitis
- Characteristic butterfly rash over nose and cheeks in less than 50% of patients
- Fatigue
- Fever
- Fingertip lesions
- Malaise
- Ocular manifestations
- Splinter hemorrhages
- Weight loss
- Depending on organ system affected:
  - Abdominal pain
  - Anemia
  - Endocarditis
  - Hair loss
  - Lymph node enlargement
  - Lung and joint issues
  - Myocarditis
  - Pleuritic chest pain
  - Psychosis
  - Reynaud's phenomenon
  - Seizures

Diagnosis

Labs
- Antinuclear antibody test positive in about 95% of patients
- Antiphospholipid antibodies
- BMP
- CBC often showing anemia, leukopenia, and thrombocytopenia
- ESR
- Lupus erythematous cell test

Diagnostic Testing
- Chest x-ray
- EKG

Treatment

- Avoidance of fatigue (e.g., naps if mild symptoms)
- Antimalarials such as chloroquine (see Appendix 8.1) depending on severity of illness
- Corticosteroids (see Appendix 8.1) to reduce inflammation
- Immunosuppressants such as hydroxychloroquine (see Appendix 8.1) used based on severity of disease
- NSAIDs (see Table A.2) to reduce inflammation and pain
- Sun protection
- Topical glucocorticoid for isolated skin lesions

Nursing Interventions

- Monitor for neurologic symptoms such as headaches, blurred vision, and seizures, as some patients have neurologic involvement.
- Monitor for peripheral numbness and tingling.
- Monitor for signs and symptoms of anemia, such as fatigue and pallor.
- Monitor for signs and symptoms of gastrointestinal bleeding with long-term NSAID use, including blood in the stool.

Patient Education

- Avoid large crowds.
- Avoid certain medications known to cause drug-induced lupus-like syndrome.
- Monitor for black, tarry stools related to long-term NSAID use.
- Notify provider of any new symptoms.
- Rest as needed to avoid fatigue.
- Take medications as prescribed.
- Wear sunscreen and/or long sleeves and pants when outdoors.

POP QUIZ 8.4

The nurse is caring for a patient with SLE admitted to the medical-surgical unit. On the morning lab draw, the nurse notes a hemoglobin of 10.5 g/dL and a hematocrit of 31%. Is the nurse concerned by this finding? Why or why not?

Appendix 8.1 Immune System Medications

Indications	Mechanism of Action	Contraindications, Precautions, and Adverse Effects
Antihistamines (diphenhydramine)		
• Used in treatment of acute allergic reaction and mild to moderate anaphylaxis	• Bind to H1 receptor sites, blocking histamine from binding • Do not block the release of histamines	• Use cautiously in patients with asthma and COPD. • Use cautiously in combination with other sedating medications such as opioids. • Adverse reactions include drowsiness, dizziness, and seizures.
Antimalarials (chloroquines)		
• Used in treatment of moderate to severe SLE	• Mechanisms of action of anti-inflammatory and immunomodulatory effects of chloroquines unknown • Several possible mechanisms of action, such as reduced cytokine production, inhibition of immune effector cell, and inhibition of platelet function	• Dose reductions may be necessary in patients with liver or kidney disease. • Use cautiously in patients with ocular disease. • Medication is contraindicated in patients with chloroquine sensitivity and in patients with psoriasis. • Adverse reactions are Stevens–Johnson syndrome, vision changes, and cardiac arrhythmias.
Epinephrine		
• Treatment of anaphylaxis	• Nonselective adrenergic agonist, leading to potent vasoconstriction	• There are no absolute contraindications to epinephrine in acute life-threatening emergencies. • Use with caution in patients with cardiac disease, because epinephrine causes a sharp increase in blood pressure and is a potent vasoconstrictor. • Adverse reactions include stroke and pulmonary edema.

(continued)

Appendix 8.1 Medications *(continued)*

Indications	Mechanism of Action	Contraindications, Precautions, and Adverse Effects
Immunosuppressants (azathioprine, mycophenolate mofetil, hydroxychloroquine)		
• Treatment of SLE	• Suppress the immune system by interfering with the synthesis of DNA • Reduce cytokine production	• Dose reduction may be needed in patients with renal impairment. • Use cautiously in patients with ocular disease. • Use cautiously in patients with psoriasis. • Use with caution in patients who have cardiac arrhythmias. • Adverse reactions include cardiomyopathy, visual impairments, and bronchospasm.
Metronidazole		
Use for treatment of *Clostridium difficile* infection	• Amebicidal, bactericidal, and trichomonacidal agent	• Medication is contraindicated in patients with renal impairment or cardiac disease. • Use cautiously in patients with ethanol ingestion. • Medication is contraindicated in the first trimester of pregnancy. • Adverse reactions include angioedema, confusion, and hypertension.

RESOURCES

Eggleton, J., & Nagalli, S. (2021, November 25). 25). *Highly active antiretroviral therapy (HAART)*. https://www.ncbi.nlm.nih.gov/books/NBK554533/

Haque, M., McKimm, J., Sartelli, M., Dhingra, S., Labricciosa, F.M., Islam, S., Jahan, D., Nusrat, T., Chowdhury, T. S., Coccolini, F., Iskandar, K., Catena, F., & Charan, J. (2020). Strategies to prevent healthcare-associated infections: A narrative overview. *Risk Management and Healthcare Policy*, *2020*, 1765–1780. https://doi.org/10.2147/RMHP.S269315

Lewis, S. L., Dirksen, S. R., Heitkemper, M. M., Bucher, L., & Harding, M. M. (2017). *Medical-surgical nursing: Assessment and management of clinical problems* (10th ed.). Elsevier.

Longe, J. L. (Ed.). (2018). *The Gale encyclopedia of nursing and allied health* (4th ed.). Gale. https://link.gale.com/apps/doc/CX3662600342/GVRL?u=kcls_main&sid=GVRL&xid=ea0319ff

Prescribers' Digital Reference. (n.d.[a]). *Chloroquine* [Drug information]. https://www.pdr.net/drug-summary/Chloroquine-Phosphate-chloroquine-phosphate-3418.2640#14

Prescribers' Digital Reference. (n.d.[b]). *Diphenhydramine hydrochloride* [Drug information]. https://www.pdr.net/drug-information/diphenhydramine-hydrochloride?druglabelid=1140

Prescribers' Digital Reference. (n.d.[c]). *Epinephrine* [Drug information]. https://www.pdr.net/drug-summary/EpiPen-epinephrine-134.6164

Prescribers' Digital Reference. (n.d.[d]). *Fluconazole* [Drug information]. https://www.pdr.net/drug-summary/Fluconazole-Injection-fluconazole-3458.3877#10

Prescribers' Digital Reference. (n.d.[e]). *Ibuprofen* [Drug information]. https://www.pdr.net/drug-summary/Ibuprofen-Tablets-ibuprofen-2618.3945

Prescribers' Digital Reference. (n.d.[f]). *Imuran* [Drug information]. https://www.pdr.net/drug-summary/Imuran-azathioprine-745

Prescribers' Digital Reference. (n.d.[g]). *Metronidazole* [Drug information]. https://www.pdr.net/drug-summary/
Flagyl-Tablets-metronidazole-2892.8330#11

Prescribers' Digital Reference. (n.d.[h]). *Plaqenil* [Drug information]. https://www.pdr.net/drug-summary/
Plaquenil-hydroxychloroquine-sulfate-1911.7193

Prescribers' Digital Reference. (n.d.[i]). *Prednisone* [Drug information]. https://www.pdr.net/drug-summary/
Prednisone-Tablets-prednisone-3516.6194

Singer, M., Deutschman, C. S., & Seymour, C. W. (2016). The third international consensus definitions
for sepsis and septic shock (Sepsis-3). *JAMA, 315*, 801–810. https://jamanetwork.com/journals/jama/
fullarticle/2492881

9

INTEGUMENTARY SYSTEM

BASAL AND SQUAMOUS CELL CARCINOMA

Overview

- *Basal cell carcinoma* is a tumor rising from epidermal tissue that is most often found on exposed areas of skin.
  - Basal cell carcinoma is the most common skin cancer. It is a slow-growing lesion (0.5 cm in 1–2 years). Patients have a good prognosis because most tumors remain localized, the tumor is slow growing, and metastasis is rare.
  - There are four types of basal cell carcinoma: morphea form, nodular, pigmented, and superficial.
- SCC are invasive tumors arising from keratinizing epidermal cells.
  - They can be highly aggressive with potential to metastasize.
  - They have a fairly good prognosis if caught early.
  - SCC often develop over a few months on skin areas with prolonged sun exposure in light-skinned people.

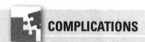

COMPLICATIONS

Complications of basal and SCC include risk of recurrence and increased risk of other types of skin cancers. While the risk of metastasis to other areas is lower than with melanoma, metastasis can occur.

Signs and Symptoms

- Basal cell carcinoma (Figure 9.1)
  - The nodular form is characterized by a papule with raised borders, superficial ulceration, and telangiectasias.
  - The superficial form is characterized by a scaly, reddened patch without ulceration, and is commonly found on the trunk.
  - The morphea form type is characterized by a pale, yellow, or white scar-like plaque with indistinct borders.
  - The pigmented form is similar in shape to the nodular form but contains melanin and appears black, brown, or blue in color.
- Squamous cell carcinoma (Figure 9.2)
  - This type is characterized most often by a crusted, erythematous patch, a nonhealing ulcer, or a firm, dark-colored nodule.
  - Lesions can also be reddened, scaly patches that are keratotic and often bleed.

Diagnosis

Diagnostic Testing

- Biopsy: definitive test
- Three common types of biopsies for assessing skin lesions:
  - Shave biopsy: The provider uses a thin blade to remove the top layers of the skin, the dermis, and epidermis.

(continued)

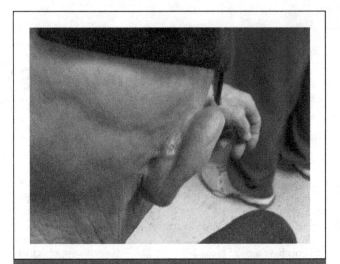

Figure 9.1 Basal cell carcinoma.

Source: Lyons, F., & Ousley, L. (2014). *Dermatology for the advanced practice*. Springer Publishing Company.

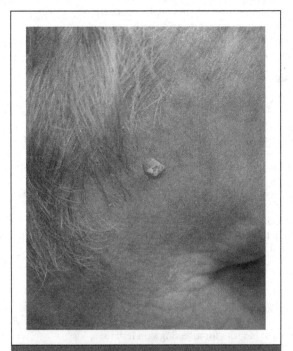

Figure 9.2 Squamous cell carcinoma.

Source: Lyons, F., & Ousley, L. (2014). *Dermatology for the advanced practice nurse*. Springer Publishing Company.

Diagnostic Testing (continued)

- Punch biopsy: A hollow, circular tool is used to remove a core of tissues, including dermis, epidermis, and superficial fat.
- Excisional biopsy: The provider removes the skin lesion, as well as healthy-appearing surrounding skin, down through the fatty layer.

Treatment

- Cryosurgery
- Electrodessication and curettage
- Mohs surgery
- Radiation
- Surgical excision

Nursing Interventions

- Address pain control needs and administer medications as ordered.
- Assist the patient with ADLs as needed, based on the location of the lesion.
- Assist the patient with ROM, depending on the location of the lesion.
- Monitor lesions and postoperative biopsy sites for bleeding.
- Monitor vital signs postoperatively.
- Provide surgical or wound care per provider order.

Patient Education

- Follow up for routine skin exams with dermatologist.
- Perform thorough skin examinations, and notify provider of any abnormalities.
- Use sunscreen when outdoors.
- Wear hats and cover exposed skin when outdoors.

 NURSING PEARL

Mohs surgery involves the excision of cancerous tissue. During this procedure, the surgeon removes the tissue one layer at a time. After each layer is removed, it is microscopically examined by a trained technician. This informs the surgeon if and where more tissue needs to be removed. This process is repeated until no more cancerous tissue is seen. Mohs surgery has the highest cure rate for most basal and SCC.

CELLULITUS

Overview

- *Cellulitis* is inflammation of skin and connective tissue as a result of bacterial entry via breaches in the skin barrier, such as from cuts, scrapes, surgical incisions, or other open wounds.
- The most common bacteria that cause cellulitis are common skin flora: *Streptococcus pyogenes* and *Staphylococcus aureus*.
- Most often, cellulitis affects the skin of the lower extremities; however, it can occur anywhere, including the arms and face.
- Risk factors for cellulitis include:
  - Diabetes
  - History of cellulitis
  - Immunosuppression
  - Impaired skin integrity due to psoriasis or other chronic integumentary illness
  - Lymphedema

 ALERT!

MRSA is a common bacterium that causes cellulitis, especially in patients who are frequently hospitalized or have chronic illnesses. Implement contact precautions for any patient with a positive wound culture.

Signs and Symptoms

- Blisters
- Drainage
- Edema
- Erythema, often expanding out from the site of initial infection
- Fever
- Inflammation
- Pain
- Tenderness
- Warmth

Diagnosis

Labs

- CBC
- CRP: may be elevated (>0.3 mg/L)
- Lactate level
- Wound culture to identify infectious organism, if present

Diagnostic Testing

- CT scan
- Ultrasound:
  - Assess for abscess.
  - Rule out DVT in the case of unilateral limb swelling.

Treatment

- Antibiotics (see Table A.1)
- Wound care to manage moisture and promote healing, performed each shift or when dressing is soiled
- Irrigation and debridement: may be necessary, depending on tissue damage

Nursing Interventions

- Administer medications as ordered.
- Assess pulse and peripheral perfusion on affected extremity.
- Assess for signs of spreading infection including redness, warmth, edema, and purulent drainage.
- Assess site frequently for signs of systemic infection.
- Elevate extremity.
- Outline areas of erythema with skin marker to determine any progression or improvement of area.
- Provide education on cellulitis prevention.
- Provide wound care, including dressing changes per provider order.

Patient Education

- Apply antibiotic cream or ointment as prescribed to surface wounds.
- Cleanse wounds daily with soap and water.
- Cover wounds with a clean dressing daily.
- Maintain adequate hygiene to prevent skin breakdown.
- Moisturize skin to prevent cracking and peeling.
- Monitor for signs and symptoms of infection.
- Promptly treat any superficial skin infections to prevent spread.

 COMPLICATIONS

If left untreated, cellulitis can affect the deeper tissues, causing necrotizing fasciitis, which is a medical emergency. Orbital cellulitis, or cellulitis affecting the area surrounding the eye, can lead to loss of vision and is also considered a medical emergency. Other complications of cellulitis include increased risk of developing cellulitis again in the future, lymphedema, and development of an abscess. In very serious cases, cellulitis can lead to amputations, bacteremia, endocarditis, sepsis, and death.

MALIGNANT MELANOMA

Overview

- *Malignant melanoma* is a neoplasm arising from the dermal or epidermal layer.
  - It is the leading cause of death from skin cancers.
  - It originates in a mole or section of skin that may appear normal at first.
- Prognosis is based on the thickness of the lesion at diagnosis and the presence of lymph node involvement. The 5-year survival rate is poor if the lesion is greater than 1.5 mm in thickness at diagnosis and if there is lymph node involvement.
- Sites most commonly associated with melanoma:
  - Back
  - Back of the hands
  - Between the toes
  - Face
  - Legs
  - Neck
  - Scalp

Signs and Symptoms

- Change in borders, color, size, or shape of an existing skin lesion
- May be pruritic or painful and bleed, ooze, or crust
- New, irregularly bordered lesion that is blue or black in color
- Nodular melanoma, which is a spherical lesion that resembles a blood blister (blue-black in color)

Diagnosis

Labs
- CBC
- Serum LDH level to assess for metastatic disease

Diagnostic Testing
- Biopsy to assess the lesion
- CT scan, MRI, or PET scan to assess for distant metastases

Treatment

- Oncology consultation for chemotherapy and radiation recommendations
- Surgical consultation for wide excision

Nursing Interventions

- Administer medications as ordered.
- Monitor lesion and biopsy site for bleeding.
- Monitor vital signs postoperatively.
- Provide analgesics in the postoperative period, PRN, if ordered.
- Provide education for wound care.
- Provide education to limit sun exposure.

COMPLICATIONS

Complications of malignant melanoma include risk of recurrence and increased risk of other types of skin cancers. The risk of metastasis is high, and distant symptoms, such as shortness of breath or weight loss, are sometimes the first sign that the melanoma has metastasized. Melanoma accounts for only about 1% of skin cancers, but it has the highest mortality rate of all skin cancers.

NURSING PEARL

Examine skin lesions for ABCDE:
Asymmetry
Border irregularity
Color variation
Diameter greater than 6 mm
Elevation/enlargement/evolving

NURSING PEARL

There is no definitive, systemic curative treatment for malignant melanoma. Most treatments are aimed at slowing disease progression and relieving symptoms.

Patient Education

Refer to Patient Education section in Basal and Squamous Cell Carcinoma section, above.
- Perform wound care per provider instructions if surgery performed.
- Take medications as prescribed by provider.

PRESSURE INJURIES

Overview

- Pressure injuries occur when skin and soft tissues are injured from prolonged pressure to one area.
- Pressure injuries most commonly occur over bony prominences such as the sacrum, heel, hip, back of head, shoulder blade, and elbow.
- Older, chronically ill, and immobile patients, as well as patients with diabetes, are at higher risk of developing pressure injuries.
- Pressure injuries can also be caused by a device putting pressure on the skin. Common devices that cause pressure injuries include nasal cannula, Foley catheter, endotracheal tube, and NG tube.
- Risk factors for pressure injuries include impaired mobility, decreased or absent sensation, confusion, poor nutrition, reduced blood flow, fragile skin, muscle volume loss, and excessive moisture.

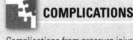

COMPLICATIONS

Complications from pressure injuries include sepsis, cellulitis, and bone and joint infections.

Signs and Symptoms

- Drainage from an open wound
- Erythema
- Nonblanchable redness
- Open wound on an area of bony prominence
- Pain or tenderness
- Purple discoloration
- Skin that feels warmer or cooler than surrounding tissue
- Tissue loss revealing deeper layers of skin

Diagnosis

Labs
- CBC to assess leukocytosis and infection
- CMP to assess nutritional status
- Wound culture to identify infectious organisms, if present

Diagnostic Testing
There is no diagnostic testing specific to diagnosing pressure injuries. A CT scan may be indicated to assess additional injuries.

NURSING PEARL

Pressure injuries depend on depth of wound and are categorized by stage or category:
- Stage 1: Nonblanchable erythema in those with lighter skin tones and blue/purple color in those with darker skin tones with no tissue loss
- Stage 2: Partial-thickness wound with damaged top layer of skin; may look like a blister
- Stage 3: Full-thickness wound extending to the subcutaneous fat
- Stage 4: Full-thickness wound with involvement of muscle or bone
- Unstageable: Obscured full-thickness skin and tissue loss; extent of tissue damage unconfirmed because it is covered by slough or eschar
- Deep tissue injury: Persistent nonblanchable deep red, maroon, or purple discoloration

Treatment

- Antibiotics (see Table A.1)
- Irrigation and debridement: may be necessary if necrotic tissue is present
- Pressure offloading from wound at all times
- Topical barrier creams or ointments
- Wound care consult for dressing recommendations based on stage of wound
- Wound VAC

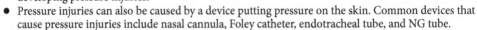

Nursing Interventions

- Ensure adequate fluid intake.
- Apply prescribed moisture barrier product.
- Apply prescribed protective/adhesive dressings to affected areas.
- Educate patient and family on basics of repositioning, keeping skin clean and dry, and signs and symptoms of infection.
- Establish turning schedule:
  - Assist patient to reposition at least every 2 hours to relieve pressure on bony prominences.
  - Use positioning wedge and pillows.
- Encourage adequate nutrition to promote wound healing.
  - Administer liquid dietary supplements.
  - Increase protein intake.
  - Obtain nutrition consult.
  - Parenteral or tube feeding nutrition may be ordered to provide additional support for wound healing.
- Ensure bony prominences are offloaded (e.g., elevate heels off bed, use heel protector boots).
- Manage moisture with wicking pads and barrier creams.
- Monitor wound by measurement and description to assess worsening of wound.
- Perform Braden scale assessments.
- Perform thorough head-to-toe wound assessments at least once per shift.
- Perform prescribed wound care, such as normal saline wet-to-dry gauze dressings for deeper wounds.
- Premedicate with pain medication before wound changes as prescribed. Provide frequent perineal hygiene, including incontinence care as soon as soiling is noted.
- Provide support surfaces and special cushions when sitting in a chair. Reposition at regular intervals while in the chair.
- Reposition movable devices such as nasal cannula and NG tube to decrease pressure points.
- Use specialty pressure redistribution surface beds to assist with offloading pressure and repositioning the patient.
- Use lift sheet instead of pulling patient up in bed to prevent shearing forces.
- Use pillow between extremities.
- Use specialty pillows to prevent breakdown on back of the patient's head.
- When cleaning skin, use a gentle cleanser and pat, rather than aggressively rub, skin.

Patient Education

- Consider obtaining a lift to assist family and caregivers with mobility and turning if immobile and requiring total care.
- Keep skin clean and dry.
  - Change pads, dressings, adult briefs, or sheets if wet or soiled.
  - Consider using wicking materials to help reduce moisture, or assistive devices such as bedside urinals or external suction catheters.
- Maintain adequate fluid and nutrition intake.
- Move and reposition frequently to alleviate pressure on bony prominences and redistribute weight.
- Notify provider if wound becomes infected.
- Perform skin checks for pressure ulcers at least daily.
- Perform wound care.
  - Obtain necessary materials if needed to perform dressing changes at home.
  - Wash hands before and after touching wound.

(continued)

Patient Education *(continued)*

- Remove the old dressing and assess wound for any new redness, warmth around site, foul smell, or discoloration.
- If possible, measure the wound to assess for any growth in width or depth.
- If ordered, apply prescribed ointment or barrier cream and dress with gauze or bandage dressing.
- If wet-to-dry dressings are prescribed, moisten gauze pad with normal saline, apply to wound, and cover with supportive pad and tape to secure (or as prescribed by provider).
- Change dressing as ordered or when dressing becomes soiled.

 POP QUIZ 9.1

A patient with a history of COPD and diabetes is admitted to the medical-surgical unit. While performing an initial assessment, the nurse notices that the patient has an area of nonblanchable erythema on the dorsum of the foot. The patient states that they have peripheral neuropathy and are not able to feel sensations in the feet very well. The discolored area feels warm to the touch. Is this finding consistent with a pressure injury? What further actions are indicated by the nurse?

PSORIASIS

Overview

- *Psoriasis* is an inflammatory, chronic skin disease that is thought to be autoimmune in nature.
- Common locations of plaques include the face, elbows, scalp, knees, lower back, and genitalia. The lesions are often bilateral.
- Periodic recurrence and improvement are common. The disease flares up in times of stress, infection, and hormone changes and goes into remission with temporary symptom relief.

Signs and Symptoms

- Psoriasis is characterized by red, scaly plaques and papules with silvery scales. Patches form from the buildup of living and dead skin.
- Plaques are dry and may be pruritic.
- There are several types of psoriasis with varying symptoms (Table 9.1).

 COMPLICATIONS

Complications of psoriasis include increased likelihood of developing cardiovascular disease, hypertension, and type 2 diabetes. Patients with psoriasis are also prone to developing inflammatory eye diseases such as blepharitis, conjunctivitis, and uveitis. Psoriasis also increases the risk of developing additional autoimmune diseases such as celiac disease and Crohn's disease.

Diagnosis

Labs
- CBC to assess leukocytosis, which may be elevated in some forms
- ESR: may be elevated in some forms of psoriasis

Diagnostic Testing
- Biopsy of plaques may be done to confirm diagnosis of psoriasis.

Treatment

- Systemic treatments (Appendix 9.1 at the end of this chapter):
  - Biologic agents such as infliximab
  - Methotrexate
  - NSAIDs (see Table A.2)
- Topical treatments (see Appendix 9.1):
  - Coal tar products
  - Medicated shampoos
  - Nonsteroidal anti-inflammatory creams

(continued)

Table 9.1 Types of Psoriasis

Type	Occurrence	Symptoms
Erythrodermic psoriasis	• Least common	• Entire body can be covered with a peeling, erythematous, pruritic rash. • May include an intense burning sensation
Guttate psoriasis	• Most commonly seen in children and young adults • Commonly preceded by a bacterial infection such as strep throat	• Small, drop-shaped, scaly lesions commonly seen on the trunk, arms, or legs
Inverse psoriasis	• May be triggered by a fungal infection	• Mainly affects the skin folds found in the axilla, groin, buttocks, and breasts • Characterized by smooth patches of red skin that are worsened by friction and sweating
Nail psoriasis	• Affects the fingernails and toenails	• Causes pitting and discoloration • Severe cases possibly characterized by crumbling of the nail and by the nail separating from the nailbed
Plaque psoriasis	• Most common form	• Causes dry, raised, red lesions covered with silvery scales • Plaques most commonly found on the elbows, knees, back, and scalp
Psoriatic arthritis	• Causes swollen, painful joints	• Joint pain sometimes first or only symptom or sign of psoriasis • Can cause stiffness and progressive joint damage that in the most serious cases may lead to permanent joint damage
Pustular psoriasis	• Rare form	• Causes pus-filled lesions • Can be widespread or occur in smaller areas on the palms of the hands or the soles of the feet

Treatment *(continued)*

- Retinoids
- Steroidal ointments
- Ultraviolet A or B light treatments

Nursing Interventions

- Administer medications as ordered.
- Advise patient to avoid sun and wear protective goggles during light treatments.
- Assist patient in applying ordered ointments.
- Assist patient with bathing and gentle debridement of plaques.
- Caution that retinoids and methotrexate are contraindicated in pregnancy; birth control must be used.
- Provide emotional support.

Patient Education

- Bathe and moisturize skin regularly.
- Contact dermatologic support groups for further emotional support.
- Maintain a skin care routine, even when disease is not prevalent.
- Manage stress with prescribed medications and/or exercise to decrease flareups.
- Monitor for signs and symptoms of infection.
- Perform wound care, if present, as prescribed.
- Take medications as prescribed.

POP QUIZ 9.2

A patient arrives to the unit with patches of red, scaly skin over bilateral elbows and knees. The patient reports no pain. The patient's blood glucose is 100, blood pressure 120/60, heart rate 75, and respiratory rate 16. What lab value would the nurse expect to be elevated based on the physical assessment? What other nursing interventions are indicated?

WOUNDS

Overview

- Wounds commonly seen in the medical-surgical setting include abrasions, infections, lacerations, and surgical wounds.
  - *Abrasions* are superficial injuries of the skin.
  - Infections occur when bacteria grow in the damaged skin area.
  - *Lacerations* are deep cuts in the skin, usually from a sharp object.
  - Surgical wounds result from surgical incisions.
- The principles of caring for wounds are similar despite the varying mechanisms of injury.

COMPLICATIONS

Complications of wound healing may include bleeding, dehiscence, delayed healing, drainage, foul odor, and erythema.

Signs and Symptoms

- Open area of skin
- Protective function of skin compromised

Diagnosis

Labs

- Blood culture
- BMP
- CBC
- Lactate
- Wound cultures to identify infectious organism, if present

NURSING PEARL

Carefully monitor for infection, including chills, fever, foul odor, erythema, and purulent drainage. If noted, notify the provider for treatment orders to decrease the severity of the infection.

Diagnostic Testing

- CT scan to assess for surgical complications
- Ultrasound to assess abscess
- X-ray

Treatment

- Antibiotics for suspected infection
- Irrigation and debridement
- Plastic surgery consult for skin graft (for large wounds)
- Surgical consult for irrigation and debridement and/or drains
- Recognizing and evaluating factors that impair wound healing (Table 9.2)
- Wound therapy consult if needed
- Wound VAC: provides increased negative pressure to promote epithelization, increase blood flow, and continuously remove drainage

Table 9.2 Factors That Impair Wound Healing	
Age	• Older patients typically heal more slowly than younger patients due to comorbidities, including chronic disease, poor nutrition, poor hydration, and hormonal changes.
Body type	• Poor circulation to adipose tissue or poor oxygen and nutritional storage in emaciated patients may impair and slow wound healing.
Chronic disease	• Chronic disease that may impair blood flow or circulation can additionally slow wound healing. This can include CAD, COPD, PVD, cancers, or diabetes.
Immunosuppression or radiation therapy	• Immunosuppression from age or medications can alter wound healing.
Laboratory values	• Alterations in nutritional labs, hemoglobin, or liver, renal, or thyroid function may slow wound healing.
Nutritional status	• Poor nutrition, including protein malnutrition, and poor hydration can result in decreased wound healing.
Vascular insufficiency	• Decreased blood supply can cause skin impairments and ulcerations while also slowing the rate of wound healing.

Source: Data from Hess, C. T. (n.d.). Checklist for factors affecting wound healing. *Advances in Skin and Wound Care, 24*(4), 192.

Nursing Interventions

- Administer analgesics before wound care as prescribed if it is anticipated to be painful for the patient.
- Apply abdominal binder as ordered for abdominal wounds.
- Assess neurologic function to identify AMS, which may indicate infection.
- Change dressings as needed or as indicated by the provider.
  - Change daily, every shift, or when dressing is soiled.
  - Wet-to-dry dressing is performed by applying gauze moistened with sterile water and covered with an ABD pad and tape to support.
- Consult case management for wound management with home care services after discharge, if indicated.
- Empty and perform drain care as ordered by provider; ensure drain tubing is patent.
- Encourage nutrition, including maximizing protein for wound healing.
- Monitor the wound for signs and symptoms of infection or other complications.
- Monitor vital signs for signs of infection, including fever, tachycardia, and hypotension.
- Offload pressure from all wounds.
- Provide emotional support.

Patient Education

- If sutures or staple closure, follow up with provider for removal. Allow wound closure strips or incision glue to fall off gradually; do not remove or pick off.
- Learn proper dressing management:
  - Change dressing using clean technique.
  - Clean hands before and after changing dressings or touching wound.
  - Assess for bleeding, drainage, and warmth around the site.
  - Obtain necessary materials for dressing change.
  - Change as ordered by provider, or if dressing becomes soiled.
- Maintain a high-protein diet to maximize wound healing.

- Monitor for signs and symptoms of infection and notify provider if present:
  - Confusion
  - Fever
  - Hypotension
- Take medications exactly as prescribed. The full course of antibiotics should always be completed. Consult provider with any medication questions.

POP QUIZ 9.3

A patient had an open cholecystectomy a month ago and has been admitted to the unit to address the surgical wound that is not healing properly. What actions will the nurse perform?

Appendix 9.1 Integumentary Medications

Indications	Mechanism of Action	Contraindications, Precautions, and Adverse Effects
Antimetabolites (methotrexate)		
• Used topically for psoriasis	• Interfere with DNA synthesis, repair, and cellular replication • Quickly replicating cells such as skin, mucous membranes, and bladder most sensitive to methotrexate	• Medication is contraindicated in pregnancy for nonmalignant conditions. • Close monitoring of patients with hepatic impairment is required. • Dose reduction may be needed in patients with renal impairment when CrCl is less than 90 mL/min. • Adverse reactions include skin necrosis, thrombocytopenia, nausea, vomiting.
Corticosteroids (prednisone)		
• Used for moderate to severe flaring psoriasis • Used topically for psoriasis	• Naturally occurring hormones that prevent or suppress inflammation and immune responses when administered at pharmacologic doses, thereby reducing inflammation	• Long-term steroid use can cause osteopenia. • Steroid use can cause hyperglycemia. • Use with caution in pregnancy. • Long-term use can cause immune suppression. • Use should be avoided in patients with Cushing's syndrome because it can aggravate the disease. • Do not abruptly discontinue dose. • Adverse reactions include visual impairment and rash.
Retinoids (retinoin)		
• Topical treatment for psoriatic lesions	• Synthetic analog of endogenous retinoids	• Medication is contraindicated in pregnancy; contraceptive requirements must be followed. • Certain brands of retinoid topical creams contain fish proteins, so use cautiously in patients with fish or shellfish allergies. • Medication can cause leukocytosis. • Medication may cause photosensitivity; avoid using on sunburn and avoid sun exposure after application. • Adverse effects include bleeding, phlebitis, and erythema.

(continued)

Appendix 9.1 Integumentary Medications *(continued)*

Indications	Mechanism of Action	Contraindications, Precautions, and Adverse Effects
Silver sulfadiazine		
• Topical treatment for bacterial infections	• Disrupts bacteria by breaking down cell membrane	• Medication is contraindicated in patients with sulfa hypersensitivity or allergy. • Medication is contraindicated in pregnancy. • Use with caution in patients with porphyria and glucose 6-phosphate dehydrogenase deficiency. • Adverse effects include skin necrosis, exfoliative dermatitis, and erythema multiforme.
TNF-alpha inhibitors (infliximab)		
• Used to suppress the immune response in patients with moderate to severe psoriasis	• Neutralize the biologic activity of the cytokine TNF-alpha	• Use cautiously in patients with hepatic impairment. • Monitor liver enzymes regularly. • Use cautiously in patients with renal impairment. • Patients can develop serious infections. Medication is contraindicated in patients with active infections. • Adverse reactions include antibody formation, abdominal pain, elevated hepatic enzymes, and hypertension.

RESOURCES

Hess, C. T. (n.d.). Checklist for factors affecting wound healing. *Advances in Skin and Wound Care, 24*(4), 192.

Lewis, S. L., Dirksen, S. R., Heitkemper, M. M., Bucher, L., & Harding, M. M. (2017). *Medical-surgical nursing: Assessment and management of clinical problems* (10th ed.). Elsevier.

Longe, J. (2018). *The Gale encyclopedia of nursing and allied health* (4th ed., Vol. 2, pp. 1131–1138). Gale. https://link .gale.com/apps/doc/CX3662600342/GVRL?u=kcls_main&sid=GVRL&xid=ea0319ff

Prescribers' Digital Reference. (n.d.[a]). *Methotrexate* [Drug information]. https://www.pdr.net/drug-summary/ Methotrexate-Tablets-methotrexate-1797.8191

Prescribers' Digital Reference. (n.d.[b]). *Prednisone* [Drug information]. https://www.pdr.net/drug-summary/ Prednisone-Tablets-prednisone-3516.6194

Prescribers' Digital Reference. (n.d.[c]). *Remicade* [Drug information]. https://www.pdr.net/drug-summary/ Remicade-infliximab-263.4292

Prescribers' Digital Reference. (n.d.[d]). *Silvadene* [Drug information]. https://www.pdr.net/drug-summary/ Silvadene-silver-sulfadiazine-2781

MUSCULOSKELETAL SYSTEM

AMPUTATION

Overview

- *Amputation* is the partial or complete removal of an extremity or limb.
- The lower extremities are the most common sites of amputation.
- Common causes of amputation include:
  - Gangrene
  - Infection
  - Malignancy in bone or soft tissue
  - Nonhealing wounds
  - Osteomyelitis
  - Trauma (motor vehicle crashes, heavy machinery workplace accidents)

Signs and Symptoms

- Avulsions
- Bleeding
- Body part wholly or partially separated from the body
- Crush injury
- Laceration
- Pain

Diagnosis

Labs

- CBC to assess for leukocytosis and anemia
- CMP
- Coagulation panel
- ESR to assess inflammatory response
- Type and screen
- Wound cultures to identify infectious organism, if present

Diagnostic Testing

Testing to determine the need for amputation may include:
- Ankle brachial index
- CT scan
- MRI
- Vascular ultrasound
- X-ray

COMPLICATIONS

Complications of amputation include poor wound healing, increased risk for emboli, bleeding, infection, and pain. After amputation, patients may experience phantom limb pain, which is pain in the part of the limb that has been amputated.

NURSING PEARL

Many amputations are the result of untreated, infected, diabetic wounds that have spread to the bone, resulting in osteomyelitis. Excellent education on the importance of foot care is a vital part of nursing care of patients with diabetes. Many patients with diabetes have neuropathy and may not realize that a wound is present because they cannot feel it. Additionally, hyperglycemia and microvascular changes seen in patients with diabetes contribute to slow wound healing.

Treatment

- Analgesics for pain control (see Table A.2)
- Antibiotics to treat infection (see Table A.1)
- Chemotherapy if amputation is related to malignancy
- Surgical removal of limb in one operation or in multiple stages
- Wound care

Nursing Interventions

- Administer medications as ordered.
- Assess pain scale and administer analgesics, PRN, as ordered.
- Assess for potential hemorrhage.
- Assess the closest proximal pulse for presence and strength and compare with the opposite extremity.
- Assist with mobility and ROM.
- Do not elevate limb itself because of the risk of flexion contractures.
- Encourage well-rounded, high-protein diet to maximize wound healing.
- Evaluate for phantom limb sensation and pain and explain to the patient. Mark bleeding and drainage on the dressing.
- Monitor for signs that indicate sufficient tissue perfusion (e.g., capillary refill less than 3 seconds, warm skin, appropriate skin color).
- Monitor site of peripheral nerve catheter or epidural, if present.
- Monitor surgical incision for signs and symptoms of infection.
- Provide education on use of assistive devices.
- Provide wound care per provider order.
- Support limb with pillows to reduce edema.
- Work with PT/OT.

Patient Education

- Comply with weight-bearing and range-of-motion precautions.
- Eat a high-protein diet to maximize wound healing.
- Maintain euglycemia to promote wound healing.
- In diabetes, perform daily skin and foot exams to check for signs of infection or skin breakdown.

 POP QUIZ 10.1

A patient has arrived to the unit after a right below-the-knee amputation. The patient complains of right foot pain. What is this a sign of, and what are the appropriate interventions by the nurse?

COMPARTMENT SYNDROME

Overview

- Compartment syndrome occurs when increased pressure within a myofascial compartment compromises the circulation and function of the tissues within that space.
- Increased compartmental pressure can result from two causes:
  - Internal: bleeding or swelling within the compartment
  - External: external restrictions (i.e., edema, a dressing, or a splint)
- Compartment syndrome is most often seen following trauma, long bone fracture, crush injuries, extensive soft tissue damage, surgery, or prolonged pressure injuries.

 COMPLICATIONS

Timely recognition and treatment of compartment syndrome is essential to avoid serious complications. Sustained, elevated pressure can lead to neurologic deficits, tissue ischemia and necrosis, infection, and delays in fracture healing. Complications of compartment syndrome may require amputation of the affected body part.

(continued)

Overview *(continued)*

- It can occur anywhere there is a muscle contained in a closed fascial space—most commonly the lower leg, forearm, foot, hand, gluteal region, and thigh. It can also develop in the abdomen after penetrating abdominal trauma or surgery.
- Acute compartment syndrome is a medical emergency. Compression of these vital structures can lead to severe tissue damage if not corrected.

Signs and Symptoms

- Delayed capillary refill
- The 6 Ps:
  - Pain out of proportion to apparent injury and/or pain with passive stretch of muscles in the affected compartment
  - Paralysis and numbness
  - Paresthesia
  - Pallor: skin that appears pale, shiny, or tight
  - Pulselessness
  - Poikilothermia
- Swelling
- Tight or stiff muscle

Diagnosis

Labs

Blood or urine testing to assess the degree of muscle damage:
- Elevated CPK
- Possible elevation of BUN
- Possible elevation of creatinine
- Presence of urine myoglobin in UA

Diagnostic Testing
- Doppler ultrasound
- CT scan or MRI, as indicated

Treatment

- Administer pain medication as ordered.
- Monitor vital signs and administer medications/fluids as ordered.
- Promptly remove any external dressing or splint (casts, bandages, dressings).
- Monitor intercompartmental pressure through needle manometry.
- Surgical fasciotomy is the standard of treatment for acute compartment syndrome in most cases to release pressure within the compartment.
  - The incision may not be closed immediately and could be left open until swelling decreases.
  - Surgical fasciotomy is contraindicated when the muscle is already dead, at which point an amputation is indicated.

 ALERT!

With acute compartment syndrome, an intra-compartmental pressure of 30 mmHg or higher is considered critical, and treatment with emergent surgical decompression should be initiated.

Nursing Interventions

- Assess for decreasing urine output, as this may indicate AKI or renal failure.
- Assess pain and administer pain medication as ordered (see Table A.2).
- Assess for symptoms of shock: hypotension, tachycardia, and increasing temperature.
- Elevate extremity no higher than heart level to facilitate venous drainage, reduce edema, and maximize tissue perfusion.
- Monitor surgical incision for signs and symptoms of infection.

(continued)

Nursing Interventions *(continued)*

- Monitor vital signs and administer medications/fluids as ordered.
- Perform peripheral vascular checks: color, sensation, motor strength, paralysis, pulses, and capillary refill.
- Perform serial musculoskeletal and neurovascular assessments to extremity.
- Prevent compartment syndrome to other high-risk extremities by removing or loosening bandages, casting, or clothing/patient gowns.

Patient Education

- Maintain range-of-motion and weight-bearing precautions.
- Monitor surgical incisions for signs and symptoms of infection.
- Follow up with provider for continued assessment of affected limb.
- Refrain from placing constricting items on affected limbs or extremities.
- Seek treatment for any worsening symptoms, including the following:
  - Increasing pain unrelieved by opioids
  - Temperature changes in affected limb
  - Worsening paresthesia
  - Worsening mobility or new-onset paralysis

 POP QUIZ 10.2

A patient with a newly placed cast on the right arm is receiving discharge instructions. What instruction should the nurse prioritize?

FRACTURE

Overview

- Fractures involve a break in bone continuity.
- Fractures are most common in the long bones, including the femur, radius, ulna, humerus, tibia, and fibula, but fractures can occur in any bone.
- Because of the surrounding tissue, musculature, and organs, femoral and pelvic fractures are associated with significant bleeding, concomitant internal injuries, and high mortality.
- There are many types of fractures (Table 10.1).

COMPLICATIONS

Complications of fractures include bone infection and avascular necrosis, compartment syndrome, breakdown of skeletal muscle, and fat embolism syndrome.

Table 10.1 Types of Fractures		
Type	**Mechanism of Injury**	**Description**
Avulsion	Forceful contraction of a muscle	Displaced bone fragment at muscle insertion point
Closed fracture	Severe direct force	Bone fractured without skin damage
Compression	Severe force to head, sacrum, or heels (i.e., from a jump); secondary to osteoporosis-related bone loss	Vertebral bones collapse; may cause displaced fragments
Greenstick	Compression force to an extremity, causing it to bend and break	Break present on one side of a long bone but does not extend through the bone
Oblique	Twisting force	Complete fracture, usually oblique angle across both of the bone's cortices

(continued)

Table 10.1 Types of Fractures *(continued)*

Type	Mechanism of Injury	Description
Open	Caused by trauma	Skin, bone, and soft tissue damage; bone may protrude through the skin
Spiral	Twisting force with the extremity planted	Fracture can resemble a corkscrew
Stress fractures	Subjected to repetitive stress (running)	Affects only one cortex of the bone
Transverse	Sharp, direct blow	Complete fracture perpendicular to the bone

Signs and Symptoms

- Abnormal movement or ROM
- Acute pain, especially following an injury
- Bruising
- Crepitus
- Discoloration
- Limb deformity
- Immobility
- Swelling
- Tenderness
- Shortened affected limb, as in femur fractures
- Inability to bear weight
- Visible bone

Diagnosis

Labs
There are no labs specific to diagnosing fracture. However, labs are indicated if surgery is necessary:
- CBC
- CMP
- Coagulation panel
- Type and cross

Diagnostic Testing
- CT scan: may be used in trauma to assess for multiple or complex breaks
- X-ray: should include joints above and below the injury site to rule out related dislocations or additional fractures

Treatment

- Analgesics as ordered for pain
- Cold therapy before and after surgery
- Consultation to orthopedic services, if indicated
- Immobilization of fractures (including joints above and below the site of injury) by casting or splinting
- Manual reduction of closed fractures
- Surgical repair of open or complex fractures
- Tetanus vaccine (see Appendix 10.1 located at the end of this chapter) and antibiotic prophylaxis for open fractures
- Traction to maintain alignment of extremity to maintain neurovascular function until operative management

Nursing Interventions

- Administer antibiotics, if ordered. Administer PRN analgesics as ordered.
- Assist patient with mobility.
- Encourage the patient to cough, deep breathe, and reposition.
- Ensure that DVT prophylaxis is ordered, either with intermittent pneumatic compression devices or medication.
- Monitor patient for constipation.
- Monitor neurovascular status of the affected limb.
- Monitor surgical incision for signs and symptoms of infection.
- Provide pin care, if present.
- Use traction, if ordered by provider.

ALERT!

Fat embolism is a rare complication of a long bone fracture. Notify the provider immediately if the patient has respiratory distress, mental status changes, fever, or petechiae, as these are signs and symptoms of fat embolism.

Patient Education

- Complete entire course of antibiotics, if prescribed.
- Keep cast clean and dry, and do not insert items into the cast.
- Learn any signs and symptoms to report to healthcare team.
- Learn appropriate use of mobility devices.
- Learn RICE interventions:
  - Rest
  - Ice
  - Compression
  - Elevation
- Maintain weight-bearing and range-of-motion precautions.
- Take pain medications as prescribed.
- Take proper fall precautions.

POP QUIZ 10.3

The nurse on the medical-surgical unit is caring for a patient who has had a total joint replacement of the left knee. What are the six Ps the nurse should focus on during the neurovascular exam?

GOUT

Overview

- *Gout* is a type of inflammatory arthritis that results from crystallized uric acid that accumulates in joints and connective tissue.
- Joints affected by gout are acutely painful, red, and swollen.
- Causes of primary gout include diet high in organ meat, seafood, or alcohol, especially beer. It is also caused by reduced renal excretion of uric acid.
- Medications, such as thiazide diuretics and cyclosporine, and conditions, such as diabetes, hypertension, polycythemia, renal disease, and hypercholesteremia, are associated with secondary gout.

COMPLICATIONS

Complications of gout include atherosclerotic disease, cardiovascular lesions, neuropathy, and renal calculi.

Signs and Symptoms

- Erythematous joints
- Joint inflammation
- Low-grade fever
- Painful or tender joints
- Skin over tophi (uric acid crystals) forming ulcers or oozing a white exudate

NURSING PEARL

Symptoms of gout often appear suddenly and peak quickly. However, severe attacks may last for days or weeks. Repetitive gout flares can lead to chronic polyarticular gout characterized by persistent, painful joints.

Diagnosis

Labs

- CBC
- Elevated CRP
- Elevated serum uric acid levels (above 7 mg/dL)
- Elevated urine uric acid levels

Diagnostic Testing

- Aspiration of synovial fluid to assess for crystals
- X-ray of affected joint(s)

Treatment

- Dietary restrictions:
  - Limit alcohol.
  - Limit foods high in purine (liver, mussels, sardines).
- Medications for prevention and treatment of acute attacks (see Appendix 10.1)
- Pain management with NSAIDs and steroids (see Table A.2)

Nursing Interventions

- Administer medications as ordered.
- Assess pain and administer analgesics as ordered.
- Ensure low-purine diet is ordered.
- Encourage resting of the affected joint.
- Encourage adequate fluid intake.
- Monitor patient's serum uric acid level.

Patient Education

- Avoid diuretics and aspirin.
- Avoid stress.
- Drink plenty of fluids.
- Maintain healthy habits, as illness exacerbates gout symptoms.
- Reduce alcohol consumption, especially consumption of beer.
- Reduce intake of foods associated with increased uric acid levels.
- Take medications as prescribed.

 POP QUIZ 10.4

A patient describes painful, tender joints and has a low-grade fever. What lab value would be elevated, and what test would confirm a diagnosis of gout?

IMMOBILITY

Overview

Immobility refers to decreased ability to move oneself and can be caused by a variety of factors, including:

- Amputation
- Balance issues
- Chronic illness
- Muscle wasting
- Pain
- Weakness

 COMPLICATIONS

Patients who experience immobility are at high risk for complications such as contractures, DVTs, PEs, pressure ulcers, or pneumonia.

Signs and Symptoms

- Flaccid extremities
- Lack of movement/inability to mobilize any part of the body
- Muscle atrophy
- With long-term immobility:
  - Atelectasis
  - Constipation
  - Contractures
  - Decreased cardiac reserve
  - Emboli
  - Loss of calcium from bones
  - Muscular atrophy and weakness
  - Osteoporosis
  - Pneumonia
  - Pressure ulcers
  - Skin breakdown
  - UTIs
  - Venous insufficiency

Diagnosis

Labs

There are no labs specific to diagnosing immobility. However, labs may be ordered to identify any underlying cause of immobility.

Treatment

- Activity as often as safely possible, being mindful of potential removal of drains, lines, or tubes; can be completed in a bed or chair (e.g., arm raises, calf pumps, leg raises)
- Activity sessions to encourage mobility
- Corresponding treatments and medications to assist in correcting underlying cause of immobility
- Identification and correction of:
  - Underlying cause of immobility, as possible
  - Complications of prolonged immobility, if present:
    - Clot preventions: SCDs, anticoagulants, IVC filter
    - Pneumonia: chest PT
    - Pressure ulcer prevention
- Physical and OT
- Repetition of skills practiced with PT (e.g., sitting at the side of the bed, standing, pivoting to a chair, ambulating)

Nursing Interventions

- Administer anticoagulation medications as ordered.
- Communicate directions and plan for mobilization effectively.
  - Secure all devices, drains, lines, and tubes prior to mobilization or ambulation.
  - Place call bell within reach if mobilizing patient out of bed to chair.
- Coordinate mobilization or ambulation attempts with additional support staff as needed (e.g., respiratory therapy, PT).
- Elevate heels to prevent skin breakdown.
- Encourage appropriate nutrition to decrease risk of pressure ulcers.
- Encourage and motivate patient, if possible, to perform physical activity and regain mobility to achieve postdischarge goal.
  - Create and encourage attainable goals.
  - Celebrate accomplishments and improvements.
  - Provide emotional and therapeutic support.

(continued)

Nursing Interventions *(continued)*

- Encourage patient to perform daily care as independently as possible (e.g., brushing teeth, washing face, brushing hair).
- Monitor vital sign changes during activity.
- Prevent pressure ulcers.
  - Change pads, dressings, adult briefs, and sheets if wet or soiled.
  - Keep skin clean and dry.
  - Monitor for new areas of skin breakdown.
  - Offload pressure on bony prominences by turning patient with pillows and elevating heels.
  - Pad bony prominences and skin that come into contact with lines, drains, or tubes to prevent skin breakdown.
  - Perform skin assessment each shift and document changes as noted.
  - Reposition frequently to alleviate pressure on bony prominences and redistribute weight.
  - Turn patient every 2 hours as ordered.

Patient Education

- Assess urinary catheter, if present, for signs and symptoms of infection and proper drainage.
- Drink plenty of water to maintain hydration.
- Maintain adequate nutrition to minimize risk of muscle wasting and osteoporosis.
- Turn, cough, and deep breathe every 2 hours.
- Perform ROM.
- Prevent constipation by drinking fluids and taking over-the-counter stool softeners.
- Report worsening wounds, fevers, signs of infection, shortness of breath, chest pain, and/or difficulty breathing to the provider.
- Routinely assess for skin breakdown.

LOW BACK PAIN

Overview

- Low back pain affects the lumbar region and is sometimes referred to as lumbar backache.
- Most low back pain is musculoskeletal; however, degenerative disk disease can also cause low back pain.

Signs and Symptoms

- Decreased motor function
- Difficulty ambulating
- Lumbar pain that may radiate down one or both legs
- Parathesis

Diagnosis

Labs

There are no labs specific to diagnosing lower back pain. However, the following labs may be ordered to rule out complications:

- Blood cultures
- CBC
- CMP
- UA and urine culture

COMPLICATIONS

Complications of low back pain include sensorimotor deficits and chronic pain. Low back pain is the leading cause of job-related disability.

ALERT!

Back pain with severe tingling, numbness, fever, weight loss, or bowel or bladder issues should be reported to a provider immediately, as these can be signs of a more serious condition such as aortic aneurysm rupture, cauda equina syndrome, infection, or malignancy.

Diagnostic Testing
- CT scan
- MRI
- Myelogram
- X-ray

Treatment

- Analgesics for pain control (see Table A.2)
- Muscle relaxers to reduce muscle spasms
- Physical/OT
- Ruling out or treating neurologic or other medical causes
- Steroid injections
- Surgical interventions such as discectomy

Nursing Interventions

- Administer pain medications, PRN, as ordered.
- Assess motor and neurologic functions.
- Assist patient in applying heat or ice to the low back.
- Encourage patient to rest in semi-Fowler's position to reduce muscle strain on the low back.
- Maintain activity restrictions postoperatively.
- Postoperatively, monitor surgical incision for signs and symptoms of infection or any indication of a CSF leak.

Patient Education

- Increase physical activity.
- Strengthen the back and core muscles.
- Use proper body mechanics when lifting heavy objects.

OSTEOARTHRITIS

Overview

- *Osteoarthritis* is a noninflammatory degenerative joint disease with slow destruction of articular cartilage.
- Weight-bearing joins such as hips and knees are primarily affected. However, other common joints that are affected include the fingers, ankles, and wrists.
- Osteoarthritis can be secondary (caused by a known injury or disease) or idiopathic (occurring without known injury or disease).

COMPLICATIONS

Complications of osteoarthritis include impaired physical mobility, increased fall risk, pain, and weakness.

Signs and Symptoms

- Crepitus in the affected joint
- Decreased ROM
- Asymmetrical inflammation
- Joint pain aggravated by activity and relieved by rest
- Joint deformity, redness, swelling, or tenderness
  - Heberden's nodes: on DIP joints due to osteophyte formation
  - Bouchard's nodes: on PIP joints
- Joint stiffness that is better in the morning and worse as the day progresses

Diagnosis

Labs
- CBC
- ESR: may be elevated in acute inflammation episodes

Diagnostic Testing
- CT scan
- MRI
- X-ray

Treatment

- Analgesic pain medications such as NSAIDs and acetaminophen (see Table A.2)
- Assistive devices such as walkers and canes to assist in mobility
- Supportive care
  - Cold therapy to improve ROB
  - Moist heat therapy to decrease muscle spasms and stiffness
  - PT
- Surgical joint replacement

Nursing Interventions

- Administer medications as ordered.
- Apply cold or heat therapy as indicated.
- Assist the patient with ambulation using assistive devices (e.g., canes for support on opposite side).
- Consult with PT for additional exercises.
- Encourage activity as tolerated, alternating with periods of rest.

Patient Education

- Avoid activities that would precipitate exacerbation.
- Maintain ROM to decrease joint stiffness.
- Modify home environment to prevent exacerbation.
- Take medications as ordered.
- Use proper body mechanics.

OSTEOMYELITIS

Overview

- *Osteomyelitis* is an infection involving bone. It may be classified based on the mechanism of infection (hematogenous vs. nonhematogenous) and the duration of illness (acute vs. chronic).
- Common sites of osteomyelitis include the femur, tibia, humerus, and vertebrae.
- It can result from an open fracture, orthopedic surgery, or an infection that travels from another part of the body.
- Patients with diabetes or ESRD who have a history of intravenous drug use or who have compromised circulation are at an increased risk of developing osteomyelitis.
- Common microorganisms that cause osteomyelitis include *Staphylococcus aureus, Streptococcus pyogenes, Pseudomonas aeruginosa,* and *Escherichia coli.*
  - *Staphylococcus aureus* accounts for approximately 90% of osteomyelitis.
- Early identification and prompt initiation of IV antibiotic therapy are needed to prevent deteriorating condition and complications.

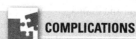 **COMPLICATIONS**

Complications of osteomyelitis include amputation, pathologic fractures, septicemia, and septic arthritis. Early identification and prompt treatment with IV antibiotic therapy is needed to prevent further complications.

Signs and Symptoms

- Bone pain
- Chills
- Decreased movement of affected extremity
- Draining wound without trauma or injury
- Edema
- Erythema
- Fever
- Malaise
- Nausea
- Tachycardia
- Warmth over the infected site
- Wound drainage

Diagnosis

Labs
- CBC
- CMP
- Lactic acid (sepsis workup)
- ESR: may be elevated
- Wound/blood cultures

Diagnostic Testing
- Imaging of the infected area:
  - CT scan
  - MRI
  - X-ray
- Bone biopsy

Treatment

- Analgesics to control pain
- Bone graft
- Cast to stabilize and protect bone
- Hyperbaric oxygen treatments, if available
- IV antibiotics to treat specific infectious organism
- Sepsis treatment, if indicated
- Surgical intervention:
  - Irrigation and drainage
  - Debridement for removal of necrotic material and culture of involved tissue and bone
  - Placement of or removal of orthopedic hardware, if applicable
  - Amputation if unable to manage infection

Nursing Interventions

- Administer antibiotics:
  - Monitor side effects.
  - Monitor dosages and trough levels.
- Assess motor and neurologic function in the affected area or limb.
- Assess and treat pain as ordered.
- Assess wound and dressing status.
  - Change wound dressing as needed/ordered.
  - Inform provider of any wound drainage changes, including color or consistency changes or new foul smell.
- Consult case manager for long-term care needs.

(continued)

Nursing Interventions *(continued)*

- Educate patient regarding administering long-term IV antibiotics at home, including PICC line and long-term port care, if needed.
- Educate patient on the use of assistive devices such as walkers.
- Encourage ROM in unaffected limbs.
- If taking PO nutrition, encourage dietary choices with high-protein and vitamin content.
- Offload pressure with repositioning, padding, and turning every 2 hours.
- Promote mobility of unaffected joints/extremities as tolerated.

Patient Education

- Complete entire course of antibiotics as prescribed, even if feeling better.
- Do not share or reuse needles if using IV medications.
- Learn actions and side effects of medications and importance of taking medications as prescribed.
- Maintain adequate nutrition to promote healing.
- Maintain euglycemia and monitor foot care if diabetic.
- Maintain range-of-motion restrictions.
- Maintain weight-bearing restrictions.
- Report to provider increased drainage, edema, pain, and redness.
- Use wound care procedures.

OSTEOPOROSIS

Overview

- Osteoporosis occurs when an imbalance between bone resorption and deposition is present.
- Osteoporosis begins after age 30 years. It progresses quickly in postmenopausal patients.
- Osteoporosis is associated with decreased estrogen, family history, immobility, nutritional deficiencies, smoking, alcohol consumption, and long-term steroid use.
- Patients with osteoporosis are at high risk for fractures. Common fracture sites include the femur, radius, ulna, and vertebrae.

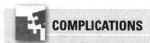

COMPLICATIONS

Complications of osteoporosis are fractures, immobility, and pain.

Signs and Symptoms

- Back pain
- Loss of height
- Kyphosis

Diagnosis

Labs

- Serum calcium and vitamin D to assess for nutritional deficiencies
- Thyroid function panel
- Testosterone levels in men

Diagnostic Testing

- DEXA scan

Treatment

- Calcium supplementation (see Appendix 10.1)
- Estrogen and progesterone to improve hormone balance
- Low-impact exercise, such as walking and weight training, to build and maintain bone mass
- Medications to prevent bone resorption, such as calcitonin (see Appendix 10.1)
- Vitamin D supplementation (see Appendix 10.1)

Nursing Interventions

- Administer medications as prescribed.
- Assist with ambulation if the patient is unsteady.
- Encourage a calcium-rich diet.
- Move the patient gently when turning and repositioning.
- Provide education about dietary sources of calcium.
- Provide education on gentle range-of-motion exercises.

Patient Education

- Increase dietary sources of calcium and vitamin D, such as almonds, calcium-fortified foods and drinks, cheese, milk, salmon, sardines, and yogurt.
- Participate in low-impact exercise such as walking or swimming.
- Set up household to reduce tripping risks to reduce chance of falls.
- Take medications as prescribed.
- Use correct body mechanics.

RHABDOMYOLYSIS

Overview

- *Rhabdomyolysis* is the rapid breakdown of muscle and release of intracellular muscle constituents into the bloodstream.
- Often, it causes myoglobinuria.
- The most common cause of rhabdomyolysis is trauma. It also occurs as a result of infection, drug use, excessive muscular contraction, DKA, heatstroke, and severe electrolyte disorders.

COMPLICATIONS

Complications of rhabdomyolysis include acute renal failure, electrolyte imbalances, and compartment syndrome. DIC is a late complication.

Signs and Symptoms

- Dark-colored urine (cola or coffee colored)
- Fever
- Malaise
- Muscle swelling
- Muscle tenderness
- Muscle weakness

Diagnosis

Labs
- Elevated CK:
  - Serum CK levels:
    - At presentation, usually at least five times the upper limit of normal, but ranging from approximately 1,500 to more than 100,000 IU/L
  - Begins to rise within 2 to 12 hours following the onset of muscle injury and reaches maximum within 24 to 72 hours
- BMP:
  - Elevated BUN and Cr
  - Hypocalcemia
  - Hyperkalemia
  - Hyperphosphatemia

(continued)

Labs *(continued)*

- Metabolic acidosis: common; increased anion gap may be present
- Severe hyperuricemia
- CBC
- ESR and CRP: likely elevated
- Toxicology screen
- UA: possible evidence of myoglobinuria from urine sample

Diagnostic Testing

There are no diagnostic tests specific to diagnosing rhabdomyolysis. However, the following may be helpful in the overall workup:

- CT scan
- MRI
- Muscle biopsy

Treatment

- Treatment focus: treating underlying cause
- Possible treatment of symptoms:
  - Aggressive IV hydration to increase GFR
  - Analgesics to treat pain
  - Dialysis in acute kidney failure
  - Diuretics

Nursing Interventions

- Early and aggressive fluid resuscitation is the major therapy.
- Administer medications as ordered.
- Apply continuous telemetry monitoring and notify provider of any arrhythmias.
- Correct metabolic and electrolyte abnormalities:
  - Hypocalcemia: calcium gluconate administration (see Appendix 10.1)
  - Hyperkalemia: administration of regular insulin, dextrose, furosemide, or sodium polystyrene (see Appendix 10.1)
  - Hyperuricemia: allopurinol administration
- Ensure PIV is patent and can tolerate high fluid volume.
- Administer FFP as ordered by provider in patients experiencing DIC.
- Monitor I/O.
- Monitor for signs and symptoms of compartment syndrome; fasciotomy will be performed if indicated.
- Monitor vital signs.
- Monitor urine output and notify provider if it falls below 30 mL/hr.
- Monitor color and clarity of urine output.
- Perform neurovascular checks if there is concern for compartment syndrome.
- Relieve pressure in compartment to increase muscle perfusion and prevent muscle breakdown and death.

Patient Education

- Maintain adequate hydration.
- Modify exercise routine to decrease risk of rhabdomyolysis.
- Seek alcohol and drug cessation therapy and support groups as appropriate.
- Take medications as prescribed.

RHEUMATOID ARTHRITIS

Overview

- *Rheumatoid arthritis* is a systemic autoimmune disease that causes inflammation of connective tissue and is characterized by joint pain and stiffness in the wrists and hands.
- It may progress over time to affect other body systems such as the heart, kidneys, and lungs.

COMPLICATIONS

Complications of rheumatoid arthritis include carpal tunnel syndrome, Raynaud's phenomenon, Sjogren's syndrome, and splenomegaly.

Signs and Symptoms

- Anorexia
- Edematous joints
- Erythema and heat complaints to joints
- Fatigue
- Fever
- Joint stiffness that is worse in the morning and better as the day progresses
- Malaise
- Ulnar deviation
- Weakness
- Weight loss

Diagnosis

Labs
- CBC:
    - WBC: may be elevated (infection or inflammation)
    - WBC: may be decreased (autoimmune)
    - Anemia: may be present
- CRP: usually elevated
- ESR: usually elevated
- Rheumatoid factor: elevated (20 IU/mL or higher)

Diagnostic Testing
- Synovial biopsy
- X-ray

Treatment

- Heat
- Ice/cold
- Medications such as TNF inhibitors, high-dose salicylates, NSAIDs, immunosuppressants, and corticosteroids (see Table A.2)
- PT to maintain ROM
- Rest
- Rheumatologist referral

Nursing Interventions

- Administer medications, including pain medications, as ordered. Around-the-clock administration of pain medications may be ordered.
- Assist with ADLs.
- Assess extremity for swelling or any developing wounds.
- Assess pain.
- Assist the patient with applying heat and ice.
- Assist the patient with range-of-motion exercises.

(continued)

Nursing Interventions *(continued)*

- Avoid large pillows under the head or knee.
- Immobilize the affected joint with a splint or brace until inflammation subsides.
- Monitor for adverse drug reactions.
- Use a bed cradle or foot cradle to keep bed linens off feet and legs until inflammation subsides.

Patient Education

- Apply heat or ice to affected joints.
- Get adequate rest.
- Maintain a well-balanced diet.
- Perform exercises to maintain ROM.
- Take medications as prescribed.

Appendix 10.1 Orthopedic Medications

Indications	Mechanism of Action	Contraindications, Precautions, and Adverse Effects
Anti-gout agents (colchicine)		
• Management of acute gout episodes	• Anti-inflammatory	• Medication is contraindicated in patients with both hepatic and renal impairment. • Use cautiously in patients with bone marrow suppression. • Use cautiously in older patients. • May pose a reproductive risk in male patients • Dose reduction may be needed if patient develops GI symptoms. • Stop treatment if patient develops symptoms of neuromuscular toxicity.
Calcium gluconate		
• To correct for hypocalcemia	• Directly repletes serum calcium levels when given IV	• Contraindicated in patients with hypercalcemia • Use with caution in patients with electrolyte disturbances. • Adverse effects include bradycardia and paresthesia. • Medication can cause extravasation injury.
Calcium carbonate		
• To supplement calcium in the body	• Acts to directly increase the calcium stores in the body	• Medication is contraindicated if patient has hypercalcemia. • Adverse effects include constipation, diarrhea, and renal calculi.

(continued)

Appendix 10.1 Orthopedic Medications *(continued)*

Indications	Mechanism of Action	Contraindications, Precautions, and Adverse Effects
Diphtheria and tetanus toxoids		
• Prophylaxis for tetanus	• Induce antibody production against *Corynebacterium diphtheriae* and *Clostridium tetani*	• Administer if 10 or more years have elapsed since the last dose. • Administer within 5 years of the last dose if the patient has a large, contaminated wound. • Medication is contraindicated in patients with thimerosal hypersensitivity and/or latex allergy. • Use with caution in patients with Guillain–Barré syndrome. • Use IM administration only. • Adverse effects are possible: fever, headache, pain at injection site.
Immunosuppressants (azathioprine, mycophenolate mofetil)		
• Treatment of rheumatoid arthritis	• Suppress the immune system by interfering with the synthesis of DNA	• Dose reduction may be needed in patients with renal impairment. • Medication is contraindicated in pregnancy in patients who are being treated for nonmalignant diseases. • Use with caution in patients with diabetes and pulmonary disease. • Adverse reactions include pancytopenia, stomatitis, and thrombocytopenia.
Muscle relaxants (cyclobenzaprine)		
• Muscle strains, spasms	• Mechanism of action similar to tricyclic antidepressants, including anticholinergic activity, potentiation of norepinephrine, and antagonism of reserpine • No direct action on the muscle	• Medication is contraindicated in patients with tricyclic antidepressant hypersensitivity, hyperthyroidism, depression, and seizure disorder. • Drug can cause drowsiness and dry mouth. • Patients may be more susceptible to sunburn. • Adverse reactions include seizures, palpitations, and hypotension. • Treatment duration beyond 2 to 3 weeks is not recommended due to CNS depression.

(continued)

Appendix 10.1 Orthopedic Medications *(continued)*

Indications	Mechanism of Action	Contraindications, Precautions, and Adverse Effects
Sodium polystyrene sulfonate		
• Used to treat hyperkalemia	• Nonabsorbed, cation-exchange polymer • Can be administered orally or rectally	• Medication is contraindicated in patients with GI obstruction. • Medication is contraindicated in patients with hypokalemia. • Use with caution so medication does not bind with other medications and decrease efficacy (space medication 3 hours apart from others). • Adverse effects include diarrhea and vomiting.
Vitamin D supplements (ergocalciferol)		
• Vitamin D deficiency	• Metabolized to calcitriol that promotes reabsorption of calcium, increases intestinal absorption of calcium and phosphorus, and increases calcium mobilization from bone to plasma	• Vitamin D supplements are contraindicated in hypercalcemia and malabsorption syndrome. • Use caution in renal failure, renal disease, and pregnancy. • Adverse effects include fatigue, headache, nausea, polydipsia, and increased urinary frequency.
Xanthine oxidase inhibitors (allopurinol)		
• Reduction of uric acid to manage gout symptoms	• Interfere with catabolism of purine, thereby reducing uric acid production	• Gout symptoms may temporarily worsen after starting allopurinol. • Use with caution if patient develops a rash. • Use with caution in patients with renal impairment and hepatic disease. • Patient should use caution if driving or operating heavy machinery, as medication can cause drowsiness. • Adverse reactions include renal failure, exfoliative dermatitis, vasculitis, and HF.

RESOURCES

Lewis, S. L., Dirksen, S. R., Heitkemper, M. M., Bucher, L., & Harding, M. M. (2017). *Medical-surgical nursing: Assessment and management of clinical problems* (10th ed.). Elsevier.

Longe, J. L (Ed.). (n.d.). *The Gale encyclopedia of nursing and allied health* (4th ed.). Gale. https://link.gale.com/apps/doc/CX3662600342/GVRL?u=kcls_main&sid=GVRL&xid=ea0319ff

Prescribers' Digital Reference. (n.d.[a]). *Allopurinol sodium* [Drug information]. https://www.pdr.net/drug-summary/Aloprim-allopurinal-sodium-847.897

Prescribers' Digital Reference. (n.d.[b]). *Colchicine* [Drug information]. https://www.pdr.net/drug-summary/Colcrys-colchicine-592

Prescribers' Digital Reference. (n.d.[c]). *Cyclobenzaprine hydrochloride* [Drug information]. https://www.pdr.net/drug-summary/Cyclobenzaprine-Hydrochloride-cyclobenzaprine-hydrochloride-3089.1153

Prescribers' Digital Reference. (n.d.[d]). *Diphtheria and tetanus toxoids absorbed* [Drug information]. https://www.pdr.net/drug-summary/Diphtheria-and-Tetanus-Toxoids-Adsorbed--For-children-6-weeks-through-6-years-of-age--diphtheria-and-tetanus-toxoids-adsorbed-3293

Prescribers' Digital Reference. (n.d.[e]). *Ergocalciferol* [Drug information]. https://www.pdr.net/drug-summary/Ergocalciferol-ergocalciferol-24306#14

Prescribers' Digital Reference. (n.d.[f]). *Imuran* [Drug information]. https://www.pdr.net/drug-summary/Imuran-azathioprine-745

Prescribers' Digital Reference. (n.d.[g]). *Kayexalate* [Drug information]. https://www.pdr.net/drug-information/kayexalate?druglabelid=2925

Prescribers' Digital Reference. (n.d.[h]). *Remicade* [Drug information]. https://www.pdr.net/drug-summary/Remicade-infliximab-263.4292

NEUROLOGICAL SYSTEM

ALZHEIMER'S DISEASE

Overview

- *Alzheimer's disease* is a degenerative disorder of the cerebral cortex that progressively worsens over time. It is a cause of dementia.
- It is characterized by brain cell atrophy with decreased levels of acetylcholine, increased ventricle size, and neuritic plaques.
- Alzheimer's disease does not have an exact cause. Research shows that it may be caused by abnormal neurologic proteins, environmental toxins, genetics, or decreased cerebral blood flow.

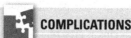

COMPLICATIONS

Complications of Alzheimer's disease include more frequent UTIs, aspiration pneumonia, falls and associated injuries, dehydration, and malnutrition. Patients with Alzheimer's disease may not be able to recognize or verbalize when they are not feeling well or are hungry or thirsty. Careful monitoring of these patients is essential to catch early signs of infection or other illness.

Signs and Symptoms

- Aphasia
- Behavioral changes
- Decreased self-care abilities
- Impaired judgment
- Memory loss
- Muscle rigidity
- Obsessive behaviors
- Restlessness

Diagnosis

Labs

- Beta amyloid protein if present (marker for diagnosis)
- CBC to rule out infection as underlying cause
- CMP to rule out electrolyte imbalance as underlying cause
- TSH to rule out thyroid imbalance as underlying cause
- UA to rule out underlying causes
- Vitamin B12 and folate levels for deficiencies

Diagnostic Testing

- CT to rule out stroke or tumor
- Definitive diagnosis only through postmortem examination of brain tissue
- Neurophysical exam focusing on history and cognitive testing

Treatment

- Antipsychotics (see Appendix 11.1 located at the end of this chapter) to treat behavioral symptoms
- Medications such as anticholinergics in early stages to improve memory

Nursing Interventions

- Administer medications as ordered.
- Assist the patient with ADLs.
- Encourage appropriate sleep/wake cycles to encourage nighttime rest.
- Give simple instructions.
- Provide a calm environment with low stimulation.
- Provide emotional support to the patient and the family.
- Speak directly to the patient in a friendly tone, even if the patient is not responsive.

Patient Education

- Avoid sleep during the day.
- Join a support group to provide emotional support.
- Keep a set schedule.
- Take medications as prescribed.
- Use a medication organizer to help keep track of medications.
- Write down important dates and appointments.

ANXIETY

Overview

- *Generalized anxiety disorder* is a mental health disorder characterized by feelings of worry, anxiety, or fear that interfere with one's daily activities.

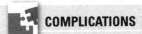

COMPLICATIONS

Patients with anxiety may have acute anxiety symptoms as well as chronic issues such as depression and substance use.

Signs and Symptoms

- Diaphoresis
- Difficulty concentrating
- Fatigue
- GI symptoms such as nausea and abdominal pain
- Insomnia
- Nervousness
- Tachycardia
- Tachypnea

Diagnosis

Labs
- Cardiac enzymes to rule out MI
- CBC to rule out other diagnosis
- CMP to rule out other diagnosis
- Liver function tests to rule out liver disease

Diagnostic Testing
- EKG to rule out MI

Treatment

- Administration of medications such as benzodiazepines and antidepressants (see Appendix 11.1)
- Counseling with a licensed mental health provider

Nursing Interventions

- Administer medications as ordered.
- Explain tests and procedures.

(continued)

Nursing Interventions *(continued)*

- Give the patient the plan for the day.
- Provide therapeutic communication.

Patient Education

- Take medications as prescribed.
- Use meditation to help achieve a calm feeling.
- Work with a mental health professional.

BRAIN TUMORS

Overview

- A *brain tumor* is a growth in the cranial cavity.
- Brain tumors can cause serious symptoms as they compress or destroy brain tissue.
- They can be benign or malignant, but symptoms are similar for both.

Signs and Symptoms

- Confusion
- Dizziness
- Headache
- Increased ICP
- Nausea
- Personality changes
- Seizures
- Varying symptoms depending on location of tumor
- Vomiting
- Visual deficits

Diagnosis

Labs

- BMP to monitor electrolytes
- CBC to monitor hydration and for bleeding disorder

Diagnostic Testing

- Brain MRI
- EEG if seizures are present
- Head CT scan

Treatment

- Chemotherapy, if malignant
- Medications to reduce ICP
- Radiation
- Surgical resection

Nursing Interventions

- Administer medications as ordered.
- Assess neurologic function.
- Assess for signs of increased ICP:
  - Blurred vision
  - Change in mental status

COMPLICATIONS

Complications of brain tumors vary widely based on the type and location of the tumor; however, the complications can be very serious and include seizures; vision loss; and increased risk of thromboembolism leading to DVT, PE, CVA, permanent disability, and death.

(continued)

Nursing Interventions *(continued)*

- Headache
- Vomiting
- Weakness
- Maintain seizure precautions.
- Monitor vital signs.

Patient Education

- Eat small, frequent meals to maintain nutrition.
- Exercise as tolerated.
- Increase activity gradually.
- Stop driving unless asymptomatic.
- Take prescribed medications as instructed.

DELIRIUM

Overview

- Delirium can present as cognitive deficits, memory loss, disorientation, or sensory disturbances in patients.
- Delirium can be hyperactive or hypoactive. It can also present with both types of symptoms.
- Patients who are experiencing severe illness and prolonged hospitalization are at risk for delirium.

Signs and Symptoms

- Behavioral changes
- New-onset disorientation in an otherwise oriented patient

Diagnosis

Labs
- CBC to determine if an infectious process is contributing to delirium
- CMP to determine if electrolyte imbalance or liver dysfunction is contributing to delirium
- Drug and alcohol levels to determine if they are contributing to delirium
- Thyroid function tests
- UA to determine if patient has infection that may be contributing to delirium

Diagnostic Testing
- Confusion assessment method tool to screen for delirium
- CT scan to rule out stroke

Treatment

- Medications to treat symptoms of delirium and underlying illness
- Regular sleep/wake cycles

Nursing Interventions

- Administer medications as ordered.
- Limit medications such as opioids and benzodiazepines.

 COMPLICATIONS

Hospital-associated delirium often increases length of stay for hospitalized patients as well as increases their risk of medical complications such as aspiration pneumonia, pressure injuries, and CAUTI. They are also at higher risk for falls and long-term cognitive impairment.

 NURSING PEARL

Mnemonic for causes of delirium:

Dementia, dehydration
Electrolyte imbalances, emotional stress
Liver failure, low oxygen
Infection, intensive care unit
Rx drugs, retention (urinary)
Injury, immobility, infection
Untreated pain, unfamiliar environment
Metabolic disorders

(continued)

Nursing Interventions *(continued)*

- Maintain appropriate sleep/wake cycles for the patient.
- Mobilize the patient during the day.
- Provide a safe environment for the patient.
- Provide devices such as hearing and vision aids.
- Reorient the patient.

Patient Education

- Maintain regular sleep/wake cycles.
- Monitor wounds for signs and symptoms of infection.
- Seek medical assistance for UTIs or other infections.

POP QUIZ 11.1

A patient has been in the hospital for hip surgery for 3 days and has a history of early dementia. The patient still works a full-time job as a cashier and does volunteer work. The patient is reporting seeing bugs on the wall and is speaking incoherently. Their family member says, "I did not think their dementia would progress so quickly." How will the nurse respond?

DEMENTIA

Overview

- *Dementia* is characterized by cognitive decline, including memory loss, personality changes, difficulty with abstract thinking, difficulty recalling words, and difficulty with ADLs.
- Patients with dementia are at increased risk of developing delirium in the setting of serious illness and lengthy hospital stay.

Signs and Symptoms

- Aggression
- Communication difficulty
- Difficulty with ADLs
- Forgetfulness
- Hallucinations
- Memory loss
- Mood changes
- Self-neglect
- Social withdrawal

COMPLICATIONS

Complications of dementia include frequent UTIs, aspiration pneumonia, falls and associated injuries, dehydration, and malnutrition. Patients with dementia may not be able to recognize or verbalize when they are not feeling well or are hungry or thirsty. Careful monitoring of these patients is essential to catch early signs of infection or other illness.

Diagnosis

Labs

- CMP to rule out electrolyte imbalance
- Thyroid tests to determine if hypothyroidism is contributing to dementia
- UA to determine if infection is underlying cause of symptoms
- Vitamin B12 to determine if deficiency is contributing to symptoms

Diagnostic Testing

- CT scan to help diagnose later stages of disease
- EEG to help diagnose later stages of disease
- MRI to help diagnose later stages of disease
- PET scan to measure metabolic activity for early diagnosis

Treatment

- Avoidance of alcohol, opiates, and benzodiazepines
- Daily exercise
- Maintenance of regular sleep/wake cycles
- Medications such as antidepressants, antipsychotics, cholinesterase inhibitors, and NMDA agonists for symptom management (see Appendix 11.1)
- Pain control

Nursing Interventions

- Administer medications as ordered.
- Balance pain control with oversedation from opiates.
- Encourage sleep at night.
- Mobilize the patient during the day.
- Reorient the patient.

Patient Education

- Avoid sleeping during the day.
- Maintain activity during the day.
- Reduce clutter and distractions in the home.
- Take medications as instructed.
- Use memory aids such as pill organizers and picture books as needed.

DEPRESSION

Overview

- *Depression* is a mental health disorder characterized by extreme loss of interest in activities and depressed mood.

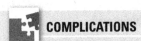 **COMPLICATIONS**

Complications of depression include unintentional weight gain or loss, worsening of physical illness, misuse of alcohol, drug use, self-harm, and suicide or suicide attempts.

Signs and Symptoms

- Agitation
- Fatigue
- Feelings of sadness, emptiness, or hopelessness
- Feelings of worthlessness or guilt
- Frequent or recurrent thoughts of death or thoughts of suicide
- Irritability
- Loss of interest in normal activities
- Reduced appetite or increased food cravings
- Restlessness
- Sleep disturbances, including insomnia or sleeping too much
- Trouble thinking, concentrating, making decisions, and remembering things
- Unexplained physical problems, such as back pain or headaches

Diagnosis

Labs

- CBC to determine anemia or infection
- CMP to determine electrolyte imbalances
- Thyroid function tests to determine if underlying hypothyroidism is contributing
- Vitamin B12 and folate levels to determine if low levels are contributing
- Toxicology studies

Diagnostic Testing

- CT scan or MRI to evaluate for underlying cause

Treatment

- Counseling with a mental health professional
- Medications such as SSRIs and SNRIs (see Appendix 11.1)

Nursing Interventions

- Administer medications as ordered.
- Assess for suicidal ideation.
- Maintain patient safety.
- Provide therapeutic communications.

Patient Education

- Be patient; many medications take weeks to begin working.
- Dial 911 if having suicidal thoughts or thoughts of self-harm and are unable to contact the provider or mental health professional.
- Notify provider, mental health professional, or a trusted friend or family member if having thoughts of self-harm or suicide.
- Take medications as instructed.

 ALERT!

If a depressed patient expresses suicidal ideation, call 911 or seek emergency assistance immediately.

ENCEPHALITIS

Overview

- *Encephalitis* is an acute and severe inflammation of the brain.
- Cerebral edema caused by inflammation causes degeneration of the brain's ganglion cells and nerve cells.
- Causes of encephalitis include adenoviruses, amoebic infection, arboviruses, enteroviruses, HIV, herpes simplex virus, mumps, and measles.

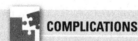 **COMPLICATIONS**

Complications of encephalitis include paralysis, seizures, mental status changes, parkinsonism, and death.

Signs and Symptoms

- Altered LOC
- Confusion
- Fever
- Headache
- Malaise
- Muscle stiffness
- Myalgias
- Photophobia
- Seizures

Diagnosis

Labs

- CBC to assess for increased WBC count
- CSF culture
- CSF testing for increased WBC, increased protein, and decreased glucose
- Serum antibodies to assess for specific causative agents

Diagnostic Testing
- Brain MRI to assess for inflammation
- EEG to show changes if encephalitis is present

Treatment

- Treatment focused on identifying and treating the underlying cause of encephalitis and decreasing ICP
- Possible transfer to higher level of care for close monitoring of neurologic status and ICP

Nursing Interventions

- Administer medications as ordered.
- Monitor for signs and symptoms of increasing ICP, such as aphasia, behavioral changes, blurred vision, decreased LOC, new or worsening headache, nausea, vomiting, and weakness.
- Provide a quiet, low-stimulation environment.
- Provide nonopioid analgesics, PRN, if ordered.

Patient Education

- Do not share needles.
- Follow local guidelines to avoid mosquito- and tick-borne illnesses.
- Practice safe sex.
- Stay up to date on vaccinations.
- Take medications as prescribed.

GUILLAIN–BARRÉ SYNDROME

Overview

- *Guillain–Barré syndrome* is an acute, progressive form of polyneuritis.
- It is almost always preceded by a viral infection.
- It is an autoimmune condition resulting in damage to peripheral nerve myelin resulting in demyelination of the peripheral and cranial nerves.

COMPLICATIONS

Complications of Guillain–Barré syndrome include paralysis, permanent muscle weakness, contractures, muscle wasting, respiratory distress, cardiac compromise, and death.

Signs and Symptoms

- Difficulty swallowing
- Difficulty talking
- Diminished deep tendon reflexes
- Loss of proprioception
- Minor febrile illness in the weeks leading up to presentation
- Paralysis of facial and oropharynx musculature
- Paralysis progressing to nerves in thorax creating respiratory distress
- Paresthesia and weakness starting in the legs and progressing up the body
- Stiffness in the legs

Diagnosis

Labs
- CSF to show increased protein levels and low blood cell count

Diagnostic Testing
- EMG
- Evoked potential studies showing decreased nerve conduction velocity

Treatment

- Intubation and hemodynamic support, requiring transfer to a higher level of care
- Plasmapheresis
- Supportive care

Nursing Interventions

- Administer oxygen to maintain oxygen saturation greater than 92%.
- Insert NGT, if ordered.
- Monitor the patient's cardiac status.
- Monitor the patient's respiratory status.
- Provide adequate nutrition.
- Provide range-of-motion exercises to reduce contractures and muscle wasting.
- Reposition the patient to prevent pressure injuries.
- Use alternative means of communication, such as nodding or blinking if the patient is aphasic.

Patient Education

- Do not drive until cleared by provider.
- Exercise as tolerated.
- Notify provider right away of symptoms such as increasing numbness or weakness, loss of bowel or bladder function, changes in vision, or dizziness.
- Participate in physical, occupational, and speech therapies.
- Set up the home environment to reduce the risk of falls.

INCREASED INTRACRANIAL PRESSURE

Overview

- *ICP* is the pressure inside the cranial cavity.
- ICP increases when there is an increased volume of cerebral blood flow, brain tissue, or CSF for which the body cannot regulate.
- The body's autoregulatory processes regulate ICP by increasing or decreasing cerebral blood flow and CSF production and absorption.
- Factors that affect ICP include tumors, cerebral edema, bleeding, or blockage of CSF.

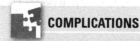

COMPLICATIONS

The complications of increased ICP are severe and include permanent brain damage, seizures, stroke, and death.

Signs and Symptoms

- Altered LOC
- Change in respiratory patterns
- Cushing's triad (bradycardia, bradypnea, and hypertension)
- Headache
- Nausea
- Pupillary changes
- Seizures
- Vomiting
- Widening pulse pressures

Diagnosis

Labs

- BMP for electrolyte disturbances
- Coagulation panel
- Magnesium

(continued)

Labs *(continued)*

- Osmolality
- Urine output to detect DI or SIADH

Diagnostic Testing
- Head CT
- ICP monitoring
- Skull x-ray

Treatment

- Hyperventilation therapy to increase carbon dioxide, which reduces cerebral edema
- Medications to treat underlying condition
- Medications such as diuretics (see Appendix 11.1) to decrease CSF
- Surgery to remove tumor or place shunt to increase CSF flow
- Higher level of care required for respiratory or cardiac distress

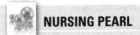

NURSING PEARL

Lumbar puncture is contraindicated in known or presumed increased ICP as it may cause a shift in CSF leading to brain herniation.

Nursing Interventions

- Assist patient to reposition in bed.
- Educate patient to not twist, move abruptly, or strain their muscles.
- Frequently monitor vital signs.
- Infuse medications slowly to allow the body time to adjust to increased volume.
- Maintain a calm and quiet environment.
- Monitor for increased ICP.
- Monitor I/O.
- Monitor neurologic status.
- Provide bed rest, with HOB elevated to greater than 30 degrees.

Patient Education

- Avoid extreme flexing or extending of the neck.
- Avoid straining when moving or having a bowel movement.
- Maintain a calm, quiet environment.
- Notify the provider immediately if changes such as worsening headache, nausea, or weakness occur.
- Remain on bedrest.

MENINGITIS

Overview

- *Meningitis* is an inflammation of the meninges (the membranous layers that surround the brain) or the subarachnoid space.
- It can be septic, which is caused by a bacterial infection, or aseptic, which is caused by a viral infection.
- Common microorganisms that cause meningitis include *Neisseria meningitidis, Haemophilus influenza, Streptococcus pneumoniae,* and *Mycobacterium tuberculosis.*

Signs and Symptoms

- Altered LOC
- Brudzinski's sign
- Fever
- Headache
- Irritability

(continued)

Signs and Symptoms *(continued)*

- Kernig's sign
- Malaise
- Myalgias
- Nausea
- Seizures
- Vomiting

NURSING PEARL

Brudzinski's sign is characterized by flexion and adduction of the leg when the neck is flexed. Kernig's sign is characterized by resistance to extension when the thigh is flexed upward toward the torso.

Diagnosis

Labs

- Blood culture to identify causative organism
- CSF to identify causative organism

Diagnostic Testing

- Lumbar puncture to determine causative organism

Treatment

- Antiepileptic medications (see Appendix 11.1) to reduce chance of seizures
- Medications to treat underlying illness, such as antibiotics for bacterial infection
- Nonopioid analgesics
- Supportive care

Nursing Interventions

- Isolate patient with droplet precautions until causative agent is identified.
- Monitor I/O, as overhydration can lead to increased ICP.
- Monitor vital signs.
- Perform frequent neurologic examinations.

Patient Education

- Avoid bright lights.
- Avoid contact with people who are sick.
- Maintain a calm, quiet environment.
- Notify nurse or provider if symptoms worsen.
- Take analgesics and antipyretics as needed.
- Take medications as instructed.
- Wash hands frequently.

MULTIPLE SCLEROSIS

Overview

- *MS* is characterized by destruction of the myelin sheaths that cover nerves.
- It is a progressive neurologic illness.
- Areas of demyelination (known as plaques) can occur in any body part but are most common on the white matter of the brain and spinal cord and on the optic nerves.
- The exact cause is unknown; it is thought to be linked to an autoimmune cause or a progressive viral illness.

COMPLICATIONS

The complications of MS include muscle stiffness, muscle spasms, depression, irritability, paralysis of the legs, forgetfulness, and difficulties with bowel or bladder function.

Signs and Symptoms

- Bowel problems ranging from constipation to fecal incontinence

(continued)

Signs and Symptoms *(continued)*

- Cognitive and/or emotional changes
- Fatigue
- Hyperreflexia
- Muscle weakness and spasticity
- Numbness and tingling in the extremities
- Urinary problems ranging from retention to incontinence
- Visual changes such as blurred vision or double vision

Diagnosis

Labs

- CSF: will have elevated proteins in MS

Diagnostic Testing

- Brain MRI to assess for plaques
- CT scan
- Evoked potentials to test nerve signals
- Lumbar puncture

Treatment

- Medications such as corticosteroids and muscle relaxants to reduce inflammation and spasticity
- Medications such as monoclonal antibodies, interferon beta 1b, and glatiramer acetate
- OT
- PT

Nursing Interventions

- Administer medications as ordered.
- Assist patient to reposition frequently to prevent pressure injuries.
- Encourage physical activity as tolerated.
- Encourage the patient to cough and deep breathe.

Patient Education

- Avoid constipation by eating a well-rounded, high-fiber diet.
- Avoid extreme heat and cold.
- Exercise as tolerated.
- Get plenty of rest.
- Notify healthcare provider if new or worsening symptoms occur.
- Take medications as instructed.
- Use mobility aids, such as a cane or walker, if needed.

MYASTHENIA GRAVIS

Overview

- *Myasthenia gravis* is an autoimmune neurologic condition characterized by muscle weakness with activity that is relieved by rest.
- The exact cause is unknown, but it is thought to be caused by acetylcholine deficiency or a defect in the postsynaptic receptor sites.

Signs and Symptoms

- Blank, expressionless face
- Difficulty chewing and swallowing

COMPLICATIONS

Complications of myasthenia gravis include myasthenia crisis with symptoms of respiratory distress, anxiety, fever, and difficulty swallowing. A cholinergic crisis may occur as a complication of anticholinesterase toxicity with symptoms including abdominal cramps, bradycardia, diarrhea, dyspnea, muscle cramps, sweating, vomiting, and respiratory distress.

(continued)

Signs and Symptoms *(continued)*

- Double vision
- Ptosis
- Skeletal muscle fatigue
- Skeletal muscle weakness relieved by rest
- Weak eye closure
- Weakened respiratory muscles

Diagnosis

Labs
- TSH

Diagnostic Testing
- Chest x-ray
- Edrophonium test
- EMG
- Neostigmine test
- Thymus scan to rule out thymoma or hyperplasia

 NURSING PEARL

In an edrophonium test, the patient is given edrophonium. The test is diagnostic for myasthenia gravis if the patient's muscles get stronger after administration of the medication. If the test is inconclusive, a neostigmine test will be performed.

Treatment

- Medications such as cholinesterase inhibitors, corticosteroids, and immunosuppressants for symptoms
- Plasmapheresis
- Thymectomy if thymoma or thymus hyperplasia is present

Nursing Interventions

- Allow for rest periods during ADLs.
- Assess for signs and symptoms of myasthenia crisis and cholinergic crisis.
- Encourage the patient to cough and deep breathe.
- Monitor the patient for decreased respiratory function.
- Provide a soft diet if the patient has difficulty chewing or swallowing.
- Schedule activities to occur after medications are given.

Patient Education

- Avoid strenuous exercise.
- Install grab bars in the bathroom for safety.
- Notify provider if starting any new medications or supplements.
- Plan activities for when energy level is high.
- Stay up to date with vaccines.
- Take medications as instructed.
- Use eye drops as instructed to treat dry eyes.
- Wash hands and avoid contact with sick people.
- Wear a medical ID bracelet.

PARKINSON'S DISEASE

Overview

- Parkinson's disease is associated with a decrease in the neurotransmitter dopamine.
- It is characterized by degeneration of the basal ganglia, substantia nigra, and corpus striatum of the brain.
- The exact cause is unknown; it is thought to be related to exposure to toxins, genetic factors, and arteriosclerotic changes.

Signs and Symptoms

- Blank, expressionless face
- Bradykinesia and, eventually, akinesia
- Decreased balance
- Decreased blinking
- Drooling
- Dysarthria
- Increased rigidity
- Pill-rolling tremors
- Poor posture
- Slow, shuffling gait
- Tremors

Diagnosis

Labs
There are no labs specific to diagnosing Parkinson's disease.

Diagnostic Testing
- CT scan or MRI to rule out stroke or tumor

Treatment

- Medications such as levodopa and anticholinergics
- PT

Nursing Interventions

- Administer medications as prescribed.
- Assist patient with mobility.
- Assist with ADLs as needed.

Patient Education

- Exercise as tolerated.
- Install grab bars in the bathroom for safety.
- Move slowly when changing positions.
- Set up the home to reduce fall risks by removing objects such as throw rugs.
- Take medications as prescribed.
- Use mobility aids, such as a cane or walker, as needed.

SEIZURE DISORDERS

Overview

- A *seizure* is caused by a sudden electrical discharge of a group of neurons.
- Seizures can be idiopathic or triggered by toxins, electrolyte imbalances, tumors, hypoxia, inflammation, or increased ICP.
- A seizure can be generalized (involving the entire brain) or partial (involving a part of the brain).
- There are three phases to a seizure:
  - The *prodromal phase* may occur hours or days before the seizure. It includes the aural phase, which happens just before the seizure begins and consists of auras such as a flash of light, mood changes, or sudden changes in smell or taste.
  - The *ictal phase* is the seizure activity itself.
  - The *postictal phase* occurs after the seizure and may include amnesia, confusion, fatigue, and difficulty arousing the patient.

Signs and Symptoms

There are many types of seizures with varying symptoms, as shown in Table 11.1.

Table 11.1 Types of Seizures	
Generalized Seizures	**Description**
Grand mal (tonic-clonic)	Convulsions, muscle rigidity, unconsciousness
Absence	Brief loss of consciousness
Myoclonic	Isolated, sporadic jerking movements
Clonic	Repetitive jerking movements
Tonic	Muscle stiffness and rigidity
Atonic	Loss of muscle tone
Partial Seizures	**Description**
Simple motor	Awareness is retained; jerking, muscle rigidity, spasms, head turning
Simple sensory	Awareness is retained; unusual sensory disturbances
Simple psychologic	Awareness is retained; memory or emotional disturbances
Complex	Awareness is lost; lip smacking; chewing; fidgeting; walking or other repetitive and involuntary, but coordinated, movements

Diagnosis

Labs
- CBC
- CMP to evaluate liver and kidney function
- CSF culture to rule out infection
- UA to rule out metabolic disorders

Diagnostic Testing
- Brain MRI
- Cerebral angiography
- EEG
- Head CT
- Lumbar puncture
- MEG

Treatment

- Medications such as anticonvulsants to prevent seizures
- Surgical resection of focal area if seizures are not responsive to medication
- Surgical resection of tumors

Nursing Interventions

- Administer benzodiazepines IV/IM if ordered by provider (see Appendix 11.1).
- Document observations such as length of seizure, type of movements, and postictal response.

(continued)

Nursing Interventions *(continued)*

- Ensure a safe environment for the patient by padding bed rails.
- Prepare to suction and/or administer oxygen if indicated.
- Protect the patient during a seizure.
- Time the patient's seizures.
- Turn the patient onto their side to protect the airway during seizure.

Patient Education

- Avoid alcohol.
- Avoid any known triggers, such as flashing lights.
- Avoid nicotine.
- Do not drive unless cleared to do so by the provider.
- Take medications as prescribed.

 POP QUIZ 11.2

A patient with a history of seizures has been admitted to the medical-surgical unit after orthopedic surgery. The patient begins to jerk and twitch but is alert. What actions should the nurse take?

SPINAL CORD INJURY

Overview

- Spinal cord injury usually results from trauma to the spinal column, which then damages the spinal cord.
- Spinal cord injury can be complete or incomplete. In a complete spinal cord injury, all voluntary motor function and sensation is lost below the level of the injury. An incomplete injury to the spinal cord leaves varying levels of motor and sensory function intact.

Signs And Symptoms

- Decreased balance
- Difficulty breathing or coughing
- Difficulty walking
- Exaggerated reflex activities or spasms
- Extreme back, neck, or head pain
- Loss of bowel or bladder control
- Loss of movement
- Loss of sensation
- Numbness and tingling
- Weakness
- Varying signs and symptoms depending on level of injury (Figure 11.1)

Diagnosis

Labs
There are no labs specific to diagnosing spinal cord injuries.

Diagnostic Testing
- CT scan
- MRI
- Spinal x-ray

Treatment

- Compression stockings to reduce DVT risk and improve venous return
- Immobilization of the spine
- Medications such as analgesics and muscle relaxants to control pain and spasms
- Surgical repair of fractures
- Surgical resection of tumors
- Higher level of care as required

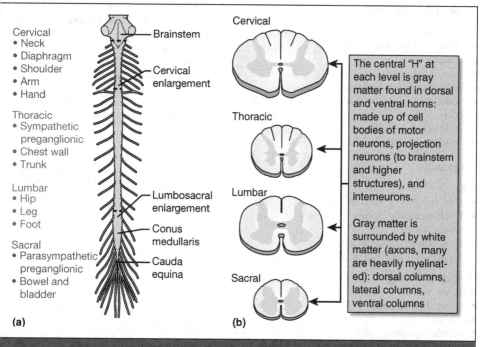

Cervical
• Neck
• Diaphragm
• Shoulder
• Arm
• Hand

Brainstem

Cervical enlargement

Thoracic
• Sympathetic preganglionic
• Chest wall
• Trunk

Lumbar
• Hip
• Leg
• Foot

Lumbosacral enlargement

Conus medullaris

Sacral
• Parasympathetic preganglionic
• Bowel and bladder

Cauda equina

(a)

Cervical

Thoracic

Lumbar

Sacral

(b)

The central "H" at each level is gray matter found in dorsal and ventral horns: made up of cell bodies of motor neurons, projection neurons (to brainstem and higher structures), and interneurons.

Gray matter is surrounded by white matter (axons, many are heavily myelinated): dorsal columns, lateral columns, ventral columns

Figure 11.1 Spinal cord regions and the areas of the body they control.

Source: Tkacs, N., Herrmann, L., & Johnson, R. (2020). *Advanced physiology and pathophysiology: Essentials for clinical practice.* Springer Publishing Company.

Nursing Interventions

- Administer medications as ordered.
- Educate the patient on bowel and bladder management.
- Encourage the patient to cough and deep breathe.
- Monitor neurologic status frequently and report changes to the provider immediately.
- Reposition the patient frequently to prevent pressure ulcers.

Patient Education

- Follow a daily bowel program.
- Modify home for safe transfers and mobility.
  Participate in PT and OT.
- Reposition frequently to prevent pressure injuries and skin breakdown.
- Self-catheterize if needed.
- Take medications as instructed.
- Use mobility devices as instructed.

 POP QUIZ 11.3

A patient with paraplegia who has a history of a spinal cord injury has no sensation or motor control below the level of the trunk. What area of the patient's spine was damaged?

STROKE

Overview

- A *stroke* results from disruption in cerebral blood flow caused by occlusion or hemorrhage.
- An *ischemic stroke* is caused by a thrombus or embolus occluding blood flow.
- A *hemorrhagic stroke* occurs when a blood vessel in the brain ruptures.

Signs and Symptoms

- Confusion
- Difficulty speaking
- Dizziness
- Loss of balance
- Sudden difficulty walking
- Sudden numbness or weakness on one side of the body
- Sudden severe headache
- Sudden vision changes

Diagnosis

Labs

- CBC to rule out infectious process
- CMP, especially glucose, as hypoglycemia can mimic a stroke
- Coagulation studies to guide treatment
- Lipid profile to guide treatment

Diagnostic Testing

- Brain MRI
- Carotid ultrasound
- CT scan
- Cerebral arteriography

Treatment

- Analgesics for treatment of headaches (see Table A.2)
- Carotid endarterectomy to remove plaques
- Medications such as antiepileptics (see Appendix 11.1), antihypertensives, and diuretics (see Appendix 11.1)
- PT and OT
- Thrombolytics such as tPA (see Appendix 11.1) given within 3 hours of the onset of symptoms of ischemic stroke to break up clots

Nursing Interventions

- Assist the patient to maintain good hydration and nutrition.
- Assist with ROM to decrease contractures and muscle wasting.
- Call for emergency assistance immediately if a stroke is suspected.
- Frequently assess neurologic status.
- Frequently assess vital signs.
- Position the patient on their side to prevent aspiration.
- Protect the patient's airway.
- Reposition the patient to reduce pressure injuries.

Patient Education

- Allow plenty of time to complete activities.
- Avoid clothing with buttons and zippers.
- Control hypertension, diabetes, and hyperlipidemia.

NURSING PEARL

Use the mnemonic FAST to remember how to quickly assess for stroke:

- **F**ace: Ask the patient to smile. Does one side of their face droop?
- **A**rms: Ask the patient to hold both arms out at shoulder height. Does one arm drift down?
- **S**peech: Ask the patient to repeat a simple phrase. Is their speech slurred or unintelligible?
- **T**ime: When was the patient's "last known normal"?

POP QUIZ 11.4

A patient on the medical-surgical unit has been admitted with hyperglycemia and cellulitis. The nurse gives the patient their medications at 10 p.m. When the nurse checks on the patient at midnight, they note that the patient is sleeping with even respirations. At 6 a.m., the nurse arouses the patient for morning medications and notices that the right side of their face is drooping and their speech is slurred. The nurse immediately calls for emergency assistance. Given the time frame of the events, is this patient eligible for tPA? Why or why not?

(continued)

Patient Education *(continued)*

- Install grab bars in the bathroom for safety, and use a shower seat if needed.
- Take medications as prescribed.
- Use mobility devices such as a cane or walker, if needed.
- Work with physical, occupational, and speech therapy.

TRANSIENT ISCHEMIC ATTACK

Overview

- A *TIA* is a temporary, short event with symptoms that are similar to a stroke.
- A TIA lasts only a few minutes, but it can be a precursor to a stroke.

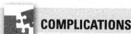 **COMPLICATIONS**

About a third of patients who experience a TIA will go on to have a stroke. Of those, about half of strokes will occur within a year of the TIA. Prompt medical attention is required to reduce the chances of progressing to a stroke.

Signs and Symptoms

- Changes in vision
- Dizziness
- Loss of balance
- Slurred or garbled speech
- Vertigo
- Weakness, numbness, or paralysis on one side of the body

Diagnosis

Labs
- Blood glucose or HbA1C to assess for diabetes, which can contribute to TIA risk
- Lipid panel to assess underlying cause of TIA

Diagnostic Testing
- Brain MRI
- Carotid ultrasound
- CT angiography

Treatment

- Medications to reduce clots, such as antiplatelets and anticoagulants (see Appendix 11.1)
- Medications to control underlying diseases that increase risk of TIA, such as hypertension, diabetes, and hyperlipidemia

Nursing Interventions

- Call for emergency assistance immediately, as TIA and stroke symptoms are similar.
- Give medications as prescribed.
- Keep the patient safe by assisting them to sit or lie down.
- Monitor vital signs.
- Perform serial neurologic exams to assess for changes.

Patient Education

- Control blood glucose.
- Exercise regularly.
- Limit alcohol intake.
- Limit cholesterol and fat intake.
- Participate in substance use treatment and/or counseling, if indicated.
- Stop smoking, if applicable.
- Take medications as prescribed, especially for hypertension and hyperlipidemia.

TRAUMATIC BRAIN INJURY

Overview

- TBI encompasses all injuries to the brain, from mild concussions to life-threatening brain injuries.

Signs and Symptoms

- Agitation
- Bradycardia
- Confusion
- Decerebrate or decorticate posturing
- Headache
- Lethargy
- LOC
- Neurologic deficits
- Pupillary changes
- Reduced LOC
- Restlessness
- Seizures
- Vomiting
- Widened pulse pressures

Diagnosis

Labs
There are no labs specific to diagnosing TBI.

Diagnostic Testing
- Brain MRI
- CT scan
- ICP monitoring
- Skull x-ray

Treatment

- Medications to decrease ICP and blood pressure
- Surgical evacuation of hematomas
- Surgical repair of fractures
- Higher level of care if needed

Nursing Interventions

- Administer medications as ordered.
- Monitor for signs and symptoms of increased ICP.
- Monitor I/O.
- Monitor neurologic status.
- Monitor vital signs.

Patient Education

- Avoid activities that make symptoms worse.
- Be patient with recovery.
- Do not return to sports until cleared by provider.
- Follow dietary recommendations for safe swallowing.
- Participate in PT, OT, and speech therapy, if needed.
- Take medications as instructed.
- Use mobility devices as needed.

Appendix 11.1 Neurologic System Medications

Indications	Mechanism of Action	Contraindications, Precautions, and Adverse Effects
Anxiolytics (benzodiazepines)		
• Management of anxiety • Treatment of seizure emergencies	• Benzodiazepines: depress CNS by potentiating GABA	• Contraindications include CNS depression, uncontrolled pain, pregnancy, lactation, grapefruit juice consumption, and concurrent use with MAOIs. • Use caution in patients with hepatic and renal impairment, pulmonary disease, or history of substance use, and in patients who are currently suicidal. • Adverse effects include respiratory depression, apnea, cardiac arrest, dizziness, and drowsiness.
Antidepressants (SSRIs, tricyclic antidepressants, SNRIs)		
• Treatment and management of depression; adjunctive treatment of anxiety conditions, chronic pain syndromes	• SSRIs: inhibit reuptake of serotonin in the CNS, potentiating the activity of serotonin • MAOIs: inhibit the enzyme monoamine oxidase, resulting in the accumulation of dopamine, epinephrine, norepinephrine, and serotonin	• Contraindications for SSRIs include pregnancy, lactation, bleeding disorders, epilepsy, and kidney, liver, or heart disease. • Contraindications for tricyclic antidepressants include QTc interval prolongation, family history of sudden cardiac death, seizure disorder, and closed-angle glaucoma. • Contraindications of MAOIs include severe renal, cardiovascular, or cerebrovascular disease, uncontrolled hypertension; CHF; concurrent drug use with SSRI, SNRIs, tricyclic antidepressants, and other medications. • Use caution in preexisting cardiovascular disease. • SSRIs have adverse effects including suicidal thoughts, neuroleptic malignant syndrome, anxiety, drowsiness, headache, weakness, and insomnia. • MAOIs have adverse effects including hypertension, seizure, ED, weight gain, nausea, vomiting, anxiety, and agitation.

(continued)

Appendix 11.1 Neurologic System Medications *(continued)*

Indications	Mechanism of Action	Contraindications, Precautions, and Adverse Effects
Antipsychotics (haloperidol, risperidone)		
• Acute and/or chronic psychosis	• Block dopamine receptors in the brain and alter dopamine release and turnover	• Contraindications include closed-angle glaucoma, head trauma, and CNS depression. • Use caution in impaired temperature regulation, cardiac disease, diabetes, respiratory insufficiency, and seizure disorder. • Adverse effects include dyskinesias, vital sign changes, and changes in LOC.
Antiplatelets (aspirin, clopidogrel)		
• For use during suspected embolic/ischemic stroke	• Prevent platelet aggregation and clot formation	• Contraindications include hypersensitivity, bleeding, and hepatic disorders. • Use caution in uncontrolled bleeding, recent surgery, alcohol misuse, and GI bleeding/ulcerative disease. • Adverse effects include generalized bleeding, GI bleeding, and Stevens–Johnson syndrome (aspirin).
Anticoagulants (enoxaparin, heparin)		
• Treatment and prophylaxis of thromboembolic disorders	• Prevent growth of existing thrombus • Prevent formation of new thrombus	• Contraindications include uncontrolled bleeding and severe thrombocytopenia. • Use caution in renal or hepatic disease, GI bleed/ulcerative disease, head injury, or bleeding disorders. • Adverse effects include bleeding.
Fibrinolytic therapy (tPA)		
• Known clot in ischemic stroke	• Breaks up and dissolves clot	• Contraindications include active internal bleeding (hemorrhagic stroke), history of CVA, recent surgery, bleeding disorders, and uncontrolled hypertension. • Use caution in patients with recent surgery or trauma, severe hepatic or renal disease, and concurrent anticoagulation therapy. • Adverse effects include generalized risk for bleeding, most notably in intracranial hemorrhage, GI bleeding, and retroperitoneal bleeding.

(continued)

Appendix 11.1 Neurologic System Medications *(continued)*

Indications	Mechanism of Action	Contraindications, Precautions, and Adverse Effects
Antiepileptics (levetiracetam, phenytoin)		
• Seizure prevention	• Decrease excitation, enhance inhibition of neurons, and/or alter electrical activity by affecting ion channels in cell membrane	• Adverse effects include CNS depression, drowsiness, diplopia, ataxia, nystagmus, cognitive function changes, and rash.
Osmotic diuretics (mannitol)		
• Reduce cerebral edema in increased ICP	• Inhibit tubular reabsorption of water and increase sodium and chloride excretion by increasing osmolarity and GFR	• Medication is contraindicated in active intercranial bleed. • Use caution in patients with HF, renal failure, cardiac or respiratory disease, pneumothorax, or surgery. • Adverse effects include seizure, coma, hyperkalemia, pulmonary edema, HF, and cardiac arrest.

RESOURCES

Lewis, S. L., Dirksen, S. R., Heitkemper, M. M., Bucher, L., & Harding, M. M. (2017). *Medical-surgical nursing: Assessment and management of clinical problems* (10th ed.). Elsevier.

Longe, J. L (Ed.). (2018). *The Gale encyclopedia of nursing and allied health* (4th ed.). Gale. https://link.gale.com/apps/pub/07UZ/GVRL?u=kcls_main&sid=GVRL

Prescribers' Digital Reference. (n.d.[a]). *Activase (alteplase)* [Drug information]. https://www.pdr.net/drug-summary/Activase-alteplase-1332.3358

Prescribers' Digital Reference. (n.d.[b]). *Coumadin (warfarin sodium)* [Drug information]. https://www.pdr.net/drug-summary/Coumadin-warfarin-sodium-106

Prescribers' Digital Reference. (n.d.[c]). *Depakote Tablets (divalproex sodium)* [Drug information]. https://www.pdr.net/drug-summary/Depakote-Tablets-divalproex-sodium-1075.5693

Prescribers' Digital Reference. (n.d.[d]). *Haldol (haloperidol)* [Drug information]. https://www.pdr.net/drug-summary/Haldol-haloperidol-942.4581

Prescribers' Digital Reference. (n.d.[e]). *Heparin Sodium Injection (heparin sodium)* [Drug information]. https://www.pdr.net/drug-summary/Heparin-Sodium-Injection-heparin-sodium-1263.107

Prescribers' Digital Reference. (n.d.[f]). *Keppra Injection (levetiracetam)* [Drug information]. https://www.pdr.net/drug-summary/Keppra-Injection-levetiracetam-1055.6058

Prescribers' Digital Reference. (n.d.[g]). *Lovenox (enoxaparin sodium)* [Drug information]. https://www.pdr.net/drug-summary/Lovenox-enoxaparin-sodium-521.2354

Prescribers' Digital Reference. (n.d.[h]). *Osmitrol (mannitol)* [Drug information]. https://www.pdr.net/drug-summary/Osmitrol-mannitol-1149

Prescribers' Digital Reference. (n.d.[i]). *Plavix (clopidogrel bisulfate)* [Drug information]. https://www.pdr.net/drug-summary/Plavix-clopidogrel-bisulfate-525.3952

Prescribers' Digital Reference. (n.d.[j]). *Phenytoin Sodium Injection (phenytoin sodium)* [Drug information]. https://www.pdr.net/drug-summary/Phenytoin-Sodium-Injection-phenytoin-sodium-1151.8322

Prescribers' Digital Reference. (n.d.[k]). *Risperdal (risperidone)* [Drug information]. https://www.pdr.net/drug-summary/Risperdal-risperidone-977

Tkacs, N., Herrmann, L., & Johnson, R. (2020). *Advanced physiology and pathophysiology: Essentials for clinical practice.* Springer Publishing Company.

12
PULMONARY SYSTEM

ACUTE RESPIRATORY DISTRESS SYNDROME

Overview

- *ARDS* is a severe lung injury that occurs when the lungs cannot maintain balance between oxygen and carbon dioxide.
- ARDS occurs as the result of diffuse alveolar damage.
- Capillaries leak, causing edema, which leads to decreased blood flow to the lungs and platelet aggregation.

Signs and Symptoms

- Accessory muscle use
- Crepitus
- Cyanosis
- Decreased breathing sounds
- Diaphoresis
- Dyspnea
- Hypertension
- Increased respiratory effort
- Restlessness
- Tachycardia
- Tachypnea
- Thick, frothy sputum
- Worsening hypoxemia despite oxygen treatment

Diagnosis

Labs

- ABG to assess respiratory status and compensation
- BMP to assess kidney and liver function
- CBC to assess the presence of leukocytosis

Diagnostic Testing

- Bronchoscopy
- Chest CT
- Chest x-ray
- Echocardiogram

Treatment

- Medications (e.g., antibiotics) to treat underlying illness
- Medications such as steroids and diuretics to treat symptoms
- Supplemental oxygen
- Transfer to higher level of care for advanced care, if needed

COMPLICATIONS

Complications of ARDS include increased risk of pneumonia, especially if the patient is mechanically ventilated; permanent lung damage; pneumothorax; and increased risk of blood clots.

Nursing Interventions

- Administer medications as ordered.
- Assist patient to obtain adequate nutrition.
- Assist with CPT to loosen secretions.
- Educate patient on coughing and deep breathing to maximize lung expansion.
- Frequently reposition patient to prevent skin breakdown and pressure injuries.
- Monitor fluid intake and output to monitor effectiveness of diuretic therapy.
- Place patient in semi-Fowler's position to improve oxygenation.
- Provide supplemental oxygen to maintain SpO_2 greater than 92%.

Patient Education

- Cough and deep breathe at least hourly.
- Eat small meals throughout the day.
- Maintain an upright position with the HOB elevated greater than 30 degrees.
- Reposition frequently.
- Take medications as prescribed.
- Use devices such as CPAP and BiPAP as needed.

ASTHMA

Overview

- *Asthma* is a chronic inflammatory disorder of the airways.
- Asthma attacks can be triggered by a variety of sources, including allergens, smoke, cold air, viral respiratory infections, and sinusitis.
- Severe asthma attacks can result in airway constriction caused by bronchoconstriction, hyper-reactivity, and edema (Figure 12.1).

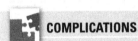 **COMPLICATIONS**

Over time, chronic airway inflammation in severe asthma can lead to airway remodeling. It leads to bronchial wall thickening and narrowing of the air passages. Airway remodeling makes breathing more difficult. Severe asthma attacks can lead to respiratory failure and death.

Signs and Symptoms

- Accessory muscle use
- Anxiety
- Audible wheezing
- Chest tightness
- Cyanosis
- Decreased breath sounds
- Dyspnea
- Hypoxia
- Increased work of breathing
- Tachycardia
- Tachypnea

Diagnosis

Labs

- ABG to assess respiratory status
- CBC with differential to assess eosinophils, which are elevated in asthma
- IgE levels: elevated in an asthma attack

Diagnostic Testing

- Chest x-ray
- Pulmonary function test

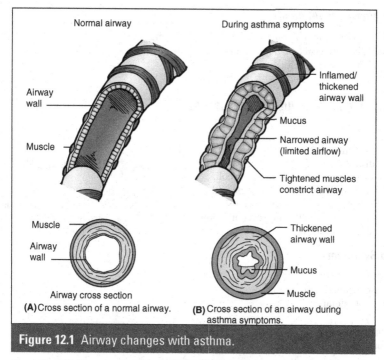

Figure 12.1 Airway changes with asthma.

Source: Tkacs, N., Herrmann, L., & Johnson, R. (2020). *Advanced physiology and pathophysiology essentials for clinical practice.* Springer Publishing Company.

Treatment

- Medications such as bronchodilators (see Appendix 12.1 located at the end of this chapter) and corticosteroids (see Table A.4)
- Supplemental oxygen

Nursing Interventions

- Administer medications as ordered.
- Administer supplemental oxygen to maintain SpO_2 greater than 92%.
- Assist patient to identify triggers.
- Educate patient and caregiver on:
  - Correct use of inhalers and spacers
  - Importance of having an asthma action plan
  - Use of a peak flow meter
- Encourage pursed-lip breathing.
- Monitor for respiratory status changes.
- Place the patient in high Fowler's position.

Patient Education

- Avoid secondhand smoke.
- Avoid contact with people who are sick.
- Identify and avoid asthma triggers.
- Receive all recommended vaccinations, including the annual flu vaccine.

 POP QUIZ 12.1

A patient is admitted to the medical-surgical unit with an acute exacerbation of asthma. What position should the nurse place the patient in to improve oxygenation?

(continued)

Patient Education *(continued)*

- Use smoking cessation materials, counseling, and treatment, as referred.
- Seek immediate medical care if lips or nails turn blue or if there is difficulty breathing.
- Take medications as prescribed.

CHRONIC OBSTRUCTIVE PULMONARY DISEASE

Overview

- *COPD* is the umbrella term for two preventable and treatable disorders that block the normal flow of air through the lungs and trap air in the alveoli.
- The two types of COPD are emphysema and chronic bronchitis. Asthma was previously considered a form of COPD; however, it is now considered a separate illness.

> **COMPLICATIONS**
>
> Complications of COPD include pulmonary hypertension, right-sided HF, weight loss due to increased nutritional needs and decreased ability to eat, and bacterial infections.

Signs and Symptoms

- Chronic bronchitis:
  - Accessory muscle use
  - Activity intolerance
  - Anxiety
  - Bronchospasm
  - Chronic, productive cough
  - Crackles
  - Cyanosis
  - Decreased breath sounds
  - Dyspnea
  - Fluid overload leading to HF, hyponatremia, and renal failure
  - Mucus plugs
  - Prolonged expiratory phase
  - Rhonchi
  - Wheezing
- Emphysema:
  - Accessory muscle use
  - Decreased activity tolerance
  - Decreased breath sounds
  - Dyspnea
  - Expiratory wheezing
  - Fatigue from increased work of breathing
  - Hyperventilation
  - Prolonged expiration

Diagnosis

Labs

- ABG to assess respiratory status
- CBC to assess for increase in RBC
- CMP to assess electrolytes and kidney and liver function
- Serum alpha-1 antitrypsin level to assess for deficiency

Diagnostic Testing

- Chest-ray
- Pulmonary function test
- Six-minute walk test to determine if patient qualifies for home oxygen

Treatment

- Antibiotics to treat or prevent infection
- Inhaled anticholinergic
- Inhaled beta-2 adrenergic agonist
- Inhaled steroids during acute exacerbation
- Supplemental oxygen

Nursing Interventions

- Administer medications as ordered.
- Administer supplemental oxygen; often, patients with COPD have a lower SpO$_2$ goal, such as 88%.
- Assist the patient to remain hydrated to thin secretions.
- Assist with CPT.
- Educate the patient on the correct use of an MDI inhaler and spacer.
- Teach the patient pursed-lipped breathing to assist with exhaling CO$_2$.
- Teach the patient to sit in a tripod position to expand lungs.

NURSING PEARL

Patients with COPD often have a lower goal for SpO$_2$ than patients without COPD. Administering excessive oxygen to a patient with COPD reduces their respiratory drive, worsening their respiratory status.

Patient Education

- Avoid contact with people who are sick.
- Eat small, frequent meals to maintain nutrition.
- Exercise as tolerated.
- Remain up to date on vaccinations.
- Rinse mouth after use of inhalers.
- Take medications as instructed.
- Use home oxygen if needed. Learn safe use of home oxygen (e.g., do not use near open flames, do not smoke).
- Use smoking cessation materials, counseling, and treatment, as referred.
- Wash hands frequently.

POP QUIZ 12.2

A patient on the medical-surgical unit is admitted with COPD exacerbation. What does the nurse teach the patient regarding optimal oxygenation?

CYSTIC FIBROSIS

Overview

CF is a genetic condition that causes thickened secretions in the lungs and digestive system, leading to lung damage, chronic respiratory infections, and pancreatic insufficiency.

Signs and Symptoms

- Bowel obstruction
- Constipation
- Exercise intolerance
- Foul-smelling, greasy stools
- Inflamed sinuses
- Persistent cough that produces thick mucus (sputum)
- Poor weight gain and growth
- Recurrent sinusitis
- Repeated lung infections
- Wheezing

COMPLICATIONS

Complications of CF are many and varied because CF affects many body systems. Complications include pancreatic insufficiency, pancreatitis, malnutrition, constipation, diarrhea, gallstones, kidney stones, bowel obstruction, diabetes, antibiotic resistance, cirrhosis, osteoporosis, arthritis, and pneumothorax.

Diagnosis

Labs
- Fecal fat test
- Genetic screening
- Sweat chloride test
- Sputum culture

Diagnostic Testing
- Chest x-ray
- Pulmonary function test

Treatment

- CPT or high-frequency chest wall oscillation vest
- Inhaled bronchodilators
- Inhaled hypertonic saline to thin secretions
- Medications to treat constipation
- Pancreatic enzymes taken with food
- Possible lung transplant
- Prophylactic antibiotics to prevent respiratory infections
- Tube feedings to increase nutrition, if needed

Nursing Interventions

- Administer medications as ordered.
- Administer pancreatic enzymes with meals and snacks.
- Administer supplemental oxygen, as needed.
- Assist patient to obtain adequate nutrition and hydration.
- Assist patient with nebulized medications.
- Educate patient on the use of inhalers and spacers for proper administration of inhaled medications.

Patient Education

- Avoid contact with people who are sick.
- Eat small, frequent meals.
- Notify provider at the first sign of respiratory infection.
- Remain up to date on vaccinations.
- Take medications as instructed.
- Use supplemental oxygen, as needed.
- Wash hands frequently.

LUNG CANCER

Overview

- Lung cancers are divided into two categories: small cell and non-small cell cancers.
- Lung cancer is the leading cause of cancer-related death in the United States.
- Table 12.1 provides descriptions of common types of lung cancers.

Signs and Symptoms

- Bone pain
- Chest pain
- Chest tightness

COMPLICATIONS

Complications of lung cancer include pleural effusion, pericardial effusion, hemoptysis, hypercalcemia from metastatic bone lesions, pulmonary hemorrhage, blood clots, and spinal cord compression.

(continued)

Table 12.1 Types of Lung Cancer

Type	Description
Adenocarcinoma	<ul><li>Peripherally located</li><li>Rarely cavitates</li><li>Slow growing</li><li>Spreads to lymph nodes early</li><li>Well-circumscribed tumor</li></ul>
Large-cell carcinoma	<ul><li>Metastasizes early</li><li>Necrotic mass</li><li>Peripherally located</li><li>Rapidly growing</li><li>Spreads extensively</li><li>Tends to cavitate</li></ul>
Small-cell carcinoma	<ul><li>Most aggressive form of lung cancer</li><li>Centrally located</li><li>Rapidly growing</li><li>Metastasizes rapidly to distant sites</li><li>Responds well to chemotherapy</li></ul>
Squamous-cell carcinoma	<ul><li>Most common form of lung cancer</li><li>Centrally located</li><li>Slow growing</li><li>Metastasizes to intrathoracic sites first</li><li>Produces early symptoms</li><li>Tends to cavitate</li></ul>

Signs and Symptoms *(continued)*

- Chronic cough
- Dyspnea
- Enlarged lymph nodes
- Fatigue
- Hemoptysis
- Joint pain
- May be asymptomatic, with symptoms first occurring from distant metastatic sites
- Shoulder or arm pain
- Superior vena cava syndrome
- Weight loss

Diagnosis

Labs

- ABG to assess respiratory status
- Calcium level to assess hypercalcemia in malignancy
- CBC
- CMP to assess liver function

Diagnostic Testing

- Biopsy of lymph node
- Biopsy of tumor
- Bronchoscopy
- Chest CT
- Chest x-ray
- PET scan

 NURSING PEARL

Superior vena cava syndrome occurs when blood flow through the superior vena cava is blocked or compressed. Symptoms include edema of the face, neck, and torso, as well as dilated veins in the chest and abdomen.

Treatment

- Chemotherapy
- Laser ablation through bronchoscopy for palliative treatment of nonresectable tumors
- Lobectomy
- Pneumonectomy
- Radiation
- Thoracentesis to relieve pleural effusion
- Wedge resection

Nursing Interventions

- Administer medications as prescribed.
- Administer supplemental oxygen PRN.
- Administer analgesics PRN as ordered.
- Assist patient to maintain adequate hydration to thin respiratory secretions.
- Encourage PO intake.
- Encourage patient to cough and deep breathe or to use incentive spirometer.
- Maintain patency and output of chest tube, if present.
- Monitor surgical incision for drainage and signs and symptoms of infection.
- Monitor vital signs.

Patient Education

- Avoid contact with people who are sick.
- Avoid strenuous activities.
- Maintain adequate hydration to thin respiratory secretions.
- Place frequently used objects nearby to maintain energy.
- Use smoking cessation materials, counseling, and treatment, as referred.
- Rest when tired.
- Stay up to date on vaccinations.
- Take medications as prescribed.

PNEUMONIA

Overview

- *Pneumonia* is characterized by acute inflammation of the lungs.
- Pneumonia can be bacterial, viral, or fungal.
- Pneumonia can occur after patients aspirate (i.e., aspiration pneumonia).

Signs and Symptoms

- Accessory muscle use
- Chest pain (pleuritic)
- Diminished breath sounds or crackles
- Dyspnea
- Fatigue
- Fever
- Increased oxygen needs
- Malaise
- Productive cough
- Tachycardia
- Weakness

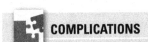 **COMPLICATIONS**

Complications of pneumonia include respiratory failure, sepsis, multiorgan failure, coagulopathy, and exacerbation of preexisting comorbidities that may lead to death.

Diagnosis

Labs
- ABG to assess respiratory status
- Blood and sputum cultures to identify causative organisms
- CBC to determine increased WBC

Diagnostic Testing
- Chest x-ray
- Thoracentesis

Treatment

- Coughing and deep breathing
- Medications to treat causes, such as antibiotics
- Medications to treat symptoms, such as bronchodilators and expectorants
- Supplemental oxygen

Nursing Interventions

- Administer medications as ordered.
- Assist patient to maintain adequate nutrition.
- Assist patient with CPT.
- Encourage coughing and deep breathing and use of incentive spirometer.
- Provide supplemental oxygen to maintain SpO_2 above 92% for most patients.

Patient Education

- Follow safe swallowing instructions.
- Maintain adequate hydration to thin respiratory secretions.
- Use smoking cessation materials, counseling, and treatment, as referred.
- Stay up to date on vaccinations.
- Take medications as prescribed.
- Use coughing and deep breathing exercises.

 ALERT!

Pneumonia is a serious complication of COVID-19. A patient may initially experience a dry cough, fever, loss of taste and smell, and shortness of breath. Patients should seek emergency care if symptoms escalate to difficulty breathing or to SpO_2 less than 95%. COVID-19 care parameters and SARS-CoV-2 variants are continually evolving. For current information on caring for patients with COVID-19, consult the National Institutes of Health (www.covid19treatmentguidelines. nih.gov) and the CDC (www.cdc.gov/ coronavirus/2019-ncov/hcp/).

PNEUMOTHORAX

Overview

- A *pneumothorax* is the presence of air in the pleural space.
- It can occur spontaneously or as a result of trauma.

Signs and Symptoms

- Absent chest wall movement
- Acute respiratory failure in cases of traumatic pneumothorax
- Asymmetrical lung expansion
- Cyanosis
- Decreased breath sounds on affected side
- Dyspnea
- Increased work of breathing
- JVD

 COMPLICATIONS

The complications of pneumothorax include pleural effusion, hemorrhage, empyema, acute respiratory failure, pneumomediastinum, arrhythmias, and cardiac arrest.

(continued)

Signs and Symptoms *(continued)*

- Pleuritic chest pain
- Tachycardia
- Tachypnea

Diagnosis

Labs
- ABG to assess respiratory status
- CBC

Diagnostic Testing
- Chest CT
- Chest x-ray

Treatment

- Chest tube to allow for drainage of fluid and promote lung expansion
- Needle aspiration of air
- Supplemental oxygen to maintain SpO_2 greater than 92%
- Surgical repair if the lung does not re-expand after insertion of the chest tube

Nursing Interventions

- Administer medications as ordered.
- Administer supplemental oxygen as needed.
- Assess and maintain chest tube integrity.
- Monitor and record chest tube output.
- Monitor for changes in respiratory status.
- Monitor vital signs.

Patient Education

- Do not dive under water until cleared by provider.
- Do not travel in a plane until cleared by provider.
- Do not travel to high altitudes until cleared by provider.
- Notify provider immediately if there are any changes in respiratory status.
- Use smoking cessation materials, counseling, and treatment, as referred.
- Take analgesics PRN, as instructed.
- Take medications as instructed.

PULMONARY EMBOLI

Overview

- A *PE* is a blockage of the pulmonary vasculature. Although the blockage is most commonly a thrombus, other embolisms include bone, fat, air, amniotic fluid, or a foreign object such as surgical cement.
- A common cause for a PE is a dislodged thrombus from a vein in the pelvis, leg, or other area of the body.

COMPLICATIONS

A massive PE can cause pulmonary hypertension, right-sided HF, ventricular hypertrophy, and death.

Signs and Symptoms

- Anxiety
- Chest pain

(continued)

Signs and Symptoms *(continued)*

- Cough with hemoptysis
- Dyspnea
- Restlessness
- Tachycardia
- Tachypnea

Diagnosis

Labs

- ABG to assess respiratory status
- D-dimer: elevated if clot is present

Diagnostic Testing

- Chest x-ray
- Echocardiogram
- Pulmonary angiography
- V/Q scan
- Ultrasound to assess for DVT

Treatment

- Medication to dissolve clot
- Supplemental oxygen
- Surgery to insert IVC filter

Nursing Interventions

- Administer supplemental oxygen.
- Monitor coagulopathies, such as PTT, if the patient is anticoagulated with a heparin drip.
- Monitor for cardiac arrythmias.
- Monitor for signs and symptoms of bleeding.
- Monitor respiratory status.

Patient Education

- Avoid long periods of immobility.
- Follow up with labs as instructed.
- Stand up and walk around when sitting for long periods, such as on a long airplane flight.
- Take medications as instructed.
- Use smoking cessation materials, counseling, and treatment, as referred.
- Wear compression stockings if instructed.

PULMONARY FIBROSIS

Overview

- *Pulmonary fibrosis* is a disease of the lungs that occurs when lung tissue becomes damaged or scarred.
- Pulmonary tissue becomes thick and stiffened as a result of this damage, leading to increased work of breathing and increased dyspnea.
- Pulmonary fibrosis can be caused by environmental toxins or radiation, can be a complication of other conditions, or can be idiopathic.

 COMPLICATIONS

Complications of pulmonary fibrosis include pulmonary hypertension, thromboembolic disease, increased risk of respiratory infections, acute coronary syndrome, hypoxia, acute respiratory failure, lung cancer, and death.

Signs and Symptoms

- Clubbing of fingernails
- Dry cough
- Dyspnea
- Fatigue
- Increased work of breathing
- Weight loss

Diagnosis

Labs

- ABG to determine low level of arterial oxygen level
- CBC to assess WBC: indicates infection if elevated
- CMP to assess kidney and liver function

Diagnostic Testing

- Bronchoscopy
- Chest CT
- Chest x-ray
- Pulmonary function tests

Treatment

- No cure; treatment to reduce symptoms
- Trigger identification and avoidance
- Preservation and optimization of remaining healthy lung tissue
- Symptom management with medications (see Table 12.1)
- Supplemental oxygen

Nursing Interventions

- Focus is on symptom management and optimizing healthy lung tissue.
- Supportive care is necessary for patients with pulmonary fibrosis.
- Provide therapeutic support to patient and family.

Patient Education

- Follow dietary instructions.
- Exercise as tolerated.
- Take medications as instructed.
- Keep up to date with recommended vaccinations, including yearly flu vaccine.
- Use smoking cessation materials, counseling, and treatment, as referred.

PULMONARY HYPERTENTION

Overview

- Pulmonary hypertension results from high pressure in the blood vessels leading from the heart to the lungs.
- Pulmonary hypertension is categorized into five groups based on cause (Table 12.2).

Signs and Symptoms

- Ascites
- Chest pain
- Dyspnea

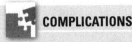

COMPLICATIONS

The most common complication of pulmonary hypertension is right-sided HF. Right-sided HF may already be present at the time of diagnosis. Right-sided HF is the most common cause of death in patients with pulmonary hypertension.

(continued)

Table 12.2 Pulmonary Hypertension Groups

Group	Type	Causes
1	Pulmonary arterial hypertension	• Congenital heart disease • Genetic mutation • Other conditions including scleroderma, lupus, HIV infection, and cirrhosis • Unknown cause in idiopathic pulmonary arterial hypertension • Use of stimulant drugs such as methamphetamines
2	Pulmonary hypertension caused by left-sided heart disease	• Left-sided heart valve disease, such as mitral valve or aortic valve disease • Failure of the lower left ventricle
3	Pulmonary hypertension caused by lung disease	• COPD • Obstructive sleep apnea • Pulmonary fibrosis
4	Pulmonary hypertension caused by chronic blood clots	• Chronic or recurrent pulmonary emboli • Other clotting disorders
5	Pulmonary hypertension triggered by other health conditions	• Blood disorders, including polycythemia vera and essential thrombocythemia • Inflammatory disorders such as sarcoidosis and vasculitis • Kidney disease • Metabolic disorders • Tumors compressing the pulmonary arteries

Signs and Symptoms *(continued)*

• Fatigue
• Heart murmur
• Hypoxia
• JVD
• Peripheral edema
• Right-sided HF

Diagnosis

Labs
• ABG to assess oxygenation status
• BNP: may be elevated
• CBC to assess for anemia

Diagnostic Testing
• Cardiac catheterization to assess pulmonary artery pressure
• Chest x-ray
• CT scan
• EKG
• Pulmonary angiography
• Pulmonary function tests
• V/Q lung scan

Treatment

- Atrial septostomy
- Heart or lung transplant in severe disease
- Medications such as anticoagulants, antihypertensives, cardiac glycosides (e.g., digoxin), and vasodilators
- Supplemental oxygen

Nursing Interventions

- Administer medications as ordered.
- Administer oxygen to maintain SpO_2 greater than 92%.
- Monitor for new cardiac arrythmias.
- Monitor labs, especially coagulopathies for drug monitoring.
- Monitor respiratory status.

Patient Education

- Exercise as tolerated. Notify provider before starting a new exercise program.
- Limit dietary sodium intake as instructed by provider.
- Limit fluid intake to 2 L/d, or as instructed by provider.
- Monitor blood pressure at home.
- Use smoking cessation materials, counseling, and treatment, as referred.
- Take medications as instructed.

PLEURAL EFFUSION

Overview

- A *pleural effusion* is a buildup of fluid in the *pleural space*, the thin space between the visceral and parietal pleura.
- A pleural effusion can be caused by a buildup of pus and necrotic tissue (empyema), blood (hemothorax), and chyle (chylothorax).

Signs and Symptoms

- Cough
- Decreased breath sounds
- Decreased chest wall movement
- Dyspnea
- Fever
- Pleuritic pain

Diagnosis

Labs
- CBC to assess for leukocytosis if infectious cause is suspected

Diagnostic Testing
- Bronchoscopy
- Chest CT
- Chest x-ray
- Pleurocentesis

Treatment

- Chest tube
- Medications to treat infectious cause
- Thoracentesis
- Thoracotomy: may be needed if thoracentesis is not effective

Nursing Interventions

- Administer medications as ordered.
- Encourage deep breathing.
- Monitor and maintain patency of chest tube.
- Provide supplemental oxygen to maintain SpO_2 greater than 92%.
- Watch for signs and symptoms of respiratory distress.

Patient Education

- Cough and deep breathe.
- Take medications as directed.
- Use a pillow to splint the chest when coughing.
- Use smoking cessation materials, counseling, and treatment, as referred.

TUBERCULOSIS

Overview

- *TB* is an infectious disease that most commonly affects the lungs, caused by the bacterium *Mycobacterium tuberculosis.*
- TB is spread from infected person to person through droplet aerosolization.

Signs and Symptoms

- Anorexia
- Chills
- Cough
- Fever
- Hemoptysis
- Night sweats
- Unintentional weight loss

Diagnosis

Labs

- Sputum culture
- Sputum smear for detection of acid-fast bacilli
- Gamma interferon TB test
- Interferon gamma release assay for TB diagnosis
- Tuberculin skin test with PPD

Diagnostic Testing

- Chest x-ray

Treatment

- Medications such as antibiotics and antituberculotics

Nursing Interventions

- Administer medications as prescribed.
- Isolate the patient in a negative-pressure room with airborne precautions.
- Use appropriate PPE when caring for the patient.

Patient Education

- Cough or sneeze into a tissue.
- Ensure that family, friends, and other close contacts are tested for TB.

(continued)

Patient Education *(continued)*

- Maintain adequate nutrition to promote healing.
- Stay home from work or school until cleared to return by provider.
- Take medications as prescribed.
- Wash hands frequently.

POP QUIZ 12.3

The nurse is preparing to admit a patient with TB to the medical-surgical floor. What type of isolation precautions are required for this patient?

Appendix 12.1 Respiratory Medications

Indication	Mechanism of Action	Contraindications, Precautions, and Adverse Effects
Anticholinergics (ipratropium)		
• Asthma, COPD, acute respiratory failure	• Block the effects of acetylcholine to help relax the muscles, causing bronchoconstriction • Reduce the production of mucus	• Medication may cause arrythmias on rare occasions; use caution in patients with known arrythmias. • Medication may cause urinary retention in patients with known BPH or urinary obstructions.
Bronchodilators (albuterol)		
• Asthma, COPD, acute respiratory failure	• Act on the beta-2 receptors of the lungs to promote smooth muscle relaxation, thereby decreasing bronchospasms	• Cardiovascular effects such as tachycardia may occur when using frequently or in high doses. • In rare cases, paradoxical bronchospasm may occur after administration.
Anticoagulants (warfarin)		
• Blood clots such as DVTs and PE	• Inhibit vitamin K availability to reduce the effects of clotting factors	• Patients taking warfarin are at high risk of bleeding; ensure bleeding and fall precautions are maintained. • Ensure patients taking warfarin have INR checked regularly and often.
Expectorants (dextromethorphan, guaifenesin)		
• Pneumonia, respiratory failure, ARDS	• Help alleviate congestion and clear mucus from airways	• Do not give for persistent or chronic cough due to smoking, asthma, or COPD.
Fibrinolytics (tPA)		
• PE, DVT	• Recombinant form of human tPA used to dissolve clots	• Use cautiously in patients who are at high risk for bleeding. • Alteplase is contraindicated for patients with uncontrolled hypertension. • For 24 hours after administration of alteplase, avoid IM injections, Foley catheter placement, IV placements, and other procedures that may cause excessive bleeding.

(continued)

Appendix 12.1 Respiratory Medications *(continued)*

Indication	Mechanism of Action	Contraindications, Precautions, and Adverse Effects
Heparin		
• PE, DVT	• Anticoagulant used to treat and prevent formation of blood clots	• Use cautiously in patients who are at high risk for bleeding. • Medication is contraindicated for patients with severe thrombocytopenia. • Monitor CBC and coagulopathies with special attention to aPTT when administering in a continuous infusion. • Use cautiously in patients with hepatic disease, as they are often at higher risk of bleeding.

RESOURCES

Lewis, S. L., Dirksen, S. R., Heitkemper, M. M., Bucher, L., & Harding, M. M. (2017). *Medical-surgical nursing: Assessment and management of clinical problems* (10th ed.). Elsevier.

Longe, J. L. (Ed.). (2018). *The Gale encyclopedia of nursing and allied health* (4th ed.). Gale. https://link.gale.com/apps/pub/07UZ/GVRL?u=kcls_main&sid=GVRL

Prescribers' Digital Reference. (n.d.[a]). *Albuterol sulfate* [Drug information]. https://www.pdr.net/drug-summary/Albuterol-Sulfate-Inhalation-Solution-0-083--albuterol-sulfate-1427.4212

Prescribers' Digital Reference. (n.d.[b]). *Alteplase* [Drug information]. https://www.pdr.net/drug-summary/Activase-alteplase-1332.3358

Prescribers' Digital Reference. (n.d.[c]). *Guaifenesin* [Drug information]. https://www.pdr.net/drug-summary/Mucinex-guaifenesin-1275.1918

Prescribers' Digital Reference. (n.d.[d]). *Heparin sodium* [Drug information]. https://www.pdr.net/drug-summary/Heparin-Sodium-and-0-9--Sodium-Chloride-heparin-sodium-1300.1856

Prescribers' Digital Reference. (n.d.[e]). *Ipratropium bromide* [Drug information]. https://www.pdr.net/drug-summary/Atrovent-HFA-ipratropium-bromide-1743.318

Prescribers' Digital Reference. (n.d.[f]). *Warfarin sodium* [Drug information]. https://www.pdr.net/drug-summary/Coumadin-warfarin-sodium-106.4534

Tkacs, N. C., Herrmann, L. L., & Johnson, R. L. (Eds.). (2020). *Advanced physiology and pathophysiology: Essentials for clinical practice*. Springer Publishing Company.

13

REPRODUCTIVE SYSTEM

BREAST CANCER

Overview

- *Breast cancer* is the most common cancer in women. About 129 out of 100,000 women are diagnosed each year.
- Breast cancer is rare in men, but one out of 100,000 men will be diagnosed every year.
- Types of breast cancer include:
  - Inflammatory
  - In situ
  - Invasive: ductal or lobular
  - Paget's disease of the nipple
  - Papillary

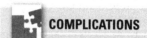

COMPLICATIONS

Complications of breast cancer include body image disturbance, lymphedema, metastasis, and postoperative infection.

Signs and Symptoms

- Asymmetrical breasts
- Erythema in inflammatory cancer
- Lump or thickening in breast
- Nipple discharge or retraction

Diagnosis

Labs

There are no labs specific to diagnosing breast cancer. However, the following labs may be used for risk factors and treatment planning:

- Breast cancer gene mutations BRCA1/BRCA2: relate to higher risk of developing breast cancer
- Cancer antigen 15-3 to monitor treatment response
- Cancer antigen 27.29 to monitor treatment response and recurrence
- CMP to determine liver or bone metastasis
- Estrogen and progesterone receptors
- HER2

Diagnostic Testing

- Bone scan
- Chest x-ray
- CT scan
- Mammogram
- Needle biopsy/fine-needle aspiration
- PET scan
- Ultrasound

Treatment

- Chemotherapy
- Endocrine therapy
- Radiation therapy
- Surgery
  - Lumpectomy
  - Mastectomy: simple or radical
  - Prophylactic oophorectomy if *BRCA1* or *BRCA2* mutation

Nursing Interventions

- Administer medications as ordered.
- Encourage proper nutrition.
- Encourage verbalization of body image change, especially after mastectomy surgery.
- Monitor adverse effects of chemotherapy.
- Monitor adverse effects of radiation therapy.
- Provide emotional support.

Patient Education

- Conduct breast self-examinations.
- Continue yearly mammograms.
- Learn ways to manage lymphedema if lymph nodes were removed:
  - Compression sleeve on affected extremity
  - Decongestive therapy: a massage-like technique to move subcutaneous fluid
  - Elevation of the arm
  - Isometric exercises
  - Protection of extremity:
    - ○ Do not take blood pressure from this side.
    - ○ Do not use IVs on operative side.
    - ○ Do not perform injections or blood draws from affected side.
    - ○ Protect the side from cuts.
- Maintain postsurgical home care: dressing changes and drain care, if present.
- Take medications as prescribed.

COMPLICATIONS

Lymphedema can occur after a mastectomy and lumpectomy, causing swelling in the affected arm. Instruct the patient on applying compression bandages to the arm and advise them to take special care if cuts occur on the affected arm.

POP QUIZ 13.1

A patient is being discharged with a JP drain after a mastectomy. What are the actions of the nurse?

CERVICAL CANCER

Overview

- *Cervical cancer* is a malignant tumor of the cervix.
- Types of cervical cancer include:
  - Carcinoma in situ
  - Dysplasia
- Invasive carcinoma

Signs and Symptoms

- Irregular vaginal bleeding and discharge
- Pelvic pain
- Weight loss in advanced disease

COMPLICATIONS

Complications of cervical cancer include bladder and rectum involvement. Metastasis to bones, lungs, and liver may occur in late stages.

Diagnosis

Labs

There are no labs specific to diagnosing cervical cancer.

Diagnostic Testing

- Cystoscopy
- HPV test (screening test)
- Pap smear: abnormal results
- Pelvic examination

Treatment

- Chemotherapy
- Conization
- Cryosurgery
- Laser therapy
- Radiotherapy
- Surgery (hysterectomy)

Nursing Interventions

- Administer medications as directed.
- Administer PRN analgesics for pain.
- Administer antiemetic medications for nausea and vomiting.
- Monitor postsurgical complications if patient undergoes surgery.
- Provide emotional support.

Patient Education

- Follow up with provider regularly to ensure cancer has been controlled.
- Monitor for postsurgical infections.
- Take medications as prescribed.

 ALERT!

A risk factor for cervical cancer is infection with HPV. The HPV vaccine is recommended for patients age 9 to 26 years to protect against cervical cancer.

CYSTOCELE AND RECTOCELE

Overview

- *Rectocele* is a protrusion of the rectum into the vagina.
- *Cystocele* is a protrusion of the bladder into the vagina.

 COMPLICATIONS

A major complication of cystocele and rectocele is complete fecal incontinence.

Signs and Symptoms

- Constipation
- Incontinence of bowel and bladder
- Pelvic pressure
- Visible protrusion into vagina

Diagnosis

Labs

- UA and culture to rule out infection

Diagnostic Testing

- Pelvic examination

Treatment

- Estrogen therapy (Appendix 13.1 at the end of this chapter)
- Pelvic floor muscle exercises

(continued)

Treatment *(continued)*

- Surgical correction, including hysterectomy
- Vaginal pessary

Nursing Interventions

- Administer medications as ordered for pain and constipation.
- Encourage pelvic floor muscle–strengthening exercises.
- Encourage periods of rest with legs elevated to relieve pelvic strain.
- Provide perineal care if post surgery.

Patient Education

- Avoid heavy lifting or intercourse until cleared by surgeon, if post surgery.
- Avoid straining during urination or defecation.
- Drink plenty of fluids to avoid constipation.
- Perform pelvic floor exercises
- Take medications as prescribed.

NURSING PEARL

Encourage patients exhibiting symptoms to rest to relieve pelvic pressure, as symptoms are aggravated by lengthy periods of standing.

POP QUIZ 13.2

A patient presents with a rectocele and requests nonsurgical interventions. What types of medications and therapies will the provider order to relieve symptoms?

ENDOMETRIOSIS

Overview

Endometriosis is an abnormal growth of cells of the uterine endometrial tissue outside of the uterus.

Signs and Symptoms

- Abnormal uterine bleeding
- Dyspareunia
- Dysuria
- Infertility
- May be asymptomatic
- Pelvic pain

Diagnosis

Labs
- CA-125: will be detected in endometriosis

Diagnostic Testing
- Laparoscopy to obtain tissue for analysis
- Pelvic and rectal exam
- Transvaginal ultrasound

Treatment

- Hormonal contraceptives (see Appendix 13.1)
- NSAIDs for antiprostaglandin action (see Table A.2)
- Surgery in rare cases

COMPLICATIONS

Complications of endometriosis are chronic pelvic pain, infertility, and ruptured cysts.

Nursing Interventions

- Administer medications as prescribed.
- Encourage adequate nutrition.
- Provide emotional support.

Patient Education

- Get enough rest.
- Follow a nutritious diet.
- Take medications as prescribed.

OVARIAN CANCER

Overview

Ovarian cancer is a malignancy of the ovary. It often is detected at later stages of the disease because early symptoms are overlooked.

Signs and Symptoms

- Abdominal or pelvic pain
- Bloating
- Feeling of fullness
- Urinary frequency and urgency

Diagnosis

Labs
- CA-125: may be elevated

Diagnostic Testing
- Color Doppler imaging
- Pelvic examination
- Transvaginal ultrasound

Treatment

- Chemotherapy
- TAH/BSO

Nursing Interventions

- Administer medications as prescribed, including pain medication and antiemetics.
- Assess the need for IV fluids if patient has persistent nausea and vomiting.
- Encourage adequate nutrition.
- Manage nausea and vomiting.
- Monitor postsurgical wounds to avoid infection, if applicable.
- Provide emotional support.

Patient Education

- Maintain nutrition by eating small, frequent meals.
- Call provider for signs and symptoms of infection from surgery site, if applicable.
- Take medications as prescribed.

COMPLICATIONS

Early diagnosis and treatment is imperative to prevent formation of scar tissue on the outside and inside of fallopian tubes.

PELVIC INFLAMMATORY DISEASE

Overview

PID is the inflammation of the pelvic area, including fallopian tubes, ovaries, and uterus.

Signs and Symptoms

- Cervical discharge
- Dysuria
- Fever
- Irregular bleeding
- Pelvic pain

Diagnosis

Labs
- CBC: may show elevated leukocytes
- CRP: elevated

Diagnostic Testing
- Pelvic exam to evaluate cervical exudate for WBCs
- Transvaginal ultrasound

Treatment

- Antibiotics (see Appendix 13.1)
- IV fluids if unable to tolerate oral fluids

Nursing Interventions

- Administer all medications as prescribed.
- Apply heating pad to lower abdomen for comfort.

Patient Education

- Complete entire course of antibiotics as prescribed.
- Use appropriate prophylactics (condoms) during sex after completion of antibiotic therapy.

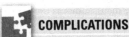 **ALERT!**

It is important for the patient to notify their sexual partner about the need for testing and that both people are treated before having any kind of intercourse, to prevent reinfecting each other.

UTERINE CANCER

Overview

- Uterine cancer includes cancerous tumors (adenocarcinoma and sarcoma) and benign tumors (fibroids and polyps).
- Endometrial cancer is the most common uterine cancer.

COMPLICATIONS

Complications of uterine cancer include breast cancer, colon cancer, and intestinal obstruction.

Signs and Symptoms

- Abdominal tenderness
- Pelvic pain
- Unusual vaginal bleeding

Diagnosis

Labs
There are no labs specific to diagnosing uterine cancer.

Diagnostic Testing

- Endometrial biopsy
- Pelvic exam
- Transvaginal ultrasound

Treatment

- Hysterectomy to remove tumor
- Radiation therapy
  - Brachytherapy
  - External radiation
- Therapies using medication
  - Chemotherapy
  - Hormone therapy
  - Immunotherapy

Nursing Interventions

- Adhere to safety precautions regarding brachytherapy (time, distance, shielding).
- Administer medications as prescribed.
- Assess patient's pain and treat with pharmacologic and nonpharmacologic medications/treatments as ordered.
- Assist with symptom management if chemotherapy is prescribed (e.g., antiemetics, adequate nutrition, encouraging patient to rest).
- Provide emotional support and encourage patient to verbalize feelings related to the diagnosis.
- Provide postoperative care including surgical site care and dressing changes.

Patient Education

- Follow up with provider and gynecologist for exams as directed.
- Notify the provider if signs and symptoms of infection occur postoperatively.
- Refrain from sexual intercourse for approximately 6 weeks postoperatively.
- Take medications as prescribed.

UTERINE PROLAPSE

Overview

Uterine prolapse occurs when the muscles in the pelvis are weakened, allowing the uterus to descend into the vagina.

Signs and Symptoms

- Frequent UTIs
- Low back pain
- Pressure in pelvic area
- Urinary frequency or urgency

Diagnosis

Labs

- UA to rule out UTI

Diagnostic Testing

- Pelvic examination

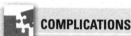 **COMPLICATIONS**

Complications of uterine prolapse include infection and necrosis of the cervix and uterus.

Treatment

- Pelvic floor muscle–strengthening exercises
- Surgical correction including hysterectomy
- Vaginal pessary

Nursing Interventions

- Administer medications as ordered for pain and constipation.
- Check for proper placement of pessary as needed.
- Encourage periods of rest with legs elevated to relieve pelvic strain.
- Encourage pelvic floor muscle–strengthening exercises.
- Provide perineal care postoperatively.

Patient Education

- Drink plenty of fluids to avoid constipation.
- Follow up with provider for pessary checks as needed.
- Perform pelvic floor muscle–strengthening exercises.
- Take all medications as prescribed.

 POP QUIZ 13.3

A patient has been prescribed a vaginal pessary. What are the indications to notify the provider after insertion?

Appendix 13.1 Reproductive Medications

Indications	Mechanism of Action	Contraindications, Precautions, and Adverse Effects
Ceftriaxone		
• Used to treat PID	• Bactericidal	• Medication is contraindicated in patients with cephalosporin hypersensitivity and penicillin sensitivity. • Educate patients on completing entire course of antibiotic. • Medication may cause diarrhea.
Clindamycin		
• Used to treat PID	• Binds with RNA of bacteria to inhibit protein synthesis resulting in antibacterial action	• Medication can cause a yeast or fungal infection or can cause diarrhea. • Use with caution with hepatic disease.
Doxycycline		
• Used to treat PID • Used to treat resistant organisms	• Bacteriostatic/antibiotic	• Do not use in patients with sulfite hypersensitivity or HIV, or in patients who are pregnant. • Medication may cause infertility.

(continued)

Appendix 13.1 Reproductive Medications *(continued)*

Indications	Mechanism of Action	Contraindications, Precautions, and Adverse Effects
Estrogen		
• Used to treat GU symptoms	• Replaces estrogen hormone that naturally decreases with age	• Medication is contraindicated in patients with ovarian cancer. • Do not use in geriatric patients. • Do not use in patients with a history of angioedema, breast cancer, hypercalcemia, or liver disease. • Use with caution in patients with diabetes and hypothyroidism. • Adverse reactions include depression, migraine headaches, PE, and thromboembolism.

RESOURCES

Centers for Disease Control and Prevention. (2020, October). *Male breast cancer incidence and mortality, United States—2013–2017* [U.S. Cancer Statistics Data Briefs, No. 19]. Department of Health and Human Services, Centers for Disease Control and Prevention. https://www.cdc.gov/cancer/uscs/about/data-briefs/no19-male -breast-cancer-incidence-mortality-UnitedStates-2013-2017.htm

Karimi-Zarchi, M., Dehshiri-Zadeh, N., Sekhavat, L., & Nosouhi, F. (2016). Correlation of CA-125 serum level and clinico-pathological characteristic of patients with endometriosis. *International Journal of Reproductive Biomedicine, 14*(11), 713–718. https://www.ncbi.nlm.nih.gov/pmc/articles/PMC5153578/

Lewis, S., Bucher, L., & Heitkemper, M. (2017). *Medical-surgical nursing* (10th ed.). Elsevier.

MedLine Plus. (n.d.). *Uterine cancer.* https://medlineplus.gov/uterinecancer.html

National Cancer Institute. (n.d). *Cancer stat facts: Female breast cancer.* U.S. Department of Health and Human Services, National Cancer Institute. https://seer.cancer.gov/statfacts/html/breast.html

Nettina, S. M. (2019). *Lippincott manual of nursing practice* (11th ed.). Wolters Kluwer.

Prescribers' Digital Reference. (n.d.[a]). Ceftriaxone [Drug information]. https://www.pdr.net/drug-summary/ Ceftriaxone-ceftriaxone-1723.4059

Prescribers' Digital Reference. (n.d.[b]). Clindamycin [Drug information]. https://www.pdr.net/drug-summary/ Clindamycin-in-5-Percent-Dextrose-Clindamycin-in-5-Percent-Dextrose-24130#10

Prescribers' Digital Reference. (n.d.[c]). Estrogen [Drug information]. https://www.pdr.net/drug-summary/ Estrace-Vaginal-Cream-estradiol-1947

Prescribers' Digital Reference. (n.d.[d]). *Doxycycline* [Drug information]. https://www.pdr.net/drug-summary/ Doxycycline-doxycycline-24308#14

14

UROLOGICAL AND RENAL SYSTEMS

BENIGN PROSTATIC HYPERPLASIA

Overview

- *BPH* is expansion of the prostate and its surrounding tissue.
  - About half of all men between ages 51 and 60 years have BPH.
  - Roughly up to 90% of men older than 80 years have BPH.
- There is not a known cause, but it is thought to be linked to hormonal changes.
- As the prostate enlarges, it compresses the urethra, resulting in decreased urine flow.

> **COMPLICATIONS**
>
> Complications of BPH include bladder damage, bladder stones, kidney damage, urinary retention, and UTIs.

Signs and Symptoms

- Bladder distention
- Dribbling urine
  Nocturia
- Urinary frequency: about every 1 to 2 hours
- Urinary retention: feel of bladder fullness, even after passing urine
- Weak urine stream

Diagnosis

Labs

- CMP to assess kidney function
- PSA to help rule out prostate cancer
- UA to determine if blood, infection, glucose, or protein is present

Diagnostic Testing

- Cystoscopy to look at urethra or bladder
- Digital rectal exam to feel wall of prostate gland to look for enlargement, tenderness, lumps, or hard spots
  MRI or CT to provide a clear image of the prostate and surrounding area
  - Sometimes done if surgery is necessary to reopen the flow of urine
  Transrectal ultrasound to look at the size and shape of the prostate
- Urine diagnostic tests:
  - Postvoid residual to measure urine left in the bladder after urinating
  - Uroflowmetry to measure how fast the urine flows
  - Urodynamic pressure flow study to measure pressure in the bladder

Treatment

Medications such as finasteride and tamsulosin to assist in facilitating urinary flow (Appendix 14.1, which is located at the end of this chapter)

(continued)

Treatment *(continued)*

- Prostatectomy
- PUL
  - Less invasive procedure and faster healing time
  - Uses a needle to place tiny implants into the prostate to lift and compress the enlarged prostate to unblock urethra
- TURP
- Urinary catheter
- Water vapor thermal therapy: uses water vapor to destroy prostate cells squeezing urethra

Nursing Interventions

- Administer medications as ordered.
- Educate patient regarding TURP:
  - Resectoscope inserted through tip of penis to trim excess prostate
  - Three-way urinary catheter present postoperatively to maintain urine flow
  - Urine potentially bloody postoperatively
- Insert and maintain urinary catheter if ordered.
- Maintain three-way catheter, if ordered.
- Monitor for signs and symptoms of surgical complications in the postoperative period.
- Monitor urine output and color.
- Perform bladder ultrasound to assess urinary retention.
- Perform voiding trial after urinary catheter is removed.

Patient Education

- After prostate surgery:
  - Avoid caffeine.
  - Avoid drinking fluids at night to avoid nocturia.
  - Avoid prolonged sitting, vigorous activity, heavy lifting, or straining.
  - Do not have sex until cleared by provider.
  - Monitor for signs and symptoms of bleeding.
  - Stay hydrated to prevent urinary stasis and constipation.
  - Take stool softeners as needed.
- Take medications as prescribed.

 POP QUIZ 14.1

A patient is admitted for TURP and is concerned about having stitches in the penis area. What education is needed for this patient?

BLADDER CANCER

Overview

- *Bladder cancer* is a common type of cancer that most often begins in the urothelial cells that line the inside of the bladder.
- Most bladder cancers are diagnosed early.
  - Early-stage bladder cancer is highly treatable.
- Bladder cancer is likely to reoccur, even if completely removed.
  - Frequent follow-up and monitoring are required.
- SCC and adenocarcinoma are less common types of bladder cancers.

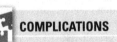 **COMPLICATIONS**

Complications of bladder cancer include hydronephrosis, urethral stricture, and urinary incontinence

Signs and Symptoms

- Back pain
- Frank or occult hematuria

(continued)

Signs and Symptoms *(continued)*

- Frequent urination
- Painful urination

Diagnosis

Labs

- Urine cytology

Diagnostic Testing

- CT urogram to examine structures of the urinary tract
- Cystoscopy to look at bladder and urethra:
  - Can also obtain a biopsy during this procedure
- After confirmation of cancer:
  - Bone scan
  - Chest x-ray
  - CT scan
  - MRI
  - PET

Treatment

- Chemotherapy
- Immunotherapy
- Intravesical therapy (infusion of medication into bladder)
- Radiation therapy
- Surgeries:
  - Bladder reconstruction
  - Cystectomy
  - Ileal conduit/reservoir
  - TURBT
- Targeted therapy (to treat advanced cancer when other options have not succeeded)

Nursing Interventions

- After surgery, assess incision or stoma site.
- Assess for signs of return of bowel functions.
- Manage patient's pain.
- Monitor for bladder distention following a partial cystectomy.
- Monitor for signs and symptoms of infection.
- Monitor urine flow, which is continuous after surgery.
  - Notify physician if urine output is less than 0.5 mL/kg/hr.
- Monitor vital signs, and notify provider of any that are abnormal.

Patient Education

- If stoma is present, assess its appearance daily and as needed and report any changes/concerns to the provider.
  - Stoma should be a beefy red. Pale or dusky appearance is a concern and should be reported to the provider right away.
- Seek immediate care for:
  - Altered mental status
  - Dysuria
  - Fever/chills
  - Hematuria
  - Inability to urinate

(continued)

Patient Education *(continued)*

- Persistent nausea/vomiting
- Uncontrolled pain
- Take medications as prescribed.
- Talk with the oncologist about chemotherapy and radiation treatment side effects and management of side effects.
- When taking pain medication, do not drive until cleared by provider.

EPIDIDYMITIS

Overview

- *Epididymitis* is inflammation of the coiled tube (epididymis) at the back of the testicle.
- It is often caused by bacterial infection, including STIs or trauma.

Signs and Symptoms

- Blood in semen
- Discharge from penis
- Pain in lower abdomen or pelvis
- Painful urination
- Swollen, red, or warm scrotum
- Testicle pain or tenderness, usually on one side, that comes on gradually
- Urgent or frequent urination

Diagnosis

Labs
- BMP to look for abnormalities
- CBC
- UA with C&S

Diagnostic Testing
- STI testing
- Ultrasound to check blood flow to testicles
  - Higher than normal blood flow may indicate epididymitis.

Treatment

- Antibiotics (see Table A.1)
- Surgery
  - Part or all of the epididymis may need to be removed in an epididymectomy.

Nursing Interventions

- Apply ice to scrotum as needed for pain.
- Assess for signs of return of bowel function.
- Manage patient's pain.
- Monitor for signs and symptoms of infection.
- Monitor vital signs.
- Use scrotal support by placing a pillow or towel under the scrotum to reduce pain.

 NURSING PEARL

Advanced epididymitis can cause testicular swelling and other changes that resemble testicular torsion. To differentiate between the two conditions, consider the onset of the patient's symptoms. Epididymitis is an infection that develops gradually, while testicular torsion has a sudden onset.

 COMPLICATIONS

Complications of epididymitis include abscess in the scrotum and, rarely, reduced fertility.

Patient Education

- Apply cold pack to scrotum as tolerated.
- Avoid lifting heavy objects.
- Avoid sex until cleared by provider.
- Keep scrotum elevated when lying down.
- Take medications as prescribed.
- Wear an athletic supporter.

GLOMERULONEPHRITIS

Overview

- *Glomerulonephritis* is an inflammation of the glomeruli.
- The kidneys slowly lose their ability to remove waste and excess fluid from the blood to make urine.
- Acute glomerulonephritis is most often a complication of a respiratory streptococcal infection or, less commonly, a streptococcal skin infection.
- Other causes include Berger's disease and lipid nephrosis.
  - Most patients fully recover from acute glomerulonephritis; however, some may progress to chronic renal failure.
- Chronic glomerulonephritis is a progressive disease that results in sclerosis and scarring and leads to renal failure.

COMPLICATIONS

Most cases of glomerulonephritis resolve with treatment and time. However, in rare cases, acute glomerulonephritis can lead to permanent kidney damage, requiring dialysis and kidney transplant.

Signs and Symptoms

- Acute glomerulonephritis
  - Dyspnea
  - Edema of the abdomen, face, feet, and hands
  - Fatigue
  - Hematuria
  - Hypertension
  - Increased serum BUN
  - Increased serum creatinine
  - Oliguria
  - Proteinuria
- Chronic glomerulonephritis: often develops slowly without symptoms; late-stage symptoms include:
  - Dyspnea
  - Edema
  - Fatigue
  - Hypertension
  - Malaise
  - Nausea
  - Pruritis
  - Vomiting

Diagnosis

Labs
- CBC to assess for leukocytosis and underlying infection
- CMP to assess BUN, creatinine, and GFR
- 24-hour urine to show low CrCl
- UA to show proteinuria, hematuria, WBCs, and casts

Diagnostic Testing
- Renal biopsy

Treatment

- Antibiotics to treat infection (see Table A.1)
- Antihypertensives
- Corticosteroids to reduce inflammation that can lead to scar tissue
- Dialysis
- Diuretics to reduce fluid overload
- Fluid restriction
- Possible kidney transplant if ESRD develops
- Sodium and potassium restriction

Nursing Interventions

- Monitor daily weight.
- Monitor fluid intake and output.
- Monitor labs, especially BMP for kidney function and electrolytes.
- Monitor patient on continuous telemetry if severe potassium derangement is present.
- Replace electrolytes as ordered.

Patient Education

- Adhere to dietary restrictions, including limiting sodium, potassium, and protein if instructed.
- Adhere to fluid restriction as instructed.
- Follow up with labs as instructed.
- Take daily weights.
- Take medications as instructed.

KIDNEY DISEASE

Overview

- CKD involves gradual loss of kidney function (eGFR < 60 mL/min/1.73 m^2 persisting for 3 months or more).
- CKD is the irreversible loss of kidney function, which can progress to ESRD.
- Advanced CKD can cause dangerous levels of fluid, wastes, and electrolytes to build up in the body.
- CKD is usually asymptomatic until stages IV and V.
- The main causes of kidney disease are diabetes and hypertension.

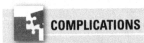

COMPLICATIONS

Complications of CKD include electrolyte abnormalities (hyperkalemia, hyperphosphatemia), metabolic acidosis, hypertension, anemia, ESRD, and death.

Signs and Symptoms

CKD affects every body system and has many symptoms of varying degree and severity depending on the stage. Signs and symptoms may include any of the following:

- Cardiovascular abnormalities:
  - CAD
  - HF
  - Hypertension
  - PAD
  - Pericarditis
- Endocrine disturbances:
  - Amenorrhea
  - Erectile dysfunction
  - Thyroid abnormalities
- GI disturbances:
  - Gastritis
  - GI bleed
  - Nausea and vomiting
- Hematologic abnormalities:
  - Anemia
  - Bleeding
  - Infection
- Integumentary complications:
  - Dry, scaly skin
  - Ecchymosis
  - Pruritis
- Musculoskeletal:
  - Calciphylaxis, a buildup of calcium in the blood vessels, skin, and visceral fat that causes painful ulcers and infection
  - Soft tissue and vascular calcifications
- Neurologic abnormalities:
  - Encephalopathy
  - Peripheral neuropathy
  - Restless leg syndrome
  - Sleep disturbances
- Pulmonary issues:
  - Pneumonia
  - Pulmonary edema
  - Uremic pleuritis
- Urinary output changes:
  - Anuria
  - Oliguria

Diagnosis

Labs

- ABG
- Albumin
- BMP
- CBC
- GFR
- Lipid profile
- UA

NURSING PEARL

Stages of CKD:

- Stage 1: Kidney damage with normal or slightly increased GFR (>90 mL/min/1.73 m^2)
- Stage 2: Mild loss in GFR (60–89 mL/min/1.73 m^2)
- Stage 3: Moderate loss in GFR (30–59 mL/min/1.73 m^2)
- Stage 4: Severe loss in GFR (15–29 mL/min/1.73 m^2)
- Stage 5: Kidney failure (ESRD) requiring dialysis (GFR <15 mL/min/1.73 m^2)

Diagnostic Testing

- Abdominal and pelvic CT scan
- KUB
- MRI
- Renal biopsy
- Renal ultrasound

Treatment

- Dialysis:
  - CRRT
  - Hemodialysis
  - Peritoneal dialysis
- Kidney transplant
- Medications to manage complications:
  - Anemia
  - Dyslipidemia
  - Hypertension
  - Metabolic/electrolyte disorders
- Nutritional therapy:
  - Fluid restriction
  - Low-protein diet of 0.6 to 0.8 g/kg/d
  - Sodium, potassium, and phosphate restriction

ALERT!

Consider consulting a dietitian or nutritionist to assist with meal planning and food options when preparing for discharge.

Nursing Interventions

- Administer medications as ordered.
- Assess AV fistula for dialysis, if applicable:
  - Assess skin color, pulse, and capillary refill of distal extremity.
  - Auscultate for bruit.
  - Palpate for thrill.
- Assess and maintain sterility of dialysis sites and lines.
- Assess EKG tracings for signs of worsening condition, electrolyte imbalances, or respiratory compromise.
- Assess vital signs for signs of worsening condition or respiratory compromise.
- Maintain strict I/O.
- Manage CRRT machine.
  - Discuss the fluid balance goals for each shift with renal team.
- Monitor fluid volume status:
  - Daily weight
  - Extra heart sounds (S3/S4, gallops, murmurs, and/or pericardial friction rubs)
  - Fluid intake from PO and/or IV fluids
  - JVD
  - Lung sounds
  - Mucous membranes
  - Peripheral edema
  - Skin turgor
  - Urine output
- Monitor neurologic status:
  - Assess for altered mental status and decreased LOC.
- Monitor and draw serial labs as ordered.
- Perform bladder scan, if needed.

Patient Education

- Avoid nephrotoxic agents (such as certain antibiotics, diuretics, contrast dye, statins, antihypertensives, or benzodiazepines) unless directed by provider.
- Avoid NSAIDs as directed by provider.
- Check blood pressure daily.
- Engage in daily physical activity.
- Follow up with scheduled outpatient appointments, dialysis sessions, and blood draws.
- Learn about renal diet modifications, including any diet requirements with fluid restrictions; high protein; or low potassium, phosphate, and sodium.
- Maintain blood sugars within target range if diabetes is present.
- Self-monitor for signs of fluid overload (such as edema in feet and ankles), worsening dyspnea, palpitations, or chest pain.

 POP QUIZ 14.2

ESRD is diagnosed after GFR decreases to what value?

 ALERT!

The National Kidney Foundation recommends that patients receiving dialysis avoid drinking more than 32 ounces of fluid per day. When teaching both patients and family, provide education on the importance of this guideline and how exceeding this fluid intake may impact clinical status.

PROSTATE CANCER

Overview

- *Prostate cancer* is a disease in which malignant cells form in the tissues of the prostate.
- Most prostate cancers are diagnosed due to screening by either PSA blood test or rectal exam.
- Most prostate cancers are adenocarcinomas.
- Other cancers that start in the prostate are:
  - Small cell carcinomas
  - Neuroendocrine tumors
  - Sarcomas

COMPLICATIONS

Complications of prostate cancer include erectile dysfunction, infertility, and pain.

Signs and Symptoms

- Decreased urine output
- Hesitancy
- Incomplete bladder emptying
- Nocturia
- Urgency and frequency

Diagnosis

Labs
- PSA
- Serum acid phosphate levels

Diagnostic Testing
- Digital rectal exam to feel wall of prostate gland to look for enlargement, tenderness, lumps, or hard spots
- Ultrasound-guided transrectal biopsy: most common method of diagnosis to find out grade of the cancer (Gleason score)
- MRI with biopsy

(continued)

Diagnostic Testing (continued)

- After confirmation of cancer:
  - CT scan
  - MRI
  - PET
  - Bone scan

Treatment

- Varies depending on stage of cancer
- Radical prostatectomy to remove the prostate, surrounding tissue, and seminal vesicles
- TURP
- Pelvic lymphadenectomy (removal of lymph nodes in the area)
- Radiation
- Chemotherapy
- Hormonal therapy (ADT)
- Targeted therapy

Nursing Interventions

- Assess for signs and symptoms of infection.
- Assess for signs of returning of bowel function after surgery.
- Assess incision sites.
- Manage pain.
- Monitor vitals.

Patient Education

- Do not drive until cleared by provider when taking pain medication.
- If taking hormone therapy, talk with oncologist about side effects.
- Seek immediate care for signs of infection (redness, erythema, unusual or increased drainage, increased pain, fever, altered mental status).
- Take medications as prescribed.
- Talk with oncologist about chemotherapy and radiation treatment side effects and management of side effects.

PYELONEPHRITIS

Overview

- *Pyelonephritis* is an infection of the urinary tract that begins in the urethra or bladder and travels to one or both of the kidneys.
- A kidney infection requires prompt medical attention.
  - Untreated kidney infections can cause permanent kidney damage or sepsis.

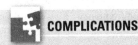 **COMPLICATIONS**

Complications of pyelonephritis include acute kidney failure, infection spreading to other organs around the kidneys, and kidney abscess.

Signs and Symptoms

- Back, flank, abdomen, and groin pain
- Burning sensation or pain when urinating
- Cloudy, foul-smelling urine
- Fever, chills
- Frequent urination
- Hematuria

(continued)

Signs and Symptoms *(continued)*

- Nausea and vomiting
- Painful urination

Diagnosis

Labs

- Blood cultures to assess if infection has spread to the blood
- CBC
- CMP
- UA with C&S

Diagnostic Testing

- CT scan to assess urinary tract and kidneys and look for blockage
- Digital rectal exam to assess prostate as appropriate, as a swollen prostate can block the neck of the bladder
- Kidney ultrasound to look at kidneys and ureters to assess for wounds, stones, or blockages
- Voiding cystourethrogram, which is an x-ray with contrast, of the bladder when full and while urinating to assess for problems in the urethra and bladder

Treatment

- Antibiotics
- Consultation with nephrologist or urologist to address underlying cause in case of frequent infections
- Possible admittance to the hospital for IV antibiotics and IV hydration

NURSING PEARL

After treatment, urine cultures are used to ensure the infection does not return. If it does, 2 more weeks of medicine is offered. If the infection returns again, a 6-week course of antibiotics may be indicated. Surgery may be needed if a block in the urinary tract or a congenital anomaly is found.

Nursing Interventions

- Administer medications as ordered (phenazopyridine, antibiotics).
- Apply heating pad to abdomen, back, or side to ease pain.
- Consult with nephrologist and urologist for further evaluation and treatment because surgery could be indicated to repair a structural abnormality.
- Monitor patient for signs and symptoms of further deterioration/sepsis.
- Monitor fluid intake and output.
- Monitor vital signs for patient deterioration.
- Provide IV hydration.
- Provide pain medications as ordered.

Patient Education

- Avoid products that may irritate the urethra, such as douches or sprays.
- Hydrate well to increase urination and flush bacteria from the urethra.
- Know that phenazopyridine changes the color of the urine to an orange-red.
  - Remember that this medication treats only urinary symptoms, not the infection itself.
- Seek immediate care for any uncontrolled pain, persistent nausea/vomiting, fever/chills, altered mental status, or urinary changes, such as dysuria, hematuria, or inability to urinate.
- Take antibiotics until the full course is completed, even if symptoms resolve.
- Take medications as prescribed.
- Know that urinating after sex may help to flush bacteria out of the urethra.
- Wipe front to back to avoid contamination and infection.

RENAL CALCULI

Overview

- *Renal calculi* are mineral deposits that form within the kidney and often cause severe pain and damage to urinary structures as the body attempts to move the stone through the urinary tract.
- Stones are a leading cause of hematuria.
- Depending on size and location, most stones can be excreted without intervention.

 COMPLICATIONS

Obstructive calculi can cause altered elimination, infection, or ischemia. While 90% of stones can pass through the urinary tract without invasive measures, surgical intervention may be required to remove or break up large-diameter stones (5 mm or greater).

Signs and Symptoms

- Dysuria
- Fever, chills
- Hematuria
- Nausea, vomiting
- Pain in flank (often unilateral), groin, lower abdomen, or back
- Restlessness and irritability
- Urinary retention, weak or interrupted stream of urine
- Urinary urgency

Diagnosis

Labs
- 24-hour urine collection (urine pH, calcium, citrate, magnesium, oxalate, phosphate, sodium, sulfate, uric acid, and total volume)
- BMP
- CBC
- Kidney stone analysis
- UA
- Urine culture with sensitivity

Diagnostic Testing
- CT scan of the abdomen and pelvis with or without contrast
- KUB x-ray
- Renal ultrasound

Treatment

- Administration of antibiotics and antiemetic medication, if indicated
- Facilitation of stone passage with ample hydration using isotonic crystalloid infusion and administration of alpha blocker (tamsulosin) to relax smooth muscle
- Measures to facilitate and monitor stone passage
- Pain management, including nonpharmacologic measures such as repositioning and pharmacologic measures such as administration of opioid analgesics and NSAIDs as needed
- Preparation of patient for procedure if indicated:
  - Cystoscopy
  - ESWL
  - Percutaneous nephrolithotomy
  - Ureteroscopy

Nursing Interventions

- Assess intake and output, strain all urine, and evaluate for urinary retention.
  - Report passage of any stones to medical provider.
  - Observe for hematuria, and alert provider to any increase in bleeding.
- Assess for signs of infection, and monitor hemodynamic status.

Nursing Interventions *(continued)*

- Encourage PO intake to increase hydration to facilitate passing of stone.
  - If patient is unable to tolerate PO intake due to nausea/vomiting, administer antiemetic medications as ordered and provide IV fluids to maintain hydration.
  - Aim to achieve urine output of 3,000 to 4,000 mL/24 hr.
- Facilitate ambulation.
- Monitor pain and administer medications as ordered.
- Promote dietary changes (see Patient Education for specifics), if applicable.

Patient Education

- Complete entire course of antibiotics as ordered.
- Learn risk factors for stone recurrence and adhere to appropriate dietary changes as indicated.
- Learn suggested therapies and dietary changes for stone composition (if known):
  - Calcium stones: limited sodium and protein intake, increased fluid intake, prescription of ammonium chloride to acidify urine, thiazide diuretics as indicated for treatment of hypercalciuria
  - Cystine stones: limited protein intake, increased fluid intake, increased intake of fruits and vegetables, addition of medication to alkalize urine (potassium citrate)
  - Struvite stones: decreased sodium intake, increased fluid intake, antibiotic administration, and surgical removal often indicated as these stones are often larger and usually associated with underlying infection
  - Uric acid stones: limited protein intake, low-purine diet (limiting or eliminating high-purine foods such as organ meats, red meat, seafood such as sardines, and certain alcohols such as beer and distilled liquors), prescription of xanthine oxidase inhibitor (allopurinol), addition of vitamin C supplement
- Know that phenazopyridine changes the color of urine to an orange-red.
  - Remember that this medication treats only urinary symptoms, not the infection.
- Seek immediate care for any uncontrolled pain, persistent nausea/vomiting, fever/chills, or urinary changes, such as dysuria, hematuria, or inability to urinate.
  - Monitor bleeding and return for further care if gross hematuria occurs.
  - Know that some hematuria is to be expected as stones are passed through the urinary tract.
- Take medications as prescribed.

 POP QUIZ 14.3

A patient arrives complaining of severe lower back pain radiating to the groin. The patient's UA is positive for hematuria. What interventions should the nurse anticipate?

TESTICULAR CANCER

Overview

- Testicular cancer occurs in the testicles, which are located outside the scrotum.
- Testicular cancer is rare but is the most common cancer in American males between ages 15 and 35 years.
- Testicular cancer is highly treatable when diagnosed early.
- In general, there are two types of testicular cancer.
  - *Seminoma* is found in all age groups but is more common in older men and is typically less aggressive.
  - *Nonseminoma* develops earlier in life and grows rapidly.
    - Nonseminoma cancers include choriocarcinoma, embryonal carcinoma, teratoma, and yolk sac tumor.

 COMPLICATIONS

Complications of testicular cancer involve side effects of chemotherapy treatment, including pulmonary toxicity, kidney damage, and nerve damage. Testicular cancer can also cause infertility.

Signs and Symptoms

- Back pain
- Dull ache in abdomen or groin
- Enlargement or tenderness of breasts
- Feeling of heaviness in scrotum
- Lump or enlargement of either testicle
- Pain or discomfort in testicle or scrotum
- Sudden collection of fluid in the scrotum

Diagnosis

Labs
- Tumor markers to assess the level of cancer involvement before and after treatment

Diagnostic Testing
- CT to assess abdomen, chest, and pelvis for spread of cancer
- Testicular ultrasound to assess testicles and scrotum for abnormalities

Treatment

- Chemotherapy: may be recommended before/after surgery
- Radiation therapy: sometimes used in seminoma
  - Radiation therapy: may be recommended after surgery
- Radical inguinal orchiectomy to remove the testicle if cancer is suspected
- Surgery to remove nearby lymph nodes
- Type and stage of testicular cancer: will determine treatment

Nursing Interventions

- Assess incision if postoperative.
- Assess for signs of return of bowel function after surgery.
- Manage patient's pain.
- Monitor I/O.
- Monitor for signs and symptoms of infection.
- Monitor vital signs.

Patient Education

- Eat a nutritious diet.
- Know that radiation or chemotherapy may lower sperm count and impact fertility.
  - Talk with provider or oncologist about options for preserving sperm before treatment begins.
- Seek immediate care for:
  - Altered mental status
  - Dysuria
  - Fever/chills
  - Hematuria
  - Inability to urinate
  - Persistent nausea/vomiting
- Stop smoking, if applicable, and limit alcohol intake.
- Take medications as prescribed.
- Talk with oncologist about chemotherapy and radiation treatment, side effects, and management of side effects.
- Talk with oncologist about support groups available in the community to provide emotional support.

TESTICULAR TORSION

Overview

- *Testicular torsion* is a urologic emergency in which the spermatic cord twists, leading to restricted arterial blood flow to the testicle.
- Testicular torsion must be identified and corrected emergently, as vascular compromise and ischemia can lead to tissue necrosis within 4 to 6 hours.
- Most cases of testicular torsion occur spontaneously, presenting with acute atraumatic, unilateral groin pain.
- In rare cases, torsion may be associated with exertion, trauma, or malignancy.
- Most cases of testicular torsion occur in adolescence, though this condition may present in patients of any age.

 COMPLICATIONS

Prompt identification and treatment of testicular torsion is key in preserving viability of the affected testicle. Compromised testicular circulation can lead to permanent damage within 4 to 6 hours of onset. If untreated, tissue necrosis will necessitate testicular amputation.

Signs and Symptoms

- Abdominal pain
- Nausea and/or vomiting
- Prehn's sign (pain when elevating the scrotum)
- Sudden-onset unilateral groin/testicular pain
- Testicular changes: swelling, erythema, edema, hardening, "high-riding" or retracted testicle

 NURSING PEARL

Advanced epididymitis can cause testicular swelling and other changes that resemble testicular torsion. To differentiate between the two conditions, consider the onset of the patient's symptoms. Epididymitis is an infection that develops gradually, while testicular torsion has a sudden onset.

Diagnosis

Labs

Emergent intervention may be prioritized over obtaining diagnostic labs; however, the following may be indicated:

- Preoperative labs:
  - CBC
  - CMP
  - Coagulation panel
  - Type and screen in case blood transfusion is needed
- UA
- Urine culture with sensitivity testing

Diagnostic Testing

- Color doppler ultrasonography to assess testicles and check blood flow

Treatment

- Urgent urologic consultation is required within 4 to 6 hours of symptom onset to expedite detorsion interventions and prevent complications related to prolonged vascular compromise.
- Bedside manual detorsion may be attempted if urologic intervention is delayed.
- Emergent orchiopexy is performed if manual detorsion is unsuccessful.
- Orchiectomy, or surgical removal of the testicle, is performed for nonviable testicle.

Nursing Interventions

- Assess pain and administer medications as prescribed.
- Monitor strict urinary output.
- Monitor vital signs and assess for patient deterioration.
- Prepare patient for emergent surgical intervention, if indicated.
- Provide emotional support.

Patient Education

- Avoid sexual stimulation until cleared by urologist to resume sexual activity.
- Seek immediate care for any recurrence of severe testicular pain, changes such as swelling or hardening of the testis, or any signs of infection such as fever/chills, erythema, dysuria, altered mental status, and abdominal pain.
- Take medications as prescribed.
- Talk with provider about available emotional support and resources regarding psychosocial impact of physiologic and cosmetic changes and risk for impaired body image.

POP QUIZ 14.4

A teenage patient calls and reports a sudden onset of scrotal pain, swelling, and erythema. What condition should the nurse suspect?

URINARY RETENTION

Overview

- *Urinary retention* is the acute or chronic inability to completely empty the bladder, which may be related to dysfunction of bladder musculature or obstructive causes, such as prostate enlargement or renal calculi.
- While urinary retention may occur in any patient due to a variety of causes, acute obstructive urinary retention is more likely to occur in older patients between the ages of 60 to 80 years.
  - It is most often related to an acute exacerbation of prostate enlargement.
- Chronic urinary retention is more likely to be neurologic in nature and is often associated with diabetic neuropathy or spinal injury.
  - Older patients with BPH also commonly experience chronic urinary retention, placing this population at greater risk for the development of urinary infections.
- Urinary retention increases likelihood of developing acute renal failure, UTIs, and urosepsis.

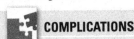

COMPLICATIONS

Urinary retention should be evaluated by assessing postvoid residual volumes via bladder ultrasound. A residual volume of 300 mL or greater suggests urinary retention, indicating possible need for catheterization.

Signs and Symptoms

- Bladder distention (palpable or detected with ultrasound)
- Dysuria
- Frequent urination in small amounts
- Lower abdominal pain
- Nocturia
- Feeling of needing to urinate after completing urination
- Urgency
- Urinary hesitancy
- Weak or interrupted urinary stream

Diagnosis

Labs
- BMP
- CBC
- PSA (in patients older than 50 years or if enlarged prostate is palpated)
- UA
- Urine culture with sensitivity testing

Diagnostic Testing

Postvoid residual obtained by ultrasound alone may be diagnostic; however, the following may be indicated to further investigate retention:

- CT scan of the abdomen and pelvis
- MRI
- Urodynamic testing (cystometry, EMG)
- Ultrasound
- Voiding cystourethrogram

Treatment

- Insertion of a urinary catheter is required for bladder decompression:
  - Advancement of the catheter may be difficult due to an enlarged prostate or other urologic conditions; catheterization may be deferred to urology to minimize urethral/genital trauma.
  - Ongoing management often involves intermittent catheterization, which is preferred because chronic indwelling catheters increase infection risk.
  - Some circumstances may contraindicate urethral catheterization by the RN, such as a patient with recent urologic surgery.
- Surgical placement of a suprapubic catheter may be required in cases where urethral catheterization is contraindicated or not possible.
- Treatment may include that of underlying conditions such as BPH, UTI, renal failure, and malignancy.
- For patients with BPH, treatment may include medical management with finasteride and tamsulosin to assist in facilitating proper urinary flow.

 NURSING PEARL

Patients with urinary retention related to an enlarged prostate may require placement of a larger coudé catheter with a curved tip to enable the catheter to bypass the prostate and facilitate urinary drainage.

Nursing Interventions

- Administer medications, such as alpha blockers or 5-alpha reductase inhibitors, as prescribed (see Appendix 14.1).
- Assess bladder volume using ultrasound, and reassess postvoid residual volume.
- Assess urine volume and quality, noting any hematuria or foul odor.
- Maintain strict I/O.
- Perform abdominal/GU assessment and discuss voiding pattern with patient.
- Perform urethral catheterization using sterile technique, if indicated or ordered by provider.
- Strain urine if renal calculi suspected.

Patient Education

- If discharged with indwelling catheter:
  - Clean around the insertion site twice daily with soap and water.
  - Empty the drainage bag every 3 to 6 hours or when two-thirds full.
  - Ensure catheter is secured to the leg to limit movement and pulling.
  - Keep the drainage bag below waist level and avoid kinking/obstructing tubing.
  - Use a leg-bag if ambulatory and connect to a standard drainage bag overnight.
  - Seek immediate care for signs of infection, such as fever, pain, or altered mental status.
  - Seek immediate care if catheter dislodges, if urine is leaking around catheter, if urine quality changes (hematuria, gross sediment), or if urine is no longer draining.
- Practice aseptic and intermittent self-catheterization if indicated.
- Seek further care if experiencing:
  - Altered mental status
  - Dysuria

(continued)

Patient Education *(continued)*

- Fever
- Flank pain
- Inability to void
- Increased urinary frequency
- Suprapubic fullness/discomfort

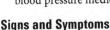

URINARY INCONTINENCE

Overview

- Urinary incontinence is loss of bladder control that may range from occasional, minor leaks of urine to frequent, small-to-moderate amounts of urine.
- Urinary incontinence is more common in older adults.
- The muscles in the bladder and urethra become weaker with age.
- Urinary incontinence may also be affected by certain drinks, foods, and medications that act as diuretics, including alcohol, artificial sweeteners, blood pressure medications, caffeine, and spicy foods.

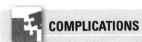

COMPLICATIONS

Complications of urinary incontinence include skin issues, personal/social issues, and UTIs.

Signs and Symptoms

Symptoms depend on the type of urinary incontinence:

- Functional incontinence: physical or mental impairment making a patient unable to reach the bathroom in time
- Mixed incontinence: more than one type of urinary incontinence, usually a combination of stress and urge incontinence
- Overflow incontinence: frequent or constant dribbling of urine because bladder does not empty completely
- Stress incontinence: urine leaks when pressure is exerted on the bladder, usually related to coughing, sneezing, laughing, lifting heavy objects, or exercising
- Urge incontinence: sudden, intense urge to urinate followed by an involuntary loss of urine: can be caused by infection or by something more serious, such as a neurologic disorder or diabetes

Diagnosis

Labs

- UA and C&S to assess for infection

Diagnostic Testing

- History and physical examination to determine diet, fluid intake habits, and incontinence description
- Postvoid residual with a catheter or ultrasound to assess for blockages or problems with bladder nerves and/or muscles
- Pelvic ultrasound to assess bladder and urethra for further testing

Treatment

Treatment depends on the type of urinary incontinence.

- Train bladder to minimize the frequency of voiding to about every 2.5 to 3.5 hours.
  - Patient is instructed to hold off urinating for about 10 minutes after they have the urge to urinate. The goal is to lengthen the time between trips to the toilet and then gradually increase that time.
- Double void (i.e., urinate, wait a few minutes, and urinate again to make sure the bladder is emptied completely).

Treatment *(continued)*

- Electrical stimulation may be used to strengthen the pelvic floor muscles.
- Manage fluid and diet to regain control of the bladder.
- Provide interventional therapies:
  - Injections, such as of botulinum toxin, into the bladder muscle
  - Nerve stimulators inserted under the skin near the sacrum or the vagina, stimulating the sacral nerves and thus helping to control an overactive bladder or urge incontinence
  - Synthetic bulking material injected around urethra to keep urethra closed: this method has not been shown to be as effective as more invasive methods
- Administer medications:
  - Anticholinergics to calm an overactive bladder
  - Alpha blockers to relax the bladder neck
- Use devices only as necessary due to increased risk of UTIs:
  - Pessary: a flexible silicone ring that is inserted into the vagina and worn all day: acts to support the urethra and prevent leakage
  - Urethral insert: a small, tampon-like disposable device that is inserted into the vagina and acts as a plug: removed before urination
- Provider may use urinary catheter for the short term if the patient's bladder is not emptying correctly. Long-term use of a urinary catheter can lead to a UTI.
- Refer to physical therapist as needed for pelvic floor strengthening if pelvic floor dysfunction is a contributing factor.
- Schedule voiding times every 2 to 4 hours to avoid waiting until urgency is felt.
- Perform surgery:
  - Artificial urinary sphincter is implanted around the bladder neck: patient presses a valve implanted under the skin that deflates and allows urine to flow to void.
  - Bladder neck suspension: helps support the urethra and bladder neck.
  - Sling procedures: mesh made from a patient's tissue or synthetic is used to create a pelvic sling under the urethra to help the urethra to close. This helps to treat stress incontinence.

Nursing Interventions

- Assess patient and vital signs regularly and assess for infection.
- Assess surrounding skin for signs of maceration and protect skin integrity as necessary.
  - Consider using barrier cream on skin if patient is wet or urinating often to protect surrounding skin.
- Assess voiding pattern and evaluate urinary retention.
  - The patient may require a urinary catheter if retaining urine.
- Consider having a bedside commode nearby for patients who get up frequently to void.
- Document input and output.

Patient Education

- Avoid alcohol, caffeine, and spicy foods; consider seeing a dietician.
- Avoid consuming large amounts of liquids.
- Avoid douching because it can increase risk for infection.
- Cleanse around vagina and rectum to prevent infection.
- Clean around catheter at insertion site and 6 inches down tubing, and empty bag as indicated.
  - Do not let urinary catheter bag overfill: empty as needed and record output if indicated.
- Discuss signs and symptoms of infection and when to call the healthcare provider.
- Eat adequate fiber to avoid constipation.
- Obtain and use a bedside commode at home if getting up frequently at night to void.
- Take medications as prescribed.
- Keep a voiding log if needed.
- Use barrier cream for surrounding skin.
- Stop smoking, if applicable.

URINARY TRACT INFECTIONS

Overview

- UTIs are among the most common infections affecting the GU system, occurring when microorganisms enter the urinary tract.
- Infections are classified by location and may be further categorized as complicated versus uncomplicated infections.
  - Upper UTIs refer to infection in the kidneys, while lower UTIs refer to infection of the bladder and urethra.
    - *Cystitis* refers to bacterial infection of the bladder, usually as a result of urethral colonization by fecal or vaginal flora (most commonly *Escherichia coli*). While most patients presenting with cystitis complain of typical urinary symptoms (such as dysuria and increased frequency), older adults often present with more nonspecific symptoms, such as lethargy and altered mental status.
    - *Pyelonephritis* is a bacterial infection of the kidneys that most often occurs as the result of ascending infection from the lower urinary tract. Patients with pyelonephritis usually experience flank pain, fever, and nausea/vomiting, and this condition may progress to sepsis.
  - Uncomplicated UTIs are more likely to occur in women and are usually caused by perineal bacteria.
  - Complicated UTIs are more likely to occur in patients with urologic abnormalities and may be related to iatrogenic causes, such as catheterization.
    - A complicated UTI refers to any UTI with features suggesting that infection likely extends beyond the bladder, with signs of systemic illness such as fever, chills, flank pain, costovertebral angle tenderness, and pelvic or perineal discomfort.
    - This includes infections involving the parenchyma (pyelonephritis and prostatitis).
    - Those with urologic abnormalities and recurrent UTIs are at increased risk for multidrug-resistant infections. Providers must look to urine culture and specificity to guide antibiotic treatment.
- UTI is responsible for nearly 25% of all cases of sepsis.
  - Nurses must be vigilant for signs of worsening infection, such as the development of systemic symptoms (including altered mental status, fevers, tachycardia, and tachypnea).

> **COMPLICATIONS**
>
> Patients with comorbidities and previous GU conditions, including internal stents or enlarged prostates, are at a higher risk for complicated UTIs. These patients may require multiple antibiotics and hospital admission to treat the infection.

Signs and Symptoms

- Abdominal, suprapubic, and/or flank pain
- Altered mental status
- Cloudy urine
- Dysuria
- Fever, chills
- Foul-smelling urine
- Hematuria
- Nausea, vomiting
- Urinary frequency and urgency
- Urinary retention
- Weakness, lethargy

> **ALERT!**
>
> Older adult patients with UTIs often present with altered mental status, although this is not considered a classic symptom of UTI.

Diagnosis

Labs

- Lab tests are dependent upon presentation, as minor symptoms may require little to no lab testing.
- Patients presenting with more severe or broad symptoms may require a more thorough workup.
  - BMP
  - Blood cultures (if urosepsis is suspected)

(continued)

Labs (continued)

- CBC
- HCG (urine or serum, if applicable)
- PSA (if applicable)
- Screening for STIs (genital cultures, HIV antibody testing, RPR, hepatitis panel)
- UA with C&S

Diagnostic Testing

- Radiographic imaging is often not required for diagnosis of urinary or genital complaints.
- More severe symptoms may require:
  - CT scan of the abdomen and pelvis
  - KUB x-ray
  - Ultrasound (abdominal, transvaginal, or scrotal)

Treatment

- Antibiotic therapy (see Table A.1)
  - Most uncomplicated UTIs can be managed in the outpatient setting and treated with a brief course of oral antibiotics.
  - Complicated UTIs are more likely to reoccur, and treatment becomes more challenging if drug-resistant pathogens have invaded the urinary tract.
    - Patients often require hospital admission to receive IV antibiotics and to monitor patient response and progression.
    - Treatment plan may need to be altered if no improvement occurs within 24 to 48 hours.
    - Complicated UTIs are more likely to progress to urosepsis.
    - Antibiotic choice should always be guided by urine culture and sensitivity results to limit proliferation of MDROs.
    - Recurrent infections are often treated based on previous urine culture results until most recent results are finalized.
    - Patients with recurrent UTIs are often treated only when symptomatic.
- Antipyretics, such as acetaminophen (see Table A.2)
- Pain management, such as a limited course of phenazopyridine hydrochloride for topical analgesia of the urinary tract mucosa (see Appendix 14.1)
  - Phenazopyridine changes the color of the urine to an orange-red.
  - Remind patient that this medication treats only urinary symptoms, not the infection itself.
- Fluid resuscitation with isotonic crystalloid, if indicated

 ALERT!

CAUTI are the most common hospital-acquired infections. Reducing unnecessary catheterizations, using proper sterile technique, and removing indwelling catheters as soon as possible all assist in reducing rates of CAUTI.

Nursing Interventions

- Administer antibiotics as ordered.
- Assess voiding pattern and evaluate for urinary retention.
- Continually reassess readiness for urinary catheter removal, and discontinue catheter as soon as appropriate.
- Institute fall precautions for all patients, especially older adults.
- Monitor I/O.
- Monitor for signs of worsening infection.
- Monitor vital signs, especially noting for fever, hypotension, or tachycardia.
- Perform catheterization as indicated for specimen collection, using aseptic technique.
  - Depending on institutional guidelines, this may involve replacing a long-term indwelling catheter prior to specimen collection.
- Provide perineal care and proper catheter care as indicated.

Patient Education

- Wipe skin from front to back after voiding.
- Avoid douching.
- Follow up regarding urine culture results.
- For long-term indwelling catheters, practice proper cleansing and catheter care.
  - Wash hands before touching the catheter.
  - Use mild soap and water to cleanse the genital area.
    - ○ Retract foreskin (if needed) to cleanse penis around the urethra.
    - ○ Separate the labia to cleanse around the urethra.
  - Continue cleaning the catheter itself from where it enters the body to 6 inches down tubing.
  - Dry the skin and the catheter itself.
  - Ensure the catheter is reattached to a securing device to limit catheter movement and prevent shearing.
- Maintain adequate hydration and nutrition.
- Seek immediate care for any uncontrolled pain, persistent nausea/vomiting, fever/chills, altered mental status, or urinary changes, such as dysuria, hematuria, or inability to urinate.
- Take all medications as prescribed, and be sure to complete the full course of antibiotics.
- Use gentle soaps when cleansing.
- Void after intercourse.

POP QUIZ 14.5

An older adult patient with a chronic indwelling urinary catheter starts complaining of flank pain. The nurse notes that the patient has a fever and altered mental status. What should the nurse suspect as the most likely cause of the patient's symptoms? What diagnostic tests should the nurse anticipate?

Appendix 14.1 Medications for Renal System

Indications	Mechanism of Action	Contraindications, Precautions, and Adverse Effects
Diuretics: loop (furosemide)		
• Fluid overload • Renal dysfunction	• Secretion of electrolytes and water by preventing resorption and increasing urine output	• Contraindications include hypersensitivity and cross sensitivity with sulfonamides (thiazide diuretics). • Use caution in hypokalemia, digoxin therapy, cardiac disease, and arrhythmia. • Adverse effects include hypokalemia, dehydration, hypomagnesemia, and hyponatremia.
Urinary analgesics (phenazopyridine hydrochloride)		
• Symptomatic relief of lower urinary tract discomfort	• Mechanism of action is unknown; azo dye provides topical analgesic effect on urinary tract mucosa	• Contraindicated in patients with impaired renal function and those with G6PD deficiency. • Educate patients that drug causes urine discoloration (red-orange stain). • Limit use to 2 days. • Medication may cause GI discomfort, so administer with meals.

(continued)

Appendix 14.1 Medications for Renal System *(continued)*

Indications	Mechanism of Action	Contraindications, Precautions, and Adverse Effects
5-Alpha reductase inhibitors (finasteride)		
• Symptomatic treatment of BPH, reducing symptoms, decreasing risk of urinary retention, and decreasing likelihood of requiring surgical interventions such as TURP and prostatectomy	• Act as an analog of testosterone to competitively inhibit type II 5-alpha reductase, thereby inhibiting conversion of testosterone into 5-alpha-dihydrotestosterone, an isoenzyme that stimulates prostate tissue development	• Use with caution in patients with hepatic disease. • Therapy is expected to result in a decreased serum PSA concentration. • Any increase from baseline PSA in patients using finasteride should be considered a possible signal of prostate cancer development. • Medication includes potential for increased incidence of high-grade prostate cancer.
Alpha blockers (tamsulosin hydrochloride)		
• Treatment of signs and symptoms of BPH, medical expulsive treatment of renal calculi	• Selective antagonist of alpha-1 receptors, assisting to mediate smooth muscle contraction, causing relaxation of the bladder neck and prostate	• Drug is a sulfa derivative and contraindicated in patients with sulfa allergy. • Use with caution in patients with history of hypotension and heart disease, as it may contribute to orthostatic hypotension. • There are significant drug–drug interactions, so assess interactions with concurrent therapies.
Alpha-1 agonists (phenylephrine)		
• Provide localized vasoconstriction when injected for priapism	• Mediate vasoconstriction through localized stimulation of alpha-adrenergic receptors	• Though localized effect is intended, systemic effects may occur (hypertension, tachycardia, reflex bradycardia, palpitations, and arrhythmias). • Use with caution in patients with cardiac disease. • Contraindicated in patients with poorly controlled hypertension or concurrent use of MAOIs.

(continued)

Appendix 14.1 Medications for Renal System *(continued)*

Indications	Mechanism of Action	Contraindications, Precautions, and Adverse Effects
Anticholinergics (e.g., oxybutynin, tolterodine, darifenacin)		
• Used for an overactive bladder with symptoms of urge urinary incontinence • Antispasmodic medication	• Act as a smooth muscle relaxer and antispasmodic • Bladder muscle relaxant that suppresses the urge to void by delaying the initial desire to void • Anticholinergics block acetylcholine from binding to its receptors in the nerve cells, blocking signals and decreasing involuntary muscle movement and nerve impulses to control urination	• Lower doses may be indicated in patients with hepatic impairment and renal impairment. • This medication can exacerbate symptoms in dementia. • Contraindicated in patients with Parkinson's disease, as this medication may cause cognitive impairment. • Contraindicated in pregnancy and breastfeeding. • Use cautiously in older adult patients, as this population is more susceptible to side effects such as sedation. • Drug may be contraindicated in some patients with an enlarged prostate. • Drug may also cause anticholinergic actions in the CNS, parotid glands, and GI tract. • Anticholinergic side effects may include dry mouth, blurred vision, constipation, urinary retention, dizziness (due to drop in blood pressure), cognitive problems (confusion), heart rhythm disturbances, and drowsiness. • Patients with high blood pressure, HF, and high heart rate should not take this medication.

RESOURCES

Alawamlh, O., Goueli, R., & Lee, R. K. (2018). Lower urinary tract symptoms, benign prostatic hyperplasia, and urinary retention. *The Medical Clinics of North America, 102*(2), 301–311. https://doi.org/10.1016/j.mcna.2017.10.005

Aune, D., Mahamat-Saleh, Y., Norat, T., & Riboli, E. (2018). Body fatness, diabetes, physical activity and risk of kidney stones: A systematic review and meta-analysis of cohort studies. *European Journal of Epidemiology, 33*(11), 1033–1047. https://doi.org/10.1007/s10654-018-0426-4

Clinic, M. (2021, March 31). *Calciphylaxis.* https://www.mayoclinic.org/diseasesconditions/calciphylaxis/symptomscauses/syc20370559#:~:text=Calciphylaxis%20(kal%2Dsih%2Dfuh,that%20can%20lead%20to%20death

Clinic, M. (2022, February 6). *Epididymitis.* https://www.mayoclinic.org/diseases-conditions/epididymitis/symptoms-causes/syc-20363853#:~:text=Epididymitis%20is%20an%20inflammation%20of,that%20usually%20comes%20on%20gradually

Clinic, M. (2022, February 26). *Urinary incontinence.* https://www.mayoclinic.org/diseases-conditions/urinary-incontinence/symptoms-causes/syc-20352808

Gawlik, K., Melnyk, B., & Teall, A. (2021). *Evidence-based physical examination.* Springer Publishing Company.

Griffin, B. R., Liu, K. D., & Teixeira, J. P. (2020, March). Critical care nephrology: Core curriculum 2020. *American Journal of Kidney Diseases, 75*(3), 435–452.

Han, H., Segal, A. M., Seifter, J. L., & Dwyer, J. T. (2015). Nutritional management of kidney stones (nephrolithiasis). *Clinical Nutrition Research, 4*(3), 137–152. https://doi.org/10.7762/cnr.2015.4.3.137

Howe, A. S., Vasudevan, V., Kongnyuy, M., Rychik, K., Thomas, L. A., Matuskova, M., Friedman, S. C., Gitlin, J. S., Reda, E. F., & Palmer, L. S. (2017). Degree of twisting and duration of symptoms are prognostic factors of testis salvage during episodes of testicular torsion. *Translational Andrology and Urology, 6*(6), 1159–1166. https://doi.org/10.21037/tau.2017.09.10

Medscape. (2022, February 26). *Urinary incontinence.* https://emedicine.medscape.com/article/452289-overview

Mellick, L. B., Sinex, J. E., Gibson, R. W., & Mears, K. (2019). A systematic review of testicle survival time after a torsion event. *Pediatric Emergency Care, 35*(12), 821–825. https://doi.org/10.1097/PEC.0000000000001287

National Cancer Institute. (2021). *Normal prostate and benign prostatic hyperplasia. Understanding prostate changes: A health guide for men.* https://www.cancer.gov/types/prostate/understanding-prostate-changes

National Cancer Institute. (2022, February 6). *Prostate cancer.* https://www.cancer.gov/types/prostate

National Kidney Foundation. (n.d.). *Fluid overload in a dialysis patient.* https://www.kidney.org/atoz/content/fluid-overload-dialysis-patient

National Center for Biotechnology Information. (2022, February 6). *Kidney disease.* https://www.ncbi.nlm.nih.gov/books/NBK568778/

Northwestern Medicine. (2022, February 26). *Types of urinary incontinence.* https://urogynecology.nm.org/urinary-incontinence.html

Prescriber's Digital Reference. (n.d.). *Phenazopyridine hydrochloride* [Drug information]. https://www.pdr.net/drug-summary/Pyridium-phenazopyridine-hydrochloride-3457

Prescriber's Digital Reference. (n.d.). *Phenylephrine hydrochloride* [Drug information]. https://www.pdr.net/drug-summary/Vazculep-pheylephrine-hydrochloride-3539.412

Prescriber's Digital Reference. (n.d.). *Tamsulosin hydrochloride* [Drug information]. https://www.pdr.net/drug-summary/Flomax-tamsulosin-hydrochloride-2893.5649

Serlin, D. C., Heidelbaugh, J. J., & Stoffel, J. T. (2018). Urinary retention in adults: Evaluation and initial management. *American Family Physician, 98*(8), 496–503.

Urology Health. (2022, February 6). *Benign prostatic hyperplasia.* https://www.urologyhealth.org/urology-a-z/b/benign-prostatic-hyperplasia-(bph)

15

PROFESSIONAL AND LEGAL ISSUES

CARING PRACTICES

Overview

- *Nursing* is the art and science of caring.
- Nurses deliver holistic, patient-centered care in a compassionate, professional manner.
- Nurses consider the physical, psychologic, social, and spiritual aspects of all patients to determine the best care.
- Care that is balanced with the patient's preferences, values, and beliefs is optimal.
- Nurses focus on the protection, promotion, and optimization of health and human autonomy.
- The nursing process is used to plan the patient's care:
  - Assessment
  - Diagnosis
  - Planning
  - Implementation
  - Evaluation

COLLABORATION

Overview

- The nurse provides care for the patient in an interdisciplinary fashion, collaborating with providers and other interdisciplinary teams (e.g., pharmacists, occupational/physical/speech therapists, social workers):
  - Initiates referrals if indicated
  - Participates in interprofessional rounds
  - Values interprofessional expertise to care for the patient
- Clinical pathways and disease navigators assist in the collaboration of teams for wraparound care.

 ALERT!

Effective communication among the healthcare team is crucial to avoid mismanaged care. The nurse must ensure effective communication using enhanced modes such as a standard change of shift process and interdisciplinary rounds.

DELEGATION

Overview

- The nurse is responsible for delegating patient care tasks to the appropriate personnel using critical thinking.
- The RN delegates to another RN, to a licensed practical nurse, or to unlicensed assistive personnel.
- The RN takes into consideration nursing board and facility rules and regulations when delegating.

 POP QUIZ 15.1

The nurse on the unit is preparing a patient for surgery. What would the nurse consider when asking a nurse assistant to take and record the patient's vital signs?

(continued)

Overview *(continued)*

- Five rights of delegation are considered when assigning a task:
  - Right task
  - Right circumstances
  - Right person
  - Right directions and communication
  - Right supervision and evaluation

EVIDENCE-BASED PRACTICE

Overview

- *EBP* is a method that uses the best research or quality improvement data to improve patient outcomes.
- EBP is a six-step process:
  - Formulate clinical question.
  - Research the topic.
  - Sort and review peer-reviewed research.
  - Implement the evidence in practice.
  - Evaluate the change.
  - Share the outcomes of the change.
- The nurse must combine their own expertise with EBP to make the best decisions about the patient's care plan.

 NURSING PEARL

The clinical question is formulated using the PICOT format:

Patients/Population
Intervention
Comparison
Outcome
Time

ETHICS

Overview

- The American Association of Nurses' *Code of Ethics for Nursing* encompasses responsibilities for nurses.
- *Ethics* is the study of an issue with moral deliberation and decision-making.
- Nurses encounter ethical dilemmas in caring for patients, including issues concerning access to care, informed consent, and treatment goals.
- Nurses advocate for the right to informed decision-making and self-determination for patients.
- Nurses collaborate with interprofessional teams for optimal outcomes in ethical discussions.
- Nurses maintain professional boundaries and prevent breaches in privacy when caring for patients.

 POP QUIZ 15.2

A patient on the medical-surgical unit has decided to change their code status to Do Not Resuscitate after 2 years of chemotherapy for malignant cancer. Their family wishes to rescind the order when the patient becomes disoriented. The family states that they do not want the patient to leave them. What is the nurse's action?

FACILITATION OF LEARNING

Overview

- Nurses have a unique connection with their patients that allows them to effectively educate regarding health issues for best outcomes.

(continued)

Overview *(continued)*

- The teaching plan is congruent with the nursing process:
  - Assessing the patient's needs and learning style
  - Diagnosing the patient's learning needs
  - Setting goals with the patient
  - Implementing patient teaching
  - Evaluating the teaching
- Patient education should be comprehensive.
- Nurses should take advantage of educational technology.
- Nurses should use the "teach back" method when administering care to ensure that the patient understands the education.

POP QUIZ 2.1

A patient is learning how to self-inject insulin for the first time. The patient states, "I'm a hands-on person." How would the nurse determine the best way to teach this skill?

LAW

Overview

- Legal issues for nurses include both professional-centered and patient-centered concerns.
  - Professional-centered concerns:
    - Ensuring standards of care are met
    - Maintaining proper state licensure
  - Patient-centered concerns:
    - Ensuring end-of-life wishes are legally obtained through documents such as DNRs and medical power of attorney
    - Ensuring informed consent is obtained
    - Ensuring patients are safe, to include limited use of restraints
    - Protecting the privacy of patients, such as by following HIPAA laws

APPROPRIATE RESPONSES TO CULTURAL AND DIVERSITY CONCERNS

Overview

- Nurses must address individual needs for advocacy as part of their patient's care, including age, race and ethnicity, gender, income, and sexual orientation.
- Nurses must address cultural aspects of care, including values, spirituality, and religion.
- Language translation assistance from a medically certified translator should be used as needed in all aspects of care:
  - Face-to-face translators
  - Phone or video translators
  - Written educational materials and consent forms in the patient's language

ALERT!

Reducing health disparities begins with the nurse. A nurse must assess their own cultural aptitude and develop cultural competence to administer care safely and effectively.

RESOURCES

American Nurses Association. (2021). *Nursing: Scope and standards of practice* (4th ed.). Author.

Glasgow, M. E. S., & Dreher, H. M. (2020). *Legal and ethical issues in nursing education: An essential guide.* Springer Publishing Company.

Lewis, S., Bucher, L., Heitkemper, M., & Harding, M. (2017). *Medical-surgical nursing* (10th ed.). Elsevier.

Wolters, K. (2017). *5 Strategies for providing effective patient education.* https://www.wolterskluwer.com/en/expert-insights/5-strategies-for-providing-effective-patient-education

16

POP QUIZ ANSWERS

CHAPTER 2

Pop Quiz 2.1

The patient has physical symptoms of a MI. The nurse would relieve the pain and dilate the coronary arteries with nitroglycerin (if not contraindicated) or morphine administration per order and apply oxygen to increase the pulse oximetry to greater than 92%. The nurse should anticipate orders to administer aspirin, obtain an EKG, obtain IV access, and prepare the patient for labs and further interventions.

Pop Quiz 2.2

The nurse should notify the provider, obtain IV access, and prepare to administer immediate-acting antihypertensive medications to decrease the blood pressure and to decrease the risk of rupture of the aneurysm. The nurse should also reassess vital signs and relay the information to the provider. Emotional support should be provided to the patient.

Pop Quiz 2.3

The nurse should auscultate an apical heart rate to confirm. The nurse should further assess for symptoms of low heart rate such as chest pain, dizziness, lightheadedness, syncope, and shortness of breath. A full set of vital signs should be evaluated in comparison with previous vital signs to determine if there is a significant change.

Pop Quiz 2.4

The nurse should educate the patient to stop massaging the leg immediately, elevate the leg, and assess for pulses in the leg.

Pop Quiz 2.5

The patient would have weight gain, peripheral edema, and dyspnea. To alleviate these symptoms, the provider would order a diuretic, such as furosemide, to remove the excess fluid. The provider would also order fluid restriction and low-sodium diet.

CHAPTER 3

Pop Quiz 3.1

The nurse should notify the provider. Urine output greater than 4.5 L/24 hr is considered polyuria for this patient.

Pop Quiz 3.2

The patient is showing signs of hypoglycemia. The nurse should check the patient's blood glucose. If the patient is hypoglycemic, the nurse should notify the provider and treat the hypoglycemia immediately by providing the patient with a source of oral glucose, such as juice, if they are awake and alert. If the patient cannot safely swallow, the nurse should give glucose via other means as directed by the provider. Once the patient is euglycemic, the nurse should discuss the order for insulin glargine with the provider.

Pop Quiz 3.3

The nurse should expect potassium to be low. Exogenous insulin causes intracellular potassium shifts, which can lead to hypokalemia.

Pop Quiz 3.4

The nurse should notify the provider, monitor blood glucose frequently, obtain IV access in anticipation of the possible administration of IV dextrose, and administer dextrose-containing continuous IV fluids if ordered to maintain euglycemia.

Pop Quiz 3.5

The patient is potentially experiencing a thyroid storm, which is a rare but life-threatening complication of Graves' disease. The nurse should contact the provider immediately for emergency assistance and prepare the patient by obtaining IV access and applying cardiac monitoring and supplemental oxygen.

CHAPTER 4

Pop Quiz 4.1

The nurse should provide a nightlight and adequate lighting to prevent injury due to decreased vision, be aware that the patient is sensitive to glare, and provide large-print teaching materials.

Pop Quiz 4.2

The bruise indicates that the patient is having possible vision problems. The nurse should investigate with the patient further regarding ability to see with simple vision questions. The nurse should verify glucometer results and insulin syringe numbers/dose, and notify the provider regarding obtaining HA1C level to determine if the current insulin regimen is sufficient. Finally, the nurse should educate the patient regarding diabetic retinopathy symptoms.

Pop Quiz 4.3

The nurse can speak clearly to allow the patient to read lips. If this is not effective, the nurse can use written communication or provide listening devices. The nurse should allow the patient to teach-back the education to ensure understanding.

Pop Quiz 4.4

The nurse should place the patient in a 90-degree position, suction remaining water from the mouth, and notify the provider before administering anything else by mouth to determine if the patient is an aspiration risk. The nurse should anticipate a speech therapy order for diagnostic swallow evaluation.

CHAPTER 5

Pop Quiz 5.1

The most likely diagnosis for this patient is respiratory acidosis.

Pop Quiz 5.2

This rare polymorphic ventricular tachycardia can occur in a patient with low magnesium.

Pop Quiz 5.3

The nurse should suspect that the patient has hypomagnesemia. Hypomagnesemia can cause psychosis and a positive Chvostek's sign, which this patient is exhibiting. The nurse would notify the provider and anticipate administration of IV magnesium.

Pop Quiz 5.4

The nurse should notify the provider. All signs of increasing fluid volume and respiratory distress should be reported to the provider as soon as possible.

CHAPTER 6

Pop Quiz 6.1

The nurse should place the patient in a position of comfort, often in a semi-Fowler's position, supine with hips and knees flexed.

Pop Quiz 6.2

The patient is recommended to follow a gluten-free diet. The safest products note that they are gluten-free on the packaging.

Pop Quiz 6.3

The nurse should educate the patient to maintain a low-fat diet and to avoid high-fat or fried foods. Low-fat foods are those with no more than 3 g of fat per serving. Low-fat foods will be easier for the patient to digest and are less likely to cause gas, bloating, or diarrhea. After surgery, the patient should not eat more than 30% of their calories from fat. The nurse should consider a referral to a dietitian or nutritionist.

CHAPTER 7

Pop Quiz 7.1

The nurse explains that the patient should consume foods rich in iron such as dark leafy greens, dried fruits, legumes, red meat, pork, poultry, and seafood. The patient should also increase foods containing vitamin C, such broccoli, kiwis, melons, and oranges.

Pop Quiz 7.2

The patient could be suffering an MI or a PE, both possible complications of DIC.

Pop Quiz 7.3

The nurse would expect the patient to present with anemia, thrombocytopenia, and elevated or normal WBCs with enlarged lymph nodes.

Pop Quiz 7.4

Hallmark signs of bone pain in the ribs, spine, and pelvis are characteristic of multiple myeloma, not Hodgkin's disease.

Pop Quiz 7.5

The likely cause is pathologic fracture of the bone due to bone degradation from multiple myeloma.

CHAPTER 8

Pop Quiz 8.1

The patient should first be educated regarding sharing needles and the danger of transmission. Per institutional policy, the patient can be referred to needle exchange programs, substance use support groups, and/or substance use treatment programs.

Pop Quiz 8.2

The nurse should notify the provider and activate the emergency response, if applicable. The nurse should administer epinephrine per the facility's emergency protocol and/or provider order. An emergency response team can assist in care if the patient progresses into severe anaphylaxis requiring a higher level of care.

Pop Quiz 8.3

The nurse should draw blood cultures first, before the antibiotics are started.

Pop Quiz 8.4

The nurse is not concerned by this finding. These labs indicate mild anemia, which is a common finding in patients with SLE.

CHAPTER 9

Pop Quiz 9.1

Yes, this patient is experiencing a Stage 1 pressure ulcer. The nurse would notify the provider. The nurse would keep the area elevated and apply appropriate barrier dressings. The nurse would also educate the patient that examination of the feet is important if peripheral neuropathy is present.

Pop Quiz 9.2

WBCs may be elevated, as well as ESR, which may indicate psoriasis. If clinically indicated, the provider may order a biopsy of the sites to confirm the diagnosis. It would be appropriate to supply the patient with information regarding psoriasis and provide emotional support.

Pop Quiz 9.3

The nurse will examine the wound, document measurements, and perform a thorough assessment so progression of wound healing can be monitored. The nurse will assess for signs and symptoms of further complications of infection, such as foul odor and drainage. The nurse will anticipate orders to determine if antibiotics are warranted or to prepare the patient for irrigation and debridement. The nurse will also provide a clean dressing to the site per wound orders. The nurse will provide emotional support to the patient.

CHAPTER 10

Pop Quiz 10.1

The patient is experiencing phantom limb pain. The nurse will provide patient education concerning this condition. Because the patient is postoperative, a complete assessment, including vital signs, will be done. The nurse will assess the pain level and administer prescribed analgesics. Also, the nurse will assess the surgical dressing/wound for complications and provide emotional support.

Pop Quiz 10.2

The nurse should educate the patient to immediately notify the provider if the patient notices numbness and tingling to the right extremity. This can indicate compartment syndrome.

Pop Quiz 10.3

The six Ps are pain, paralysis, paresthesia, pallor, pulselessness, and poikilothermia.

Pop Quiz 10.4

The patient's uric acid blood test result would be elevated. The nurse would prepare the patient for a joint aspiration for synovial fluid analysis to confirm the diagnosis of gout.

CHAPTER 11

Pop Quiz 11.1

The nurse will explain to the patient's family member that this sudden onset of symptoms is caused by hospital delirium and is not related to early-onset dementia. The nurse will explain to the patient and family that dementia has a slow progression, but delirium has a rapid onset and can last up to a few weeks. The nurse will provide emotional support.

Pop Quiz 11.2

The nurse should maintain the patient's airway, then turn the patient to the side to further protect the airway, ensure suction is set up and working to be prepared if seizure worsens, assess vital signs, notify the provider, document the length and severity of the seizure, administer any medications per provider orders, and provide emotional support to the patient.

Pop Quiz 11.3

The thoracic spine is responsible for sensation and motor function at or below the trunk.

Pop Quiz 11.4

The patient is not eligible for tPA. The patient's "last known normal" was 8 hours before the patient was noted to be having stroke-like symptoms. The window for tPA administration is 3 hours.

CHAPTER 12

Pop Quiz 12.1

The nurse would place the patient in the high Fowler's position to improve oxygenation.

Pop Quiz 12.2

Pursed-lip breathing helps reduce respirations and improves the expiratory phase of breathing. Tripod positioning lowers the diaphragm to open lung space.

Pop Quiz 12.3

Airborne precautions include placing the patient in a negative-pressure, single-occupancy room. Also, all staff are to wear HEPA masks when entering the patient's room.

CHAPTER 13

Pop Quiz 13.1

The nurse will provide teaching concerning the JP drain. They will demonstrate emptying of the drain and have the patient return the demonstration. The nurse will instruct the patient to record output and to call the provider if there is increased output, increased bleeding, or signs and symptoms of infection. The nurse will instruct the patient to follow up with the provider for removal of the drain.

Pop Quiz 13.2

The provider will order stool softeners and pelvic floor muscle exercises. The nurse should explain to the patient that they should not strain to produce stool, as this will aggravate muscle weakness. Pelvic floor exercise must be performed on a regular basis to increase the strength of the pelvic floor and relieve pain and pressure.

Pop Quiz 13.3

The patient should report to the provider any vaginal bleeding, foul-smelling discharge, pelvic pain, swelling, fever, or difficulty urinating.

CHAPTER 14

Pop Quiz 14.1

Preoperative teaching is needed for this patient, including education on surgical approach (through the penis) and what to expect after surgery (three-way catheter with bloody urine). The patient should be reassured that no stiches are needed but taught that they may experience soreness and painful urination after surgery.

Pop Quiz 14.2

ESRD is diagnosed after GFR drops below 15 mL/min/1.73 m^2.

Pop Quiz 14.3

This patient is experiencing signs of possible renal calculi. The nurse should expect orders for additional diagnostic testing, including a CT scan of the abdomen and pelvis or a KUB x-ray, and administration of IV fluids and pain medication.

Pop Quiz 14.4

The sudden onset of scrotal pain should prompt the nurse to suspect that this patient has developed testicular torsion. Testicular torsion is the sudden twisting of the spermatic cord. It is a urological emergency and requires prompt surgical intervention to prevent long-term complications.

Pop Quiz 14.5

The nurse should suspect that this patient has developed a complicated UTI. The nurse should notify the provider and expect that there will be an order to collect a UA and urine culture with sensitivity testing from the catheter sampling port. Depending on institutional guidelines, the nurse should remove and place a new catheter prior to collection. The nurse should expect further orders for lab studies such as a CBC, BMP, lactate level, and blood cultures. Radiographic imaging such as an abdominal CT or renal ultrasound may be indicated to investigate flank pain. A head CT scan may also be indicated due to mental status changes.

CHAPTER 15

Pop Quiz 15.1

The nurse would consider if the task is appropriate for the nurse assistant according to their training. The nurse would ensure that the vital signs are taken and recorded correctly.

Pop Quiz 15.2

The nurse would advocate for the decision that the patient made before becoming disoriented. The nurse would collaborate with an interprofessional care team and meet with the family to further discuss the patient's ultimate wishes.

Pop Quiz 15.3

The nurse would first assess the patient's learning style. Because the patient stated that they like to learn by doing, the nurse would instruct the patient to give the shot while offering guidance. The nurse would then ask the patient to "teach back" the skill and would evaluate the patient's teaching.

APPENDIX A: COMMON MEDICATIONS FOR MEDICAL-SURGICAL PATIENTS

Table A.1 Common Antibiotics and Antifungals for Medical-Surgical Patients

General Indications	General Mechanism of Action	General Contraindications, Precautions, and Adverse Effects
Aminoglycosides (gentamicin, streptomycin, neomycin)		
Common indications among aminoglycosides: • Bacteremia and sepsis • Bone and joint infections • Community-acquired pneumonia • Empiric treatment for febrile neutropenia • Infective endocarditis • Intraabdominal infections • Lower respiratory tract infections • Nosocomial pneumonia • Ophthalmic infections • Surgical infection prophylaxis **Specific indications for gentamycin:** • Complicated UTIs • Meningitis and ventriculitis • PID • Pyelonephritis • Skin and skin structure infections **Specific indications for streptomycin:** • Gram-negative bacillary bacteremia, meningitis or lower respiratory tract infections in combination with other antimicrobials • UTI • Drug susceptible tuberculosis **Specific indications for neomycin:** • Adjunctive therapy for hepatic encephalopathy or coma • Infectious diarrhea	• Inhibit bacterial protein synthesis, causing bactericidal effect	• Medication is contraindicated for organisms resistant to aminoglycosides. • Use caution in administering to patients with inflammatory bowel disease, as there is a high likelihood for developing pseudomembranous colitis or *Clostridium difficile*. • Adverse effects include nephrotoxicity, ototoxicity, neurotoxicity, nausea, vomiting, auditory disturbances, headache, skin irritation, rash, anemia, and elevated liver enzymes. • Monitor closely for nephrotoxicity or neurotoxicity, including ototoxicity in all aminoglycoside medications. Nephrotoxicity or ototoxicity development requires dose adjustment or discontinuation.

(continued)

Table A.1 Common Antibiotics and Antifungals for Medical-Surgical Patients *(continued)*

General Indications	General Mechanism of Action	General Contraindications, Precautions, and Adverse Effects
Antiprotozoals, respiratory (pentamidine)		
• Pneumocystis pneumonia • Leishmaniasis • Oral inhalation antifungal agent used for various fungal infections	• Mechanism of action not clearly known; thought to interfere with fungal DNA and RNA replication	• Use caution if administering rapidly, as it can lead to hypotension. • Use caution in patients with renal, hepatic, or cardiac disease; asthma; or pregnancy. • Adverse effects include arrhythmia, bronchospasm, elevated AST/ALT, hypoglycemia, tremor, cough, fever, itching, diarrhea, headache, or night sweats.
Azoles (fluconazole)		
• Cutaneous leishmaniasis • Cutaneous or lymphocutaneous sporotrichosis • Skin or skin structure *Candida* infection • Talaromycosis, coccidioidomycosis, or histoplasmosis prophylaxis in HIV-infected patients • Primary pulmonary histoplasmosis • Bacterial vaginosis • Treatment and prophylaxis treatment for recurrent vulvovaginal candidiasis infections • Osteomyelitis, bone and joint infection caused by *Candida* • Infective endocarditis caused by *Candida* • Infected pacemaker, ICD (implantable cardioverter-defibrillator), or VAD (ventricular assist device), caused by *Candida* • Treatment of meningitis due to *Histoplasma capsulatum* in patients with HIV • CNS infections due to *Coccidioides,* cryptococcus, or *Candida* • Organ transplant recipients • Candida prophylaxis in bone marrow transplant or high-risk cancer patients • Pyelonephritis caused by *Candida* • UTI caused by *Candida* • Intraabdominal infections caused by *Candida* • Pneumonia caused by *Candida* • Thrush	• Alter fungal cell membrane to inhibit fungal reproduction and growth through fungistatic action	• Use caution in cardiac, hepatic, or renal conditions. • Avoid use during pregnancy except in severe, life-threatening emergencies. • Adverse effects include dizziness, rash, diarrhea, nausea, and headache.

(continued)

Table A.1 Common Antibiotics and Antifungals for Medical-Surgical Patients *(continued)*

General Indications	General Mechanism of Action	General Contraindications, Precautions, and Adverse Effects
Beta-lactam penicillin (amoxicillin)		
• Used as first-line treatment of acute bacterial sinusitis • Indicated for adults and children older than 2 years	• Inhibit final stage of bacterial cell wall synthesis by binding to penicillin-binding proteins • Lead to cell lysis	• Use caution and adjusted dosages in renal impairment. • Common side effects include nausea, vomiting, abdominal pain, rash, and diarrhea.
Carbapenems (ertapenem, meropenem)		
Indications for both ertapenem and meropenem: • Bacterial encephalitis or meningitis • Intraabdominal infections • Complicated skin and skin structure infections • Empiric treatment of febrile neutropenia • Bacteremia or sepsis • Pneumonia (CAP (community-acquired pneumonia) or nosocomial) **Additional indications for ertapenem:** • Complicated UTI and pyelonephritis • Acute pelvic infection • Surgical prophylaxis	• Inhibit cell wall synthesis by binding to penicillin-binding proteins inside bacterial cell wall, resulting in cell death to prevent organism growth	• Use caution in patients receiving carbapenem treatment who undergo concurrent hematologic testing. Positive Coombs tests have been reported in patients taking carbapenems (meropenem). • Use caution in patients with cephalosporin, penicillin, or other beta-lactam hypersensitivity, as cross sensitivity is possible. • Use caution in head injury or neurologic disease due to risk of seizure associated with carbapenem administration. • Use caution in renal failure, impairment, or dysfunction, as carbapenems are excreted by the kidneys and can result in further damage. • Use caution when administering to patients with inflammatory bowel disease due to high likelihood of developing pseudomembranous colitis and *C. difficile*. • Adverse effects include nausea, headache, diarrhea, rash, vomiting, confusion, delirium, hypoglycemia, pseudomembranous colitis, neutropenia, renal failure, and seizure.
Cephalosporins, first generation (cefazolin)		
• Upper respiratory tract infections • Skin and skin structure infections • Biliary tract infections • UTI • Infective endocarditis	• Inhibit cell wall synthesis by binding to penicillin-binding proteins inside the bacterial cell wall, resulting in cell death to prevent organism growth, causing bactericidal effect	• Do not administer in viral infections or for organisms with antimicrobial resistance to cephalosporins. • Use caution in allergy to penicillin, as cross reaction is possible.

(continued)

Table A.1 Common Antibiotics and Antifungals for Medical-Surgical Patients *(continued)*

General Indications	General Mechanism of Action	General Contraindications, Precautions, and Adverse Effects
Cephalosporins, first generation (cefazolin) (continued)		
• Surgical infection prophylaxis • Lower respiratory tract infections (pneumococcal pneumonia and community-acquired pneumonia) • Bacteremia • Bone and joint infections • Mastitis • Bacterial encephalitis or meningitis		• Use caution in renal failure, impairment, or dysfunction. Carbapenems are excreted by the kidneys and can result in further damage. • Adverse effects include headache, diarrhea, nausea, vomiting, maculopapular rash, fever, confusion, bleeding, seizures, azotemia, and renal failure. • Medication is contraindicated in cephalosporin-resistant organisms and viral infection.
Cephalosporins, second generation (cefuroxime)		
• Chronic bronchitis • Skin and skin structure infections • UTI • Treatment of bone and joint infection • Pharyngitis • Gonorrhea • Lyme disease • Acute otitis media • Bacteremia • Meningitis • Surgical infection prophylaxis • Tonsillitis • Sinusitis • Intraabdominal infections • Lower respiratory tract infections • Pneumonia (CAP and nosocomial)	• Inhibit bacterial cell wall synthesis by binding to specific penicillin-binding proteins within the cell wall, causing bactericidal effect	• Medication is contraindicated in penicillin allergy, viral infections, or bacteria with known drug resistance. • Use caution in renal failure/impairment, pseudomembranous colitis, and PKU. • Adverse effects include nausea, vomiting, flatulence, dyspepsia, dysuria, phlebitis, jaundice, Stevens–Johnson syndrome, and vasculitis.
Cephalosporins, third generation (ceftriaxone)		
• Bacteremia and sepsis • UTI • Acute bacterial otitis media • Skin and skin structure infections • Surgical incision site infections • Necrotizing infections • Intraabdominal infections • Surgical infection prophylaxis • PID • Bone and joint infections	• Inhibit bacterial cell wall synthesis by binding to specific penicillin-binding proteins within the cell wall, causing bactericidal effect	• Medication is contraindicated in penicillin allergy, jaundice, or hyperbilirubinemia in premature neonates, viral infection, or antimicrobial resistance. • Use caution in GI disease, as it may cause or worsen existing colitis.

(continued)

Table A.1 Common Antibiotics and Antifungals for Medical-Surgical Patients *(continued)*

General Indications	General Mechanism of Action	General Contraindications, Precautions, and Adverse Effects
Cephalosporins, third generation (ceftriaxone) (continued)		
• Lower respiratory tract infection • Pneumonia (nosocomial and CAP) • Infective endocarditis • Meningitis and vasculitis • Gonorrhea • Lyme disease • Congenital syphilis • Bacterial sinusitis		• Adverse effects include seizures, bronchospasm, pancreatitis, biliary obstruction, erythema multiforme, acute generalized exanthematous pustulosis, Stevens–Johnson syndrome, renal failure, thrombocytosis, elevated liver enzymes, anemia, thrombocytopenia, neutropenia, hypoprothrombinemia, jaundice, superinfection, edema, nausea, vomiting, headache, and itching.
Cephalosporin, fourth generation (cefepime)		
• Monotherapy for febrile neutropenia • Complicated UTI and pyelonephritis • Intraabdominal infections • Severe skin and skin structure infections • Pneumonia (CAP and nosocomial) • Bacterial meningitis • Infective endocarditis • Sepsis	• Inhibit bacterial cell wall synthesis by binding to specific penicillin-binding proteins within the cell wall, causing bactericidal effect	• Medication is contraindicated in penicillin allergy and antimicrobial resistance. • Use caution in colitis, GI disturbances, and renal failure. Cefepime may worsen colitis, other GI issues, and kidney function. • Adverse effects include seizure, anaphylactic shock, Stevens–Johnson syndrome, toxic epidermal necrolysis, erythema multiforme, agranulocytosis, pancytopenia, aplastic anemia, elevated liver enzymes, hypophosphatemia, hypoprothrombinemia, bleeding, colitis, vaginitis, pseudomembranous colitis, hypercalcemia, superinfection, confusion, hallucination, rash, vomiting, diarrhea, itching, nausea, headache, and fever.
Cephalosporins, fifth generation (ceftaroline, fosamil)		
• Acute bacterial skin and skin structure infections • Community-acquired pneumonia • Sepsis	• Inhibit bacterial cell wall synthesis by binding to specific penicillin-binding proteins within the cell wall, causing bactericidal effect	• Medication is contraindicated in viral infection and antimicrobial resistance. • Use caution in patients with colitis, GI disturbances, or renal impairments/failure. Condition can be worsened by ceftaroline.

(continued)

Table A.1 Common Antibiotics and Antifungals for Medical-Surgical Patients *(continued)*

General Indications	General Mechanism of Action	General Contraindications, Precautions, and Adverse Effects
Cephalosporins, fifth generation (ceftaroline, fosamil) (continued)		
		• Adverse effects include hyperkalemia or hypokalemia, bradycardia, seizure, renal failure, agranulocytosis, anaphylaxis, elevated liver enzymes, constipation, hepatitis, hyperglycemia, thrombocytopenia, pseudomembranous colitis, encephalopathy, diarrhea, rash, vomiting, abdominal pain, headache, and dizziness.
Fluoroquinolones (ciprofloxacin)		
• UTI, cystitis, and pyelonephritis	• Inhibit DNA gyrase, causing bactericidal effect	• Use caution in patients with cardiac disease or cardiac arrhythmias, CNS disorders, or history of myasthenia gravis, diabetes mellitus, renal impairments, and hepatic dysfunction.
• Lower respiratory tract infections, pneumonia (CAP and nosocomial)		
• Chronic bronchitis exacerbations		• Adverse effects include hepatotoxicity, phototoxicity, tendon rupture, neurotoxicity, hepatic dysfunction, hyperglycemia or hypoglycemia, exacerbation of myasthenia gravis symptoms, worsening colitis or GI dysfunction, nausea, vomiting, or rash.
• Skin and skin structure infections		
• Animal bite wounds		
• Enteric infections		
• Mild to moderate acute sinusitis		
• Acute prostatitis		
• Febrile neutropenia		
• Bacterial conjunctivitis		• Discontinue immediately at any sign of tendon inflammation or tendon pain. These symptoms often present before tendon rupture.
• Ophthalmic infections related to corneal ulcers		
• Acute otitis externa		
• Bone and joint infections		
• Meningococcal infection/prophylaxis		
• Intraabdominal infections		
• Peritoneal dialysis infections		
• Dental infections		
• Surgical infection prophylaxis		
• Pulmonary infections in CF		
• Infective endocarditis		
• Sepsis		
• Traveler's diarrhea		
Glycopeptides (vancomycin)		
• Infective endocarditis	• Bind to parts of bacterial cell wall, preventing synthesis	• Medication is contraindicated in viral infection and vancomycin-resistant organisms.
• Pseudomembranous colitis due to *C. difficile* infection		
• Enterocolitis		• Use caution in renal disease, hearing impairment, HF, and serious rash.
• Sepsis and bacteremia		
• Serious gram-positive infections		
• Mastitis		

(continued)

Table A.1 Common Antibiotics and Antifungals for Medical-Surgical Patients *(continued)*

General Indications	General Mechanism of Action	General Contraindications, Precautions, and Adverse Effects
Glycopeptides (vancomycin) (continued)		
• Gram-positive lower respiratory infections (CAP and nosocomial pneumonia) • Pleural empyema • Surgical infection prophylaxis • Meningitis and other CNS infections • Bone and joint infections • Septic arthritis • Prosthetic joint infections • Febrile neutropenia • Intraabdominal infections • Peritoneal dialysis related peritonitis		• Adverse effects include rash, itching, nausea, abdominal pain, fever, diarrhea, and Stevens–Johnson syndrome.
Lincosamides (clindamycin)		
• Bacteremia • Lower respiratory tract infections, including CAP and nosocomial pneumonia • Intraabdominal infections • Skin and skin structure infections • Animal bites • Diabetic foot ulcer • Gynecologic infections • Bacterial vaginosis • Acne • Mastitis • Bone and joint infections • Bacterial sinusitis • Acute otitis media • Surgical infection prophylaxis	• Bind to RNA of bacteria to inhibit protein synthesis	• Medication is contraindicated in patients with a history of enteritis, UC, and pseudomembranous colitis. • Use caution in patients with diarrhea or hepatic disease. • Adverse effects include toxic epidermal necrolysis, Stevens–Johnson syndrome, erythema multiforme, exfoliative dermatitis, proteinuria, oliguria, superinfection, fungal overgrowth, pseudomembranous colitis, edema, leukopenia, thrombocytopenia, elevated hepatic enzyme, fever, fatigue, dizziness, vomiting, nausea, headache, and itching.
Lipopeptide (daptomycin)		
• Endocarditis • Skin infections including cellulitis, diabetic foot ulcers, and surgical incision site infections. • *Staphylococcus aureus* • VRE infections	• Cell wall structure interference to cause a depolarization of membrane potential, resulting in bacterial cell death	• Medication is inactivated by pulmonary surfactant and is contraindicated in treating pneumonia. • Use with caution in patients with history of *C. difficile* and renal impairment. • Adverse effects include *C. difficile*, peripheral neuropathy, rhabdomyolysis, and serious rashes.

(continued)

Table A.1 Common Antibiotics and Antifungals for Medical-Surgical Patients *(continued)*

General Indications	General Mechanism of Action	General Contraindications, Precautions, and Adverse Effects
Macrolides (azithromycin)		
• Mild to moderate bacterial exacerbations of chronic bronchitis in patients with COPD • Acute otitis media • Bacterial conjunctivitis • CAP • Skin and skin structure infections • PID • Gonorrhea • Mycobacterium infection • Acute bacterial sinusitis • Bacterial endocarditis prophylaxis	• Inhibit protein synthesis in bacterial cells, causing bacteriostatic effect • Bactericidal in high concentrations	• Medication is contraindicated in patients with a history of jaundice or hepatic dysfunction prior to macrolide use, viral infection, and drug-resistant bacteria. • Use caution in renal impairment, cardiovascular disease, colitis, or GI disease, and in patients with a history of myasthenia gravis. • Adverse effects include photosensitivity, arrhythmia and QT prolongation, renal failure, hyperkalemia, bronchospasm, seizures, elevated liver enzymes, hyperbilirubinemia, constipation, jaundice, superinfection, anemia, dermatitis, and hypo- or hyperglycemia.
Oxazolidinones (linezolid)		
• Lower respiratory tract infections • CAP and nosocomial pneumonia • Skin and skin structure infections • Sepsis and bacteremia caused by VRE • MRSA bacteremia • MRSA-associated bone and joint infection • Septic arthritis • Prosthetic joint infections • Meningitis and other CNS infections • Febrile neutropenia • Intraabdominal infections • Peritonitis	• Inhibit bacterial protein synthesis by preventing translation and protein production, thus preventing bacterial growth	• Medication is contraindicated with concurrent use of metrizamide or iohexol during procedures requiring radiographic contrast administration. • Use caution in uncontrolled hypertension, concurrent use with MAOIs, diarrhea, pseudomembranous colitis, history of seizures, and diabetes (may cause hypoglycemia). • Adverse effects include myelosuppression, short-term decreased fertility in male patients, hypoglycemia, pancytopenia, optic neuritis, seizures, anaphylaxis, angioedema, anemia, thrombocytopenia, elevated hepatic enzymes, hypertension, hypoglycemia, pseudomembranous colitis, diarrhea, vomiting, abdominal pain, rash, itching, and tooth discoloration.

(continued)

Table A.1 Common Antibiotics and Antifungals for Medical-Surgical Patients *(continued)*

General Indications	General Mechanism of Action	General Contraindications, Precautions, and Adverse Effects
Penicillin and beta-lactamase inhibitor combinations (augmentin)		
• Used as a second-line treatment for acute bacterial sinusitis • Used in patients with high antibiotic resistance	• Inhibit final stage of bacterial cell wall synthesis by binding to penicillin-bonding proteins • Lead to cell lysis • Inhibit activity of beta-lactamases	• Medication may cause diarrhea, headache, white patches in mouth or throat, or rash. • Use caution when breastfeeding. • Medication may reduce the effects of oral contraceptives.
Penicillins (ampicillin)		
• Severe infections including bacteremia • Infective endocarditis • Respiratory tract infections • Skin and skin structure infections • GU infections • UTI • Gastrointestinal infection	• Inhibit cell wall synthesis to produce a bactericidal effect, preventing organism growth	• Medication is contraindicated in penicillin-resistant organisms. • Use caution in renal impairments, cephalosporin and carbapenem hypersensitivity, colitis and other GI disturbances, and mononucleosis. • Adverse effects include antibiotic-associated colitis, anaphylaxis, exfoliative dermatitis, seizures, rash, nausea, vomiting, leukopenia, thrombocytopenia, platelet dysfunction, anemia, elevated hepatic enzymes, pseudomembranous colitis, superinfection, or diarrhea.
Sulfonamides/trimethoprim (sulfamethoxazole/trimethoprim)		
• UTI • Pyelonephritis • Pneumocystic pneumonia • Otitis media • Acute bacterial exacerbations of chronic bronchitis	• Sulfonamides: Broad spectrum that inhibits enzymes in folic acid synthesis pathway, causing bacteriostatic effects • Trimethoprim: bactericidal • Combination antibiotic synergistic against bacteria	• Medication is contraindicated in folate deficiency, megaloblastic anemia, G6PD deficiency, severe renal impairment, and hepatic disease. • Use caution in patients with hypothyroidism, colitis or GI disturbances, HIV/AIDS, cardiac disease, and arrhythmia. • Adverse effects include megaloblastic anemia, aplastic anemia, hemolytic anemia, TTP (thrombotic thrombocytopenic purpura), angioedema, Stevens–Johnson syndrome, exfoliative dermatitis, anaphylactic reaction, anuria, hyperkalemia, rhabdomyolysis, seizures, hemolysis, leukopenia, QT prolongation, chest pain, dyspnea, nausea, vomiting, itching, fever, and chills.

(continued)

Table A.1 Common Antibiotics and Antifungals for Medical-Surgical Patients *(continued)*

General Indications	General Mechanism of Action	General Contraindications, Precautions, and Adverse Effects
Tetracyclines (doxycycline)		
• Necrotizing ulcerative gingivitis • Treatment when penicillins are contraindicated • Uncomplicated gonorrhea • Chlamydia • Psittacosis • Respiratory tract infections • Skin and skin structure infection • Severe acne • Rocky mountain spotted fever • Cholera • Psittacosis	• Bind to ribosomes of susceptible bacteria and inhibit protein synthesis • Bacteriostatic, bactericidal in high concentrations	• There are no direct contraindications. • Use caution in renal impairment/ failure, hepatic disease, colitis, and GI disease. • Adverse effects include photosensitivity, exfoliative dermatitis, enterocolitis, hepatic failure, pericarditis, anaphylaxis, hemolytic anemia, azotemia, blurred vision, dysphagia, erythema, thrombocytopenia, neutropenia, nail discoloration, headache, vomiting, diarrhea, nausea, rash, and tooth discoloration.

Note: All agents are contraindicated in the presence of hypersensitivity to the medication or one of its components.

Table A.2 Common Pain and Sedation Medications for Medical-Surgical Patients

General Indications	General Mechanism of Action	General Contraindications, Precautions, and Adverse Effects
Analgesics with antipyretic activity (acetaminophen, aspirin)		
• Fever • Mild pain or temporary relief of headache, myalgia, back pain, musculoskeletal pain, dental pain, dysmenorrhea, arthralgia, and minor aches and pains with the common cold or flu • Moderate to severe pain with adjunctive opioid analgesics • Osteoarthritis pain • Acute migraine	• Increase pain threshold by inhibiting prostaglandin synthesis through the COX pathway	• Medication is contraindicated in severe hepatic impairment or severe active hepatic disease. • Use caution in renal disease or G6PD. • Adverse effects include elevated hepatic enzymes, rash, jaundice, hypoprothrombinemia, neutropenia, angioedema, hemolytic anemia, and rhabdomyolysis.
Anticonvulsants, barbiturates (phenobarbital)		
• Status epilepticus • Maintenance for all types of seizures • Short-term treatment of insomnia • Procedural sedation • Relief of preoperative anxiety • Relief of anxiety, tension, and apprehension	• Nonselective CNS depressant with sedative hypnotic actions	• Medication is contraindicated in pulmonary disease in which obstruction or dyspnea is present, hepatic disease or hepatic encephalopathy, pregnancy, and porphyria. • Use caution in acute pain, as paradoxical reactions can occur.

(continued)

Table A.2 Common Pain and Sedation Medications for Medical-Surgical Patients *(continued)*

General Indications	General Mechanism of Action	General Contraindications, Precautions, and Adverse Effects
Anticonvulsants, barbiturates (phenobarbital) (continued)		
		• Use caution in rapid administration of IV phenobarbital, as this can cause bronchospasm. • Do not abruptly discontinue medication, as withdrawal can occur. • Adverse effects include suicidal ideation, megaloblastic anemia, bradycardia, depression, tolerance, impaired cognition, respiratory depression, confusion, elevated liver enzymes, hepatitis, jaundice, neutropenia, dependence, withdrawal if abruptly discontinued, emotional lability, rash, nausea, vomiting, fatigue, decreased libido, and ptosis.
Gabapentinoids (gabapentin)		
• Adjunct treatment of partial seizures • Neuropathic pain • Moderate to severe restless leg syndrome • ALS (amyotrophic lateral sclerosis) • Tremor • Nystagmus • Spasticity due to MS • Pruritis • Fibromyalgia • Dysautonomia following severe TBI (traumatic brain injury) • Alcohol dependence	• Unknown mechanism of action, but thought to bind with high affinity to cells within the brain, reducing pain response	• There are no contraindications to use. • Use caution in renal failure and pulmonary disease. Gabapentin is excreted in the kidneys; dose adjustments may be required for patients in renal failure or with renal impairments. Monitor patients with pulmonary disease carefully for respiratory depression. • Do not abruptly discontinue, as withdrawal symptoms can occur. • Adverse effects include hyperglycemia, withdrawal symptoms if abruptly discontinued, tolerance, depression, confusion and memory impairments, dehydration, jaundice, respiratory depression, dizziness, headache, fatigue, nausea and vomiting, tremor, decreased libido, back pain, emotional lability, skin irritation, diarrhea, and irritability.
General anesthetics (ketamine)		
• General anesthesia induction/ maintenance • Preanesthetic sedation in pediatric patients • Treatment of refractory bronchospasm in status asthmaticus	• Interrupt pathways in the brain prior to producing somesthetic sensory blockade and selectively depress the thalamo-neocortical system	• Medication is contraindicated in patients if additional blood pressure increase would be hazardous, including hypertension, hypertensive crisis, stroke, head trauma, intercranial mass, or intracranial bleeding.

(continued)

Table A.2 Common Pain and Sedation Medications for Medical-Surgical Patients *(continued)*

General Indications	General Mechanism of Action	General Contraindications, Precautions, and Adverse Effects
General anesthetics (ketamine) (continued)		
• Treatment-resistant depression in adults • Moderate to severe pain • Induction agent during rapid sequence intubation		• Use caution in glaucoma and in patients with increased ICP, alcoholism, substance use, and thyrotoxicosis. • Adverse effects include bradycardia, DI, arrhythmia, laryngospasm, apnea, ocular hypertension, increased ICP, hallucinations, delirium, hypertension, respiratory depression, confusion, withdrawal, psychosis, dysphoria, urinary incontinence, nightmares, nausea, vomiting, anxiety, and insomnia.
Nonsteroidal anti-inflammatory drugs (ibuprofen, ketorolac)		
• Relief of minor aches and pain as analgesic • Temporary fever reduction as an antipyretic • Short-term treatment of moderate pain and acute migraine (ketorolac)	• Inhibit COX 1 and 2 enzymes to decrease formation of prostaglandin precursors	• Medication is contraindicated for treatment after CABG (coronary artery bypass grafting) surgery. • Adverse effects include AKI, increased risk of cardiovascular thrombotic events and gastrointestinal bleeding, ulceration, and inflammation. • Use caution in patients with coagulation disorders, liver disease, renal impairment, and hyperkalemia. • Do not use ketorolac for longer than 5 days due to risk of serious adverse effects.
Opioids: fentanyl		
• Control of moderate to severe pain • Intraoperative or procedural management of severe pain • Postoperative main management • Management of chronic severe pain in opioid-tolerant patients requiring around-the-clock, long-term opioid treatment • Management of severe breakthrough cancer pain in opioid-tolerant patients • Short-term management of acute postoperative pain • Adjunctive management of general anesthesia maintenance and intraoperative pain control	• Bind to pain receptors in the body to decrease pain pathways and alleviate pain	• Transdermal fentanyl patches are contraindicated in patients with known or suspected paralytic ileus or GI obstruction. • Nonparenteral fentanyl is contraindicated in status asthmaticus and severe respiratory depression. • Do not stop taking medication abruptly, as it may cause withdrawal to occur. • Use caution in patients with history of alcoholism or substance use, as there is a high risk for psychologic dependence. • Use with caution in patients with respiratory disorders, as it may cause respiratory depression.

(continued)

Table A.2 Common Pain and Sedation Medications for Medical-Surgical Patients *(continued)*

General Indications	General Mechanism of Action	General Contraindications, Precautions, and Adverse Effects
Opioids: fentanyl (continued)		
• Major surgery • Sedation and analgesia prior to rapid sequence intubation • Management of dyspnea in patients with end-stage cancer or lung disease • Procedural sedation		• Use caution in patients with head trauma or neurologic disorder, as it may increase drowsiness and decrease respirations. • Adverse effects include GI obstruction, bradycardia, laryngospasm, respiratory depression, pneumothorax, apnea, chest wall rigidity, ileus, arrhythmia, constipation, hypokalemia, hypoventilation, respiratory depression, dyspnea, confusion, hallucinations, dysphoria, blurred vision, psychologic and physiologic dependence, withdrawal, rash, vomiting, abnormal dreams, drowsiness, fatigue, paranoia, anxiety, agitation, emotional lability, and nausea.
Opioids: hydrocodone		
• Treatment of chronic severe pain requiring around-the-clock long-term opioid treatment • Treatment of refractory restless leg syndrome	• Agonistic activity at the mu receptors resulting in changes in the perception of pain at the spinal cord and into the CNS	• Medication is contraindicated in patients with significant respiratory depression, acute or severe asthma, known or suspected GI obstruction, or paralytic ileus. • Use caution in substance use, depression, geriatric populations, CNS depression and/or head trauma, increased ICP, psychosis, opioid-naïve patients, seizures, cardiac disease, adrenal insufficiency, hypothyroidism, or myxedema. • Do not discontinue abruptly. • Long-term use may increase risk of infertility. • Adverse reactions include GI obstructions, seizures, apnea, SIADH, respiratory arrest, constipation, depression, dyspnea, confusion, withdrawal if abruptly discontinued, respiratory depression, hypoxia, hypotension, psychologic and physiologic dependence, infertility, nausea, tremor, anxiety, dizziness, and drowsiness.

(continued)

Table A.2 Common Pain and Sedation Medications for Medical-Surgical Patients *(continued)*

General Indications	General Mechanism of Action	General Contraindications, Precautions, and Adverse Effects
Opioids: hydromorphone		
• Relief of moderate to severe pain • Management of chronic severe pain in opioid-tolerant patients requiring around-the-clock, long-term opioid treatment	• Act at the mu receptor, causing changes in perception to pain at the spinal cord and into the CNS	• Medication is contraindicated in patients with respiratory depression, status asthmaticus (immediate-release tablets), paralytic ileus (extended-release tablets), and sulfite hypersensitivity. • Use caution in substance use, opioid-naïve patients, head trauma or CNS depression, cardiac disease, geriatric populations, adrenal insufficiency, hypothyroidism, and myxedema. • Adverse reactions include bronchospasm, GI obstruction, bradycardia, anaphylaxis, laryngospasm, apnea, respiratory arrest, ileus, constipation, depression, dysphoria, hallucinations, confusion, euphoria, withdrawal if abruptly discontinued, urinary retention, nausea, drowsiness, vomiting, fatigue, dizziness, diarrhea, anxiety, tremor, paranoia, and lethargy.
Opioids: morphine		
• Acute and chronic moderate to severe pain • Management of chronic severe pain in patients who require daily, around-the-clock long-term opioid treatment • Treatment of noninfectious diarrhea • Dyspnea in patients with end-stage cancer or pulmonary disease • Procedural sedation • Painful diabetic neuropathy • Refractory restless leg syndrome	• Act at the mu receptor, causing changes in perception to pain at the spinal cord and into the CNS	• Medication is contraindicated in significant respiratory depression in unmonitored settings, acute or severe bronchial asthma (oral solutions), respiratory depression or hypoxia, upper airway obstruction, acute alcoholism or delirium tremens (rectal route), known or suspected GI obstruction or paralytic ileus, hypovolemia, circulatory shock, cardiac arrhythmia or HF secondary to chronic lung disease, and concurrent use with MAOI therapy. • Use caution in substance use, alcoholism, opioid-naïve patients, CNS depression, head trauma, seizures or increased ICP, cardiac disease, adrenal insufficiency, hypothyroidism, and myxedema. • Do not abruptly discontinue, as withdrawal symptoms can occur.

(continued)

Table A.2 Common Pain and Sedation Medications for Medical-Surgical Patients *(continued)*

General Indications	General Mechanism of Action	General Contraindications, Precautions, and Adverse Effects
Opioids: morphine (continued)		
		• Adverse effects include ileus, bradycardia, arrhythmia, increased ICP, bronchospasm, GI obstruction, laryngospasm, depression, confusion, hypoxia, edema, euphoria, delirium, respiratory depression, dysphagia, hallucinations, psychosis, withdrawal if abruptly discontinued, physiologic dependence, adrenocortical insufficiency, drowsiness, diarrhea, constipation, headache, fever, nausea, restlessness, and vomiting.
Opioids: oxycodone		
• Treatment of severe pain • Management of chronic severe pain in patients requiring daily, around-the-clock long-term opioid management • Painful diabetic neuropathy • Restless leg syndrome	• Mu receptor agonists that change pain perceptions at the spinal cord and into the CNS	• Medication is contraindicated in patients with significant respiratory depression, patients with hypercarbia, GI obstruction, and paralytic ileus. • Use caution in opioid-naïve patients, abrupt disconsolation, CNS depression, head trauma, psychosis and increased ICP, cardiovascular disease, seizures, adrenal insufficiency, hypothyroidism, and myxedema. • Adverse effects include laryngospasm, seizure, ileus, bradycardia, GI obstruction, constipation, euphoria, dysphoria, confusion, blurred vision, dysuria, dyspnea, hypotension, hallucinations, nausea, drowsiness, vomiting, diarrhea, abdominal pain, or fatigue.
Opioids: tramadol		
• Moderate to moderately severe pain • Moderate chronic pain or moderately severe chronic pain in patients requiring continuous around-the-clock treatment for an extended period of time • Adjunctive treatment of osteoarthritis • Diabetic neuropathy • Postherpetic neuralgia • Postoperative shivering	• Agonistic activity at the central opiate receptor	• There are no direct contraindications. • Use caution in polysorbate 80 hypersensitivity, CNS depression, head trauma, seizure and increased ICP, severe pulmonary disease, biliary disease, GI obstruction or GI disease, renal or hepatic impairments, substance use, geriatric population, adrenal insufficiency, hypothyroidism, and myxedema.

(continued)

Table A.2 Common Pain and Sedation Medications for Medical-Surgical Patients *(continued)*

General Indications	General Mechanism of Action	General Contraindications, Precautions, and Adverse Effects
Opioids: tramadol (continued)		
		• Adverse effects include hepatic failure, pancreatitis, bradycardia, seizures, pulmonary edema, arrhythmia, bronchospasm, constipation, hallucinations, hypertension, hypertonia, dyspnea, urinary retention, peripheral edema, blurred vision, withdrawal with abrupt discontinuation, hepatitis, amnesia, confusion, nausea, dizziness, headache, vomiting, drowsiness, agitation, and pruritus.
Platelet aggregation inhibitors (aspirin)		
• Used for emergency management of acute coronary syndrome before or at hospital arrival • Used for secondary stroke prophylaxis • Used for long-term MI prophylaxis • Used after CABG or bypass graft surgery	• Inhibit COX 1 and 2 enzymes • Inhibit platelet aggregation • Have antipyretic, analgesic, and anti-inflammatory properties by inhibiting prostaglandins	• Adverse effects include bleeding and GI disturbances. • Medication is contraindicated in patients with asthma, rhinitis, and nasal polyps. • Use cautiously in patients with alcoholism, bleeding disorders, liver disease, renal impairment, and gastritis.
Sedatives: benzodiazepines (lorazepam)		
• Anxiety management • Short-term management of insomnia due to anxiety or transient situational stress • Procedural sedation or preoperative sedation induction • Preoperative sedation induction and/or relief of preoperative anxiety in adults • Status epilepticus • Alcohol withdrawal • Chemotherapy-induced nausea/vomiting prophylaxis • Treatment of acute agitation	• Produce CNS depression by inhibiting neurotransmitter GABA • Tranquilizer action on the CNS without affecting respiratory and cardiovascular systems	• Medication is contraindicated in sleep apnea or severe respiratory insufficiency/failure that is not mechanically ventilated, acute closed-angle glaucoma, and myasthenia gravis. • Use caution in geriatric populations, depressive disorder, CNS depression, hepatic disease, substance use, and dementia. • Adverse effects include coma, seizure, apnea, pneumothorax, arrhythmia, bradycardia, delirium, confusion, hypotension, hallucinations, memory impairment, constipation, respiratory depression, tolerance, psychologic dependence, withdrawal if abruptly discontinued, drowsiness, dizziness, weakness, headache, and tremor.

(continued)

Table A.2 Common Pain and Sedation Medications for Medical-Surgical Patients *(continued)*

General Indications	General Mechanism of Action	General Contraindications, Precautions, and Adverse Effects
Skeletal muscle relaxants (cyclobenzaprine)		
• Muscle spasms • Fibromyalgia	• Relieve muscle spasms through a central action • Similar chemical structure as amitriptyline	• Medication is contraindicated in patients with acute MI, QT prolongation, and paralytic ileus. • Use with caution in patients with hypothyroidism, seizure disorders, glaucoma, and urinary retention. • Adverse effects include sunburn after UV exposure, drowsiness, hallucinations, and hypertension. • Medication should be for short-term use only.

Table A.3 Common Intravenous Fluids for Medical-Surgical Patients

General Indications	General Mechanism of Action	General Contraindications, Precautions, and Adverse Effects
D5NS		
• Parenteral (IV) treatment for hypoglycemia and hyperkalemia • Nutritional and parenteral nutrition	• Replaces and supplements glucose, supplies energy to cells	• Medication is contraindicated in hyperglycemia and severe dehydration. • Use caution in hypernatremia, hyperchloremia, metabolic acidosis, infection, diabetes, (hepatic disease, HHS hyperosmolar hyperglycemic state), and electrolyte imbalance. • Adverse effects include hyperglycemia.
D5W		
• Parenteral (IV) treatment for hypoglycemia and hyperkalemia • Nutritional and parenteral nutrition • Oral glucose tolerance test	• Replaces and supplements glucose, supplies energy to cells	• Medication is contraindicated in hyperglycemia and severe dehydration. • Use caution in infection, diabetes, hepatic disease, HHS, and electrolyte imbalance. • Adverse effects include hyperglycemia.
Normal saline (sodium chloride, 3%, 0.9%, 0.45%)		
• Dehydration or hypovolemia, including during DKA, CPR, and shock • Hyponatremia • Mucolysis and sputum induction in patients with CF	• Regulates membrane potential of cells to help maintain water balance and homeostatic function	• There are no direct contraindications. • Use caution in hypernatremia, hyperchloremia, and metabolic acidosis.

(continued)

Table A.3 Common Intravenous Fluids for Medical-Surgical Patients *(continued)*

General Indications	General Mechanism of Action	General Contraindications, Precautions, and Adverse Effects
Normal saline (sodium chloride, 3%, 0.9%, 0.45%) (continued)		
• Treatment of nasal congestion and dryness • Nutritional supplementation • Temporary relief of corneal edema • Treatment of increased ICP (3% hypertonic solution) • Inpatient management of viral bronchiolitis		• Adverse effects include HF, encephalopathy, hypernatremia, and sodium retention.
Lactated Ringer's solution		
• Any condition requiring water replacement or electrolyte supplementation, hypotension • Any condition requiring an increase in pH level in the body	• Regulates homeostasis by supplementing water and electrolytes	• There are no true contraindications. • Use caution in alkalosis, diabetes, metabolic disturbances (hypokalemia, hypercalcemia, or metabolic acidosis), arrhythmia, hypoxemia, and pulmonary, cardiovascular, and hepatic disease. • Adverse effects include change in taste, weight gain, vomiting, stomach pain, seizures, nausea, dizziness, faintness, nervousness, confusion, blurred vision, and edema.

Table A.4 Common Steroids for Medical-Surgical Patients

General Indications	General Mechanism of Action	General Contraindications, Precautions, and Adverse Effects
Corticosteroids (prednisone)		
• Maintenance therapy of primary or secondary adrenocortical insufficiency • Congenital adrenal hyperplasia • Kidney transplant rejection prophylaxis	• Inhibit steps in the inflammatory pathway to prevent systemic infection and inflammation of the lungs and to reduce mucus production	• Patients receiving corticosteroids for an extended time or in high doses are at increased risk of immunosuppression, making them more prone to infection.
• Chronic graft-versus-host disease • Acute lymphocytic leukemia • Chronic lymphocytic leukemia • Short-term treatment of hypercalcemia secondary disease		• Avoid using in patients with Cushing's syndrome. • Use caution in untreated infection, diabetes, glaucoma, immunodepression, and liver disease.

(continued)

Table A.4 Common Steroids for Medical-Surgical Patients *(continued)*

General Indications	General Mechanism of Action	General Contraindications, Precautions, and Adverse Effects
Corticosteroids (prednisone) (continued)		

Corticosteroids (prednisone) (continued)

- Inflammatory bowel disease
- Crohn's disease
- UC
- Rheumatic conditions
- Systemic autoimmune conditions
- Hemolytic anemia
- Asthma exacerbation
- Thrombocytopenia or ITP (immune thrombocytopenic purpura)
- Myasthenia gravis
- Psoriatic arthritis
- Proteinuria in nephrotic syndrome
- Severe erythema multiforme or Stevens–Johnson syndrome
- Treatment of ACE inhibitor-induced angioedema
- Allergic disorders including anaphylaxis
- ARDS
- Pneumonia
- Hodgkin lymphoma
- Multiple myeloma
- Duchenne muscular dystrophy
- Carpal tunnel syndrome
- Autoimmune hepatitis
- Primary amyloidosis
- Exacerbation of COPD
- Idiopathic or viral pericarditis
- Interstitial nephritis
- Bell's palsy
- Transplant rejection

- Adverse effects include growth inhibition, osteoporosis, osteopenia, impaired wound healing, immunosuppression, candidiasis, fluid retention, hypernatremia, euphoria, hallucinations, hyperglycemia, nausea, weight gain, fluid retention, emotional lability, headache, hoarseness, diaphoresis, and bronchospasm.
- Medication may reduce glucose tolerance, causing hyperglycemia in diabetic patients.

RESOURCES

Mayo Foundation for Medical Education and Research. (2021, February 1). *Lactated ringer's (INTRAVENOUS route) side effects.* https://www.mayoclinic.org/drugs-supplements/lactated-ringers-intravenous-route/side-effects/drg-20489612?p=1

Prescribers' Digital Reference. (n.d.[a]). *Acetaminophen* [Drug information]. https://www.pdr.net/drug-summary/Ofirmev-acetaminophen-1346

Prescribers' Digital Reference. (n.d.[b]). *Amikacin sulfate* [Drug information]. https://www.pdr.net/drug-summary/Amikacin-Sulfate-amikacin-sulfate-676

Prescribers' Digital Reference. (n.d.[c]). *Ampicillin* [Drug information]. https://www.pdr.net/drug-summary/Ampicillin-for-Injection-ampicillin-677

Prescribers' Digital Reference. (n.d.[d]). *Ativan* [Drug information]. https://www.pdr.net/drug-summary/Ativan-Injection-lorazepam-996

Prescribers' Digital Reference. (n.d.[e]). *Azithromycin* [Drug information]. https://www.pdr.net/drug-summary/Azithromycin-azithromycin-24249

Prescribers' Digital Reference. (n.d.[f]). *Bactrim* [Drug information]. https://www.pdr.net/drug-summary/Bactrim-Bactrim-DS-sulfamethoxazole-trimethoprim-686

Prescribers' Digital Reference. (n.d.[g]). *Cefazolin* [Drug information]. https://www.pdr.net/drug-summary/Cefazolin-Sodium-cefazolin-sodium-1193

Prescribers' Digital Reference. (n.d.[h]). *Cefepime (Maxipime)* [Drug information]. https://www.pdr.net/drug-summary/Maxipime-cefepime-hydrochloride-3215.5755

Prescribers' Digital Reference. (n.d.[i]). *Ceftriaxone* [Drug information]. https://www.pdr.net/drug-summary/Ceftriaxone-ceftriaxone-1723

Prescribers' Digital Reference. (n.d.[j]). *Cefuroxime* [Drug information]. https://www.pdr.net/drug-summary/Zinacef-cefuroxime-242

Prescribers' Digital Reference. (n.d.[k]). *Ciprofloxacin* [Drug information]. PDR Search. https://www.pdr.net/drug-summary/Ciprofloxacin-Injection-ciprofloxacin-3255

Prescribers' Digital Reference. (n.d.[l]). *Clindamycin* [Drug information]. https://www.pdr.net/drug-summary/Cleocin-Phosphate-Injection-clindamycin-1865

Prescribers' Digital Reference. (n.d.[m]). *Dextrose monohydrate* [Drug information]. https://www.pdr.net/drug-summary/5--Dextrose-dextrose-monohydrate-24283

Prescribers' Digital Reference. (n.d.[n]). *Dilaudid* [Drug information]. https://www.pdr.net/drug-summary/Dilaudid-Injection-and-HP-Injection-hydromorphone-hydrochloride-490

Prescribers' Digital Reference. (n.d.[o]). *Doxycycline* [Drug information]. https://www.pdr.net/drug-summary/Doxycycline-doxycycline-24308

Prescribers' Digital Reference. (n.d.[p]). *Ertapenem* [Drug information]. https://www.pdr.net/drug-summary/Invanz-ertapenem-359

Prescribers' Digital Reference. (n.d.[q]). *Fentanyl* [Drug information]. https://www.pdr.net/drug-summary/Fentanyl-Citrate-fentanyl-citrate-2474

Prescribers' Digital Reference. (n.d.[r]). *Fluconazole* [Drug information]. https://www.pdr.net/drug-summary/Diflucan-fluconazole-1847

Prescribers' Digital Reference. (n.d.[s]). *Gentamicin sulfate* [Drug information]. https://www.pdr.net/drug-summary/Gentamicin-Injection-40-mg-mL-gentamicin-sulfate-3299

Prescribers' Digital Reference. (n.d.[t]). *Ketamine* [Drug information]. https://www.pdr.net/drug-summary/Ketalar-ketamine-hydrochloride-1999#10

Prescribers' Digital Reference. (n.d.[u]). *Merrem* [Drug information]. https://www.pdr.net/drug-summary/Merrem-meropenem-2055

Prescribers' Digital Reference. (n.d.[v]). *Morphine* [Drug information]. https://www.pdr.net/drug-summary/Morphine-Sulfate-Tablets-morphine-sulfate-1520

Prescribers' Digital Reference. (n.d.[w]). *Neomycin* [Drug information]. https://www.pdr.net/drug-summary/Neomycin-Sulfate-neomycin-sulfate-819

Prescribers' Digital Reference. (n.d.[x]). *Neurontin* [Drug information]. https://www.pdr.net/drug-summary/Neurontin-gabapentin-2477.4218

Prescribers' Digital Reference. (n.d.[y]). *Oxycodone* [Drug information]. https://www.pdr.net/drug-summary/Oxycodone-HCl-oxycodone-hydrochloride-24333

Prescribers' Digital Reference. (n.d.[z]). *Pentamidine* [Drug information]. https://www.pdr.net/drug-summary/NebuPent-pentamidine-isethionate-1408

Prescribers' Digital Reference. (n.d.[aa]). *Phenobarbital* [Drug information]. https://www.pdr.net/drug-summary/Phenobarbital-Elixir-phenobarbital-2669#10

Prescribers' Digital Reference. (n.d.[ab]). *Prednisone* [Drug information]. https://www.pdr.net/drug-summary/Prednisone-Prednisone-Intensol-prednisone-2575

Prescribers' Digital Reference. (n.d.[ac]). *Sodium chloride* [Drug information]. https://www.pdr.net/drug-summary/Sodium-Chloride-sodium-chloride-24245

Prescribers' Digital Reference. (n.d.[ad]). *Streptomycin* [Drug information]. https://www.pdr.net/drug-summary/Streptomycin-streptomycin-1600

Prescribers' Digital Reference. (n.d.[ae]). *Teflaro (ceftaroline fosamil)* [Drug information]. https://www.pdr.net/drug-summary/Teflaro-ceftaroline-fosamil-158

Prescribers' Digital Reference. (n.d.[af]). *Tobramycin* [Drug information]. https://www.pdr.net/drug-summary/Tobramycin-tobramycin-916

Prescribers' Digital Reference. (n.d.[ag]). *Vancomycin* [Drug information]. https://www.pdr.net/drug-summary/Vancocin-vancomycin-hydrochloride-802

Prescribers' Digital Reference. (n.d.[ah]). *Zohydro-ER (hydrocodone)* [Drug information]. https://www.pdr.net/drug-summary/Zohydro-ER-hydrocodone-bitartrate-3389

Prescribers' Digital Reference. (n.d.[ai]). *Zyvox (Linezolid)*. https://www.pdr.net/drug-summary/Zyvox-linezolid-2341

Prescribers' Digital Reference. (n.d.[aj]). *Cubicin* [Drug information]. *https://www.pdr.net/drug-summary/Cubicin-daptomycin-1279.6189*

Prescribers' Digital Reference. (n.d.[ak]). *Cyclobenzaprine* [Drug information]. https://www.pdr.net/drug-summary/Cyclobenzaprine-Hydrochloride-cyclobenzaprine-hydrochloride-3089.1153

Prescribers' Digital Reference. (n.d.[al]). *Durlaza-aspirin* [Drug information]. https://www.pdr.net/drug-summary/ Durlaza-aspirin-3789.4184

Prescribers' Digital Reference. (n.d.[am]). *Ketorolac* [Drug information]. https://www.pdr.net/drug-summary/ Ketorolac-Tromethamine-Tablets-ketorolac-tromethamine-1793.3935#15

Prescribers' Digital Reference. (n.d.[an]). *Sulfamethoxazole/trimethoprim* [Drug information]. https://www.pdr.net/ drug-summary/Sulfamethoxazole-and-Trimethoprim-sulfamethoxazole-trimethoprim-2663.4372#14

APPENDIX B: ABBREVIATIONS

ABC	airway, breathing, and circulation
ABG	arterial blood gas
ACE	angiotensin-converting enzyme
ACTH	adrenocorticotropic hormone and corticotropin
ADH	antidiuretic hormone
ADLs	activities of daily living
ADT	androgen deprivation therapy
AHF	antihemophilic factor
AKI	acute kidney injury
ALS	amyotrophic lateral sclerosis
ALT	alanine transaminase
AMD	age-related macular degeneration
AMSN	Academy of Medical-Surgical Nurses
ANA	American Nurses Association
ANCC	American Nurses Credentialing Center
aPTT	activated partial thromboplastin clotting time
ARB	angiotensin receptor blocker
ARDS	acute respiratory distress syndrome
ART	anti-retroviral therapy
AST	aspartate aminotransferase
ATP	adenosine triphosphate
ATT	authorization to test
AV	atrioventricular
BMP	basic metabolic panel
BNP	brain natriuretic peptide
BP	blood pressure
BPH	benign prostatic hyperplasia
BRCA1	breast cancer gene 1
BRCA2	breast cancer gene 2
BSO	bilateral salpingo-oophorectomy
BUN	blood urea nitrogen
CABG	coronary artery bypass grafting
CAD	coronary artery disease
CAP	community-acquired pneumonia
CAUTI	catheter-associated urinary tract infection
CBC	complete blood count
CBT	computer-based test
CCR5	chemokine receptor antagonists
CEA	carcinoembryonic antigen tumor maker
CF	cystic fibrosis
CHF	congestive heart failure
CK	creatine kinase
CKD	chronic kidney disease
CK-MB	creatine kinase–myoglobin binding
CLABSI	central line–associated bloodstream infection
CMP	comprehensive metabolic panel
CMSRN	Certified Medical-Surgical Registered Nurse

CNS	central nervous system
COPD	chronic obstructive pulmonary disease
CPK	creatine phosphokinase
CPT	chest physiotherapy
CrCl	creatinine clearance
CRP	c-reactive protein
CRRT	continuous renal replacement therapy
CSF	cerebrospinal fluid
CVA	cerebrovascular accident
C&S	culture and sensitivity
DEXA	dual-energy x-ray absorptiometry
DI	diabetes insipidus
DIC	disseminated intravascular coagulation
DIP	distal interphalangeal joint
DKA	diabetic ketoacidosis
DNA	deoxyribonucleic acid
DNR	do not resuscitate
DVT	deep venous thrombosis
EBP	evidence-based practice
ECF	extracellular fluid
ED	endoscopy
ED	emergency department
EEG	electroencephalogram
EGD	esophagogastroduodenoscopy
EKG	electrocardiogram
ELISA	enzyme-linked immunosorbent assay
EMG	electromyography
ERCP	endoscopic retrograde cholangiopancreatography
ESBL	extended spectrum beta-lactamase
ESR	erythrocyte sedimentation rate
ESRD	end-stage renal disease
ETT	endotracheal tube
EWSL	extracorporeal shock wave lithotripsy
FEES	fiberoptic endoscopic evaluation of swallowing
FFP	fresh frozen plasma
FI	fusion inhibitor
G6PD	glucose-6-phosphate dehydrogenase
GABA	gamma-aminobutyric acid
GERD	gastroesophageal reflux disease
GFR	glomerular filtration rate
GI	gastrointestinal
GU	genitourinary
HAART	highly active antiretroviral therapy
HAI	healthcare-associated infection
HCG	human chorionic gonadotropin
HER2	human epidermal growth factor receptor 2
HF	heart failure
HHS	hyperosmolar hyperglycemic state
HIV	human immunodeficiency virus
HOB	head of bed
HPV	human papillomavirus
HR	heart rate
HTN	hypertension
IBS	irritable bowel syndrome
ICD	implantable cardioverter-defibrillator
ICP	intracranial pressure
IM	intramuscular

INSTI	integrase strand transfer inhibitor
IOP	intraocular pressure
ITP	immune thrombocytopenic purpura
IV	intravenous
IVC	inferior vena cava filter
JVD	jugular vein distention
KPC	*Klebsiella pneumonia* carbapenemase
KUB	kidney, ureter, and bladder
LDH	lactate dehydrogenase
LLQ	left lower quadrant
LOC	level of consciousness
MAOI	monoamine oxidase inhibitor
MAP	mean arterial pressure
MDRO	multidrug-resistant organism
MEG	magnetoencephalography
MI	myocardial infarction
MRA	magnetic resonance angiography
MRI	magnetic resonance imaging
MRSA	methicillin-resistant *Staphylococcus aureus*
MS	multiple sclerosis
MSNCB	Medical-Surgical Nursing Certification Board
NGT	nasogastric tube
NMDA	n-methyl-d-aspartate
NNRTIs	non-nucleoside reverse transcriptase inhibitors
NPO	nothing by mouth
NRTI	nucleoside/nucleotide reverse transcriptase inhibitor
NSAIDs	non-steroidal anti-inflammatory drugs
NSTEMI	non-ST-elevation myocardial infarction
OCT	optical coherence tomography
OT	occupational therapy
PAD	peripheral arterial disease
PCOS	polycystic ovarian syndrome
PE	pulmonary embolism
PET	positron emission tomography
PICC	peripherally inserted central catheter
PID	pelvic inflammatory disease
PIP	proximal interphalangeal
PI	protease inhibitor
PKU	phenylketonuria
PO	by mouth
PRBC	packed red blood cell
PRN	pro re nata (as needed)
PrEP	preexposure prophylaxis
PSA	prostate-specific antigen
PT	physical therapy
PTH	parathyroid hormone
PTT	partial thromboplastin time
PUL	prostatic urethral lift
PVD	peripheral vascular disease
RBC	red blood cell
RLQ	right lower quadrant
RN	registered nurse
RNA	ribonucleic acid
RN-BC	Registered Nurse–Board Certified
ROB	retinopathy of prematurity
ROM	range of motion
RPR	rapid plasma reagin

RUQ	right upper quadrant
SCC	squamous cell carcinoma
SCD	sequential compression device
SIADH	syndrome of inappropriate antidiuretic hormone secretion
SLE	systemic lupus erythematous
SNRI	serotonin and norepinephrine reuptake inhibitor
SSRI	selective serotonin reuptake inhibitor
STEMI	ST-elevation myocardial infarction
STI	sexually transmitted infection
TAH	total abdominal hysterectomy
TBI	traumatic brain injury
TIA	transient ischemic attack
TNF	tumor necrosis factor
tPA	tissue plasminogen activator
TSH	thyroid-stimulating hormone
TTP	thrombotic thrombocytopenic purpura
TURBT	transurethral resection of bladder tumor
TURP	transurethral resection of the prostate
UA	urinalysis
UC	ulcerative colitis
UTI	urinary tract infection
VAD	ventricular assist device
VBG	venous blood gas
VRE	vancomycin-resistant enterococcus
WBC	white blood cell

INDEX

Printed in the United States
by Baker & Taylor Publisher Services